Mixed Effects Models for the Population Approach

Models, Tasks, Methods and Tools

Chapman & Hall/CRC Biostatistics Series

Published Titles

Adaptive Design Methods in Clinical Trials, Second Edition
Shein-Chung Chow and Mark Chang

Adaptive Design Theory and Implementation Using SAS and R
Mark Chang

Advanced Bayesian Methods for Medical Test Accuracy
Lyle D. Broemeling

Advances in Clinical Trial Biostatistics
Nancy L. Geller

Applied Meta-Analysis with R
Ding-Geng (Din) Chen and Karl E. Peace

Basic Statistics and Pharmaceutical Statistical Applications, Second Edition
James E. De Muth

Bayesian Adaptive Methods for Clinical Trials
Scott M. Berry, Bradley P. Carlin, J. Jack Lee, and Peter Muller

Bayesian Analysis Made Simple: An Excel GUI for WinBUGS
Phil Woodward

Bayesian Methods for Measures of Agreement
Lyle D. Broemeling

Bayesian Methods in Epidemiology
Lyle D. Broemeling

Bayesian Methods in Health Economics
Gianluca Baio

Bayesian Missing Data Problems: EM, Data Augmentation and Noniterative Computation
Ming T. Tan, Guo-Liang Tian, and Kai Wang Ng

Bayesian Modeling in Bioinformatics
Dipak K. Dey, Samiran Ghosh, and Bani K. Mallick

Benefit-Risk Assessment in Pharmaceutical Research and Development
Andreas Sashegyi, James Felli, and Rebecca Noel

Biosimilars: Design and Analysis of Follow-on Biologics
Shein-Chung Chow

Biostatistics: A Computing Approach
Stewart J. Anderson

Causal Analysis in Biomedicine and Epidemiology: Based on Minimal Sufficient Causation
Mikel Aickin

Clinical and Statistical Considerations in Personalized Medicine
Claudio Carini, Sandeep Menon, and Mark Chang

Clinical Trial Data Analysis using R
Ding-Geng (Din) Chen and Karl E. Peace

Clinical Trial Methodology
Karl E. Peace and Ding-Geng (Din) Chen

Computational Methods in Biomedical Research
Ravindra Khattree and Dayanand N. Naik

Computational Pharmacokinetics
Anders Källén

Confidence Intervals for Proportions and Related Measures of Effect Size
Robert G. Newcombe

Controversial Statistical Issues in Clinical Trials
Shein-Chung Chow

Data and Safety Monitoring Committees in Clinical Trials
Jay Herson

Design and Analysis of Animal Studies in Pharmaceutical Development
Shein-Chung Chow and Jen-pei Liu

Design and Analysis of Bioavailability and Bioequivalence Studies, Third Edition
Shein-Chung Chow and Jen-pei Liu

Design and Analysis of Bridging Studies
Jen-pei Liu, Shein-Chung Chow,
and Chin-Fu Hsiao

Design and Analysis of Clinical Trials with Time-to-Event Endpoints
Karl E. Peace

Design and Analysis of Non-Inferiority Trials
Mark D. Rothmann, Brian L. Wiens,
and Ivan S. F. Chan

Difference Equations with Public Health Applications
Lemuel A. Moyé and Asha Seth Kapadia

DNA Methylation Microarrays: Experimental Design and Statistical Analysis
Sun-Chong Wang and Arturas Petronis

DNA Microarrays and Related Genomics Techniques: Design, Analysis, and Interpretation of Experiments
David B. Allison, Grier P. Page,
T. Mark Beasley, and Jode W. Edwards

Dose Finding by the Continual Reassessment Method
Ying Kuen Cheung

Elementary Bayesian Biostatistics
Lemuel A. Moyé

Frailty Models in Survival Analysis
Andreas Wienke

Generalized Linear Models: A Bayesian Perspective
Dipak K. Dey, Sujit K. Ghosh,
and Bani K. Mallick

Handbook of Regression and Modeling: Applications for the Clinical and Pharmaceutical Industries
Daryl S. Paulson

Interval-Censored Time-to-Event Data: Methods and Applications
Ding-Geng (Din) Chen, Jianguo Sun,
and Karl E. Peace

Joint Models for Longitudinal and Time-to-Event Data: With Applications in R
Dimitris Rizopoulos

Measures of Interobserver Agreement and Reliability, Second Edition
Mohamed M. Shoukri

Medical Biostatistics, Third Edition
A. Indrayan

Meta-Analysis in Medicine and Health Policy
Dalene Stangl and Donald A. Berry

Mixed Effects Models for the Population Approach: Models, Tasks, Methods and Tools
Marc Lavielle

Monte Carlo Simulation for the Pharmaceutical Industry: Concepts, Algorithms, and Case Studies
Mark Chang

Multiple Testing Problems in Pharmaceutical Statistics
Alex Dmitrienko, Ajit C. Tamhane,
and Frank Bretz

Optimal Design for Nonlinear Response Models
Valerii V. Fedorov and Sergei L. Leonov

Patient-Reported Outcomes: Measurement, Implementation and Interpretation
Joseph C. Cappelleri, Kelly H. Zou,
Andrew G. Bushmakin, Jose Ma. J. Alvir,
Demissie Alemayehu, and Tara Symonds

Randomized Clinical Trials of Nonpharmacological Treatments
Isabelle Boutron, Philippe Ravaud, and David Moher

Randomized Phase II Cancer Clinical Trials
Sin-Ho Jung

Sample Size Calculations in Clinical Research, Second Edition
Shein-Chung Chow, Jun Shao and Hansheng Wang

Statistical Analysis of Human Growth and Development
Yin Bun Cheung

Statistical Design and Analysis of Stability Studies
Shein-Chung Chow

Statistical Evaluation of Diagnostic Performance: Topics in ROC Analysis
Kelly H. Zou, Aiyi Liu, Andriy Bandos, Lucila Ohno-Machado, and Howard Rockette

Statistical Methods for Clinical Trials
Mark X. Norleans

Statistics in Drug Research: Methodologies and Recent Developments
Shein-Chung Chow and Jun Shao

Statistics in the Pharmaceutical Industry, Third Edition
Ralph Buncher and Jia-Yeong Tsay

Survival Analysis in Medicine and Genetics
Jialiang Li and Shuangge Ma

Theory of Drug Development
Eric B. Holmgren

Translational Medicine: Strategies and Statistical Methods
Dennis Cosmatos and Shein-Chung Chow

Chapman & Hall/CRC Biostatistics Series

Mixed Effects Models for the Population Approach

Models, Tasks, Methods and Tools

Marc Lavielle
INRIA Saclay
Orsay, France

With Contributions by
Kevin Bleakley
Inria, Popix team

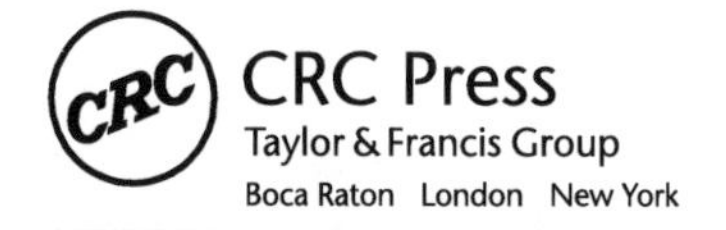

CRC Press is an imprint of the
Taylor & Francis Group, an **informa** business
A CHAPMAN & HALL BOOK

CRC Press
Taylor & Francis Group
6000 Broken Sound Parkway NW, Suite 300
Boca Raton, FL 33487-2742

First issued in paperback 2022

Version Date: 20140611

ISBN 13: 978-1-03-247735-0 (pbk)
ISBN 13: 978-1-4822-2650-8 (hbk)

DOI: 10.1201/b17203

Library of Congress Cataloging-in-Publication Data

Lavielle, Marc, author.
Mixed effects models for the population approach : models, tasks, methods and tools / Marc Lavielle.
p. ; cm. -- (Chapman & Hall/CRC biostatistics series)
Includes bibliographical references and index.
ISBN 978-1-4822-2650-8 (hardcover : alk. paper)
I. Title. II. Series: Chapman & Hall/CRC biostatistics series (Unnumbered)
[DNLM: 1. Models, Statistical. 2. Biometry--methods. 3. Population Characteristics. WA 950]

QA180.55.S7
001.4'22--dc23 2014019439

Visit the Taylor & Francis Web site at
http://www.taylorandfrancis.com

and the CRC Press Web site at
http://www.crcpress.com

à Elena, Pablo et Oriana

Contents

Preface

Population models describe biological and physical phenomena observed in each of a set of individuals, and also the variability between individuals. This approach finds its place in domains like pharmacometrics when we need to quantitatively describe interactions between diseases, drugs and patients. This means developing models that take into account that different patients react differently to the same disease and the same drug.

The adoption of the population approach in pharmacometrics is largely due to the creation of the NONMEM software in the late 1970s which enabled the use of nonlinear mixed effects models for pharmacometric data analysis. Indeed, the population approach can be formulated in statistical terms using mixed effects models. While linear mixed effects models have been around and widely used since the 1950s, nonlinear mixed effects models remain rarely used even in areas where they are particularly well-suited such as biology, agronomy, econometrics, environmental and human sciences.

Even though each of these domains has its own models and particularities, a rigorous framework for describing and representing any given model turns out to be possible. This leads to a streamlined and precise way to implement methods of interest as readily available software. The main goal of this book is to give a coherent overview of the different components that make up this framework.

First, we will see how the framework allows us to represent models for many different data types including continuous, categorical, count and time-to-event data. This opens the way for the use of quite generic methods for modeling these diverse data types. In particular, the SAEM (Stochastic Approximation of EM) algorithm is extremely efficient for maximum likelihood estimation of population parameters, and has been proven to converge in quite general settings.

Though these practical and theoretical properties are satisfying and extremely useful, the implementation of the methods themselves is rather intricate, requiring considerable knowledge of stochastic algorithms, Monte Carlo Markov chain (MCMC) methods, importance sampling techniques and so on.

To bring these methods to a much wider audience, they have therefore been implemented in the MONOLIX software and are ready-to-use for a vast array of real-world data modeling situations. One can also visually explore models in detail using MLXPLORE, or simulate using Simulx. These publicly available tools all use the same model coding language MLXTRAN and will be used throughout the book to illustrate the various tasks a modeler must perform.

All of this leads to a coherency in the overall process from models to methods, methods to tools, and tools to results. It also means that statisticians and mathematicians can be satisfied with the rigorous representation of the models and theoretical properties of the methods, and modelers with the practical capabilities of the tools.

It is not, however, the goal of the book to exhaustively cover the whole range of models and methods available for the population approach. We will limit ourselves to parametric approaches, without ignoring the fact that nonparametric approaches can perhaps be imagined in certain situations. In our treatment, Bayesian methods are not looked at as a specific approach competing with frequentist ones, but integrated into the general statistical framework. In effect, we will construct models using available information, then use these models to perform various tasks. The tasks might include maximum likelihood estimation if we only have data, posterior distribution estimation if we also have prior information, or a mixture of both if we have partial prior information.

The underlying goal of this book is to provide a rigorous approach for model description, implementation and practical use, not "recipes" for modeling or "tricks" for using software. It is intended for mathematicians and statisticians interested in modeling, and for modelers aware of the role of mathematics and statistics in models. It will be useful for training and teaching in any field where population modeling occurs. Furthermore, all the tools presented and used here (MONOLIX, MLXPLORE, Simulx, R) are free for academic and teaching purposes.

All code and data used in the text are available from the supporting website:

`http://www.math.u-psud.fr/~lavielle/book`

Acknowledgments

Now that the book is completed, I can see more clearly that it is the final result of several years of intensive work, but also the result of many crossed paths and collaborations.

Above all, I have to emphasize the luck I have had to be a part of the Orsay Mathematics Laboratory for many years now. It is a fantastic environment in which to do mathematics and also create collaborations with scientists from different disciplines. I would also like to gratefully thank Inria, which has always supported and encouraged me and my projects.

Developing new methods and algorithms constitutes undeniably the heart of my activities. But it was my collaboration with Eric Moulines followed by Bernard Delyon on the SAEM algorithm that definitively convinced me that if an algorithm could work so well in practice, its properties must be provable mathematically (the converse of which is often far from being true ...).

SAEM quickly asserted itself as an incredible estimation tool for (nonlinear) mixed effets models. In 2003, I, along with France Mentré (Inserm) and Jean-Louis Foulley (Inra), formed the MONOLIX (MOdèles NOn LInéaires à effets miXtes) working group, active for around six years, with the aim of popularizing new statistical methods for mixed effects models. I would like to personally thank all the participants of this group and especially France with whom I collaborated over several years, and who introduced me to the world of pharmacometrics and the PAGE (Population Approach Group in Europe) community.

Here, I found a fascinating and rich environment where numerous disciplines such as statistics, pharmacology and biology co-exist. I appreciated meeting several modelers from this community who were understanding of the need to develop new and innovative modeling methods and tools while also being conscious of the need for rigorous mathematics to support them.

I very quickly came to the conclusion of the necessity of implementing as software the new methods we were developing in order to make them accessible to the wider community. I give heartfelt thanks to Inria and various modeling and simulation groups (Johnson & Johnson, Novartis, Roche, Sanofi-Aventis, Astrazeneca) for having actively supported development of the MONOLIX software.

I have been lucky to be able to count on the development team of Hector Mesa, Kaelig Chatel and later Eric Blaudez, a group of exceptional engineers who have carried this project further than my highest hopes. I thank them greatly as well as the rest of the current Lixoft team that continues to develop MONOLIX as well as other new modeling tools.

Much of this book has benefited from joint research with a number of colleagues, including Gregory Batt (Inria), Kevin Bleakley (Inria), Emmanuelle Comets (Inserm), Anne Dubois (Inserm), Mats Karlsson (Uppsala University), France Mentré (Inserm), Eric Moulines (Télécom ParisTech), Rada Savic (UCSF), Eric Snoeck (Exprimo) and Benjamin Ribba (Inria). I thank you all.

Several chapters are also based on collaborations with current and past doctoral students: Célia Barthélémy, Maud Delattre, Sophie Donnet, Estelle Kuhn, Cristian Meza, Cyprien Mbogning and Adeline Samson, with whom I have had great pleasure in working.

I gratefully acknowledge support from the French national research agency, project ANR-05-blan-0274 "MONOLIX", and the Innovative Medicines Initiative Joint Undertaking under grant agreement n. 115156, "Drug and Disease Modeling Resources" (DDMoRe).

A big thanks to Kevin Bleakley for his work in translating my *frenglish* into something readable, as well as his ruthless proofreading of the manuscript.

Lastly, I would like to thank John Kimmel at Chapman & Hall for his interest in this project from the beginning and his continuous support throughout.

Marc Lavielle,
Orsay, May 2014

Part I

Introduction and Preliminary Concepts

1

Overview

1.1 The population approach

The desire to model a biological or physical phenomenon often arises when we are able to record some observations issued from it. Nothing would therefore be more natural than to begin this introduction by looking at some observed data. We will not go into the details of the data here; we use it only to illustrate in an intuitive and introductory way what we call the population approach.

The first example involves weight data for rats measured over 14 weeks for a subchronic toxicity study related to the question of genetically modified (GM) corn. To evaluate health risks associated with GM organisms, individual rats were put on diets containing different quantities of GM corn. To discover whether there is an effect due to GM food on weight, for instance, we look to find whether part of the variability observed among the growth curves can be explained by diet. For each rat, the sequence of observations is longitudinal data (Fitzmaurice et al., 2008; Molenberghs and Verbeke, 2005); the same information (weight) is measured at multiple time points (Figure 1.1).

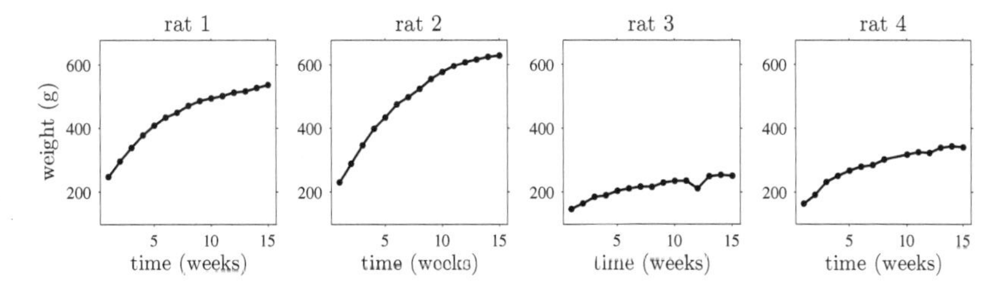

FIGURE 1.1: Weight curves for four rats.

The next set of plots displays the viral load of four patients with hepatitis C who started a treatment at time $t = 0$. Viral load data for hepatitis C carriers exhibit great clinical response variability under the same treatment (Snoeck et al., 2010). Some patients respond to treatment and their viral load decreases, while others have no response or see their viral load rise again at the treatment's end (Figure 1.2).

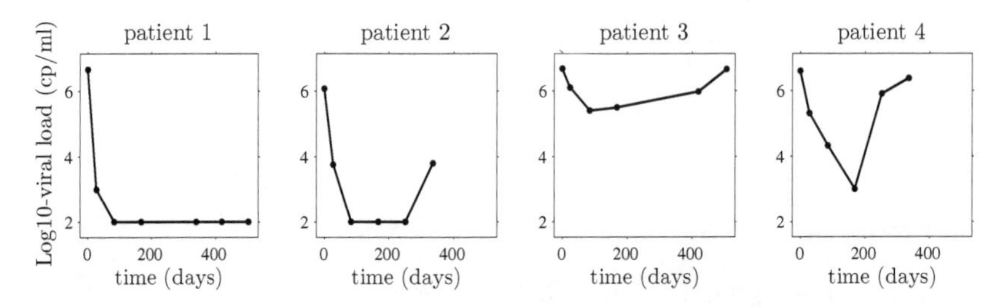

FIGURE 1.2: Viral load of four patients with hepatitis C.

In the next example (Figure 1.3), the data are fluorescence intensities measured over time in a cellular biology experiment which aims to describe the cell cycle and the creation of free radicals (Faure et al., 2013). Several repeats of the same experiment are necessary because the same experimental conditions can lead to great variability in fluorescence activity.

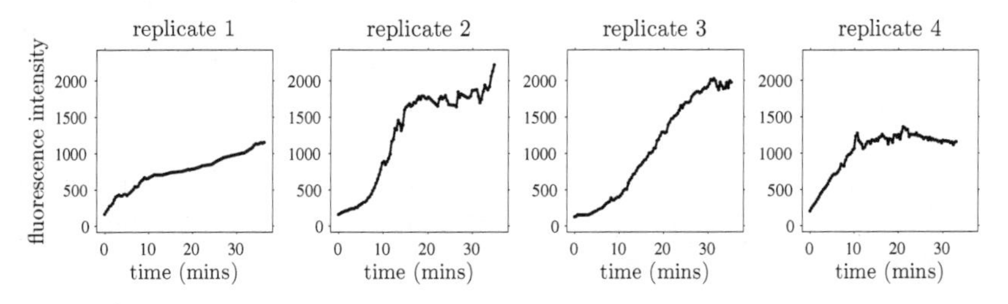

FIGURE 1.3: Fluorescence intensities from four replicates of the same experiment.

Note that repeated measurements are not necessarily always functions of time. For example, we may be interested in corn production as a function of fertilizer quantity (Makowski and Lavielle, 2006). Such studies are important in agriculture in order to provide recommendations for farmers as to optimal fertilizer use. In nature there exists variability in soil conditions, and studies need to be performed over several parcels of land (Figure 1.4).

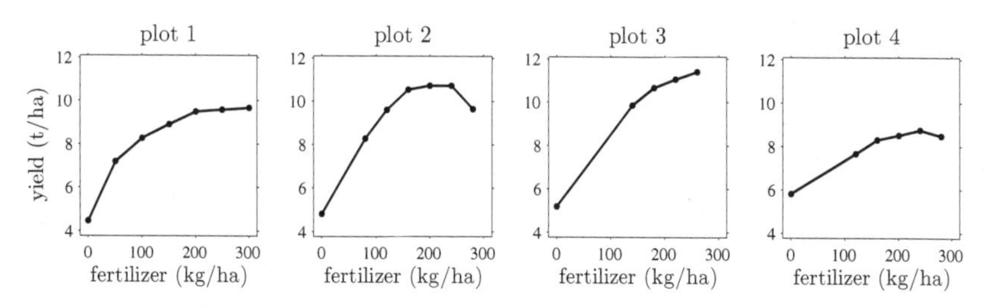

FIGURE 1.4: Corn production as a function of fertilizer quantity.

Even though these examples come from quite different domains, in each case the data is made up of repeated measurements on several individuals from a population. What we will call a "population approach" will be relevant for characterizing and modeling this data. The modeling goal is thus twofold: characterize, first, the biological or physical phenomena observed for each individual and, second, the variability seen between individuals.

In the example with rats, the model needs to integrate a growth model that describes how a rat's weight increases with time and a statistical model that describes why this process can vary from one rat to another. The goal is thus to finish with a "typical" growth curve for the population and be able to describe and explain, as much as possible, the variability in the individual's curves around this population curve.

As these are longitudinal data, a curve with weight as a function of time gives a natural graphical representation of a mathematical growth model. Thus, after looking at the data, the first step is to choose a growth model well adapted to the data. For example, we might consider a very simple growth model of the form $f(t) = a + b(1 - e^{-k\,t})$. We can then check that curves created using this model "look like" the observed growth curves for a suitably chosen set of parameters (a, b, k). In addition to its simplicity, another advantage of this model is that its parameters can be interpreted biologically: a is the rat's weight at time 0, i.e., at birth, b the maximum weight gain (as time t tends to infinity) and k a measure of the speed at which the rat grows. Obviously, other growth models are available of which some will be more adapted than others to modeling certain types of growth. This leads to the need for model selection criteria, kept out of this introductory section for simplicity, but looked at later in the book.

Beyond these technical aspects of model selection, it is important to have in mind that the selection of a model must first and foremost be guided by the usage we intend to make of it. In the above example, the model was chosen quite empirically and we have no misconceptions that it is a true biological model, i.e., the equation form of some physiological process. It is merely a reasonable approximation of what was empirically observed. Clearly, the model does not allow us to precisely characterize the rat's growth process, its limbs and organs, etc. If it is these types of complex phenomena that need to be studied, we would have to develop much more sophisticated models to describe them. If on the other hand we are only interested in a basic characterization of the phenomenon, our simple model may just do the trick; it could be useful for such things as predicting the weight of a rat at 15 or 16 weeks, or detecting rats with atypical growth patterns.

The use of such types of parametric models will allow us to formalize and quantify the concept that we have so far introduced intuitively yet informally: the *population approach.* First, defining a typical population curve means in essence defining a typical set of population parameters $(a_{\text{pop}}, b_{\text{pop}}, k_{\text{pop}})$. Then, each individual's curve can be seen as depending on its own set of individual parameters (a_i, b_i, k_i). Characterizing the *inter-individual* variability of these curves around the typical population curve thus means characterizing the inter-individual parameter variability around the typical population parameters. Figure 1.5 shows the population curve as well as the four individual's curves.[1]

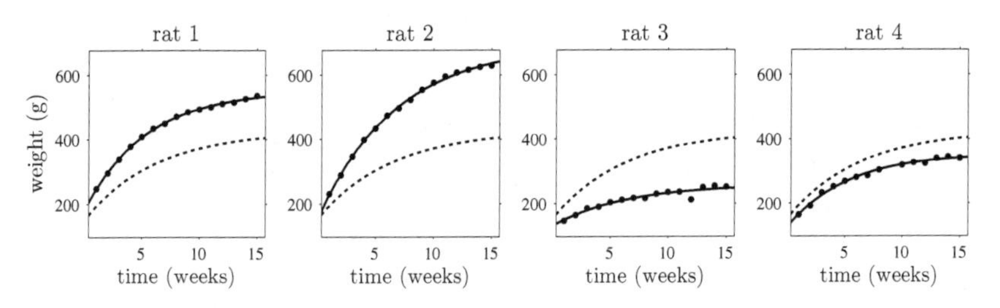

FIGURE 1.5: Weights of four rats. The observed weights are displayed with dots, the individual growth curves with solid lines, the population curves with dotted lines.

This step of modeling the inter-individual variability happens in a probabilistic framework: we consider that each individual in the sample was drawn at random from the population of interest. The individual parameters are then regarded as random variables that possess a certain distribution, precisely representing the way in which the values of these parameters are distributed within the population. Such types of statistical models based on probability distributions allow us to describe the inter-individual variability of the parameters. We would like not only

[1]Population and individual parameters have been estimated using the software MONOLIX and the methods described in Chapter 7. Modeling of this data is presented in detail in Section 8.1.

to characterize this variability, but to understand it as best as possible. Thus, in our example with rats, we can see that some rats are heavier than others, but can we say why? Do we have, for example, relevant information perhaps to explain why rats 1 and 2 are heavier and put on weight faster that rats 3 and 4? Well yes! We notice that these two rats are male while the other two are female. Gender should therefore help explain some of the variability seen here.

In addition to the population curve and the four individual growth curves, Figure 1.6 shows the typical growth curves for males and females.

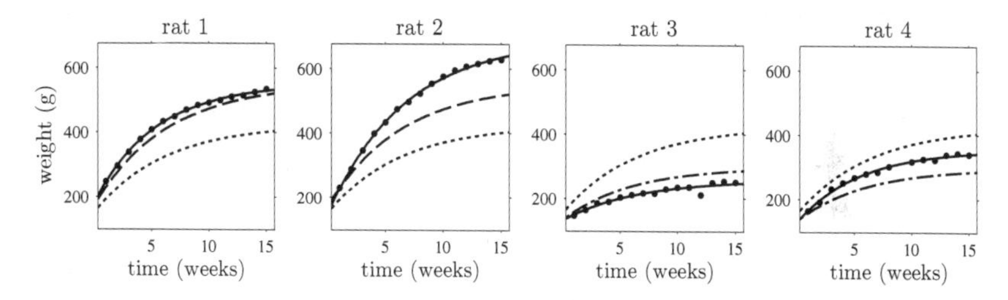

FIGURE 1.6: The typical male curve is displayed with dashed line and female curve with dash-dot line. Rats 1 and 2 are male, rats 3 and 4 are female.

This figure thus shows a decomposition of the variability of the growth curves around the typical population curve: first we decompose the population into two subpopulations, male and female, each of which possesses a typical curve. The differences between these curves represent the *inter-group* variability and already explain much of the variability observed between rats. Of course, all males (nor the females) are not the same weight, so there exists intra-group variability represented by the variability of individual curves around the group ones.

The question then naturally arises as to whether this *intra-group* variability can itself be explained by other *covariates*. In the case of a toxicological study for GM crops, for example, we can wonder if these weight differences are related to diet.

But whether we are in the context of toxicological studies, clinical trials or agronomic trials, modeling is not only for characterizing the collected data. The main goal is the building of a *population model* which applies by definition to the entire population. We therefore move from a purely descriptive treatment of the data to an inferential one. The question is then whether some characteristic observed in the sample can be generalized to the whole population. For example, can the weight difference observed between males and females be truly "explained" by a "gender effect," or can it be attributed to random sampling? In other words, would we have a good chance of reaching the same conclusions if the experiment were repeated with new individuals?

1.2 About models

1.2.1 Mixed effects models and hierarchical models

When observations (rat weights, for example) are available, the observed data have no reason to be absolutely identical to the predictions provided by the model (the growth model in our example). Indeed, the model is chosen to try to mimic the studied phenomenon; thus, the prediction it provides is not necessarily the rat's actual weight. Furthermore, the observations are subject to measurement errors; whatever the quality of the measuring device, it is not possible to measure "exactly" the weight of a rat. The model must therefore include a statistical model that can describe how observations are distributed around the values predicted by the model.

Yet another component of the model must describe the inter-individual variability of the model's parameters. The model will explain some of this variability using individual covariates such as sex, but some variability will remain unexplained and have to be considered as random. Integrating both fixed and random effects into the same model leads naturally to the use of mixed effects models.

Linear mixed effects models (Verbeke and Molenberghs, 2000; West et al., 2006), generalized linear mixed models (Dobson, 2002; McCulloch et al., 2008) and nonlinear mixed effects models (Lindstrom and Bates, 1990; Davidian and Giltinan, 1995; Pinheiro and Bates, 2009) are widely used in applications such as sociology and demography (O'Brien et al., 2008), psychophysiology (Bagiella et al., 2000), ecology and evolution (Bolker et al., 2009), genomics (Haldermans et al., 2007), portfolio risk (McNeil and Wendin, 2007), agronomy (Bürger et al., 2012), neuroimaging (Friston et al., 2005), medicine (Brown and Prescott, 2006), genetics (Ott, 1979), systems biology (Gonzalez et al., 2013) and clinical trials (Andersen and Millen, 2013). Nonlinear mixed effects models have also been an essential tool for pharmacokinetic-pharmacodynamic (PKPD) modeling for several decades (Bonate, 2011). The adoption of population approaches in pharmacometrics owes a lot to the development of the NONMEM software in the 1980's (Beal and Sheiner, 1980) as well as the pioneering work of Lewis Sheiner (Rowland, 2005). We will see in this book that mixed effects models are particularly well-suited statistical tools for population modeling of broad types of data including continuous, categorical, count and time-to-event data.

An alternative yet equivalent approach considers the model to be hierarchical; each individual data series is described by a single model, and variability between individual models is described by a population model. In the case of parametric models, this means that the observations for a given individual are described by a probability distribution that depends on a vector of individual parameters; this is the classic individual approach. The population approach is then a direct extension of this; we add a new component to the model, a probability distribution that describes variability of the individual parameters within the population.

A mixed effects model can thus be seen as a hierarchical model, i.e., as a joint probability distribution for the observations and individual parameters. This joint distribution can easily be extended to the case where other variables in the model are considered as random variables, such as covariates, population parameters or the design.

The use of hierarchical models has grown enormously since the development of Bayesian inference methods (Congdon, 2006; Gelman et al., 2003; Robert, 2007). Markov chain Monte Carlo (MCMC) methods are particularly well-suited to this type of model (Gilks et al., 1996; Robert and Casella, 2004). Hierarchical models are thus used today in a great number of domains including spatial data modeling (Banerjee et al., 2003), marketing (Allenby and Rossi, 1998), political science (Hurwitz and Peffley, 1987), climate studies (Cooley et al., 2007; New and Hulme, 2000), plant growth (Baey et al., 2013), leisure sciences (Crawford et al., 1991), sociology (Raftery, 1995), PKPD modeling (Wakefield et al., 1998) and epidemiology (Lawson, 2013).

Mixed effects models and hierarchical models turn out to be complementary approaches which lead to different representations of the same model.

1.2.2 Description, representation and implementation of models

A model can be used in the real world if it can be implemented in a software program. To do this, we need a language that can be understood by the software. Before even arriving at this point, it is important to be very clear and systematic about what a model is and how we want to use it.

It is of fundamental importance to distinguish between the description, representation and implementation of a model. Each of these three concepts uses a specific language. In the context of mixed effects models,

models that we want to implement can be decomposed into two components: the structural model and the statistical model. Both have to be described, represented and implemented with precision.

Consider first our rat growth model:

1. We start describing a model with words, i.e., a human language: "The weight of a rat increases over time with a growth rate that decreases exponentially"

2. Then we represent the model using a mathematical language: $w(t) = a + b(1 - e^{-k\,t})$

3. Lastly, we implement the model via a language understood by the software:

```
WEIGHT = a + b*(1-exp(-k*TIME))
```

We can follow the same process for the statistical model. A description of the model for the initial weight a might be, "The weight at birth is log-normally distributed in the population." This model can then be mathematically represented:

$$\log(a) \sim \mathcal{N}(\log(a_{\text{pop}}), \omega_a^2), \tag{1.1}$$

and implemented, for instance, with MLXTRAN (see Section 5.2.3), a powerful declarative language for implementing models:

```
a={distribution=lognormal, reference=a_pop, sd=omega_a}
```

This model representation is not unique. Indeed, model (1.1) could also be represented (and implemented) using an equation rather than a definition:

$$a = a_{\text{pop}} e^{\eta}, \tag{1.2}$$

where $\eta \sim \mathcal{N}(0, \omega_a^2)$. This gives us two representations of the same statistical model where the distribution of a is given explicitly in (1.1) and implicitly in (1.2). The choice of representation should be driven by the tasks we want to execute. If the model is only used to perform simulation, both representations contain all the information required. On the other hand, if the log-normal assumption needs to be tested or the probability distribution function (pdf) of a needs to be computed without using approximation, the distribution needs to be represented by an explicit definition as in (1.1).

1.3 Tasks, methods and tools

We will talk about models all the way through the book, but remember at all times that the main purpose of a model is to be *used.* We will essentially focus on two types of task *i)* modeling, in which we have data and wish to construct a model that could have generated this data or is capable of explaining its variability and *ii)* simulation, where we want to generate virtual data using a model.

Remark: This book does not pretend to cover all possible tasks one can perform with a model. Optimization of the design, for instance, is of real importance in practice but will not be considered here. There exists an extensive bibliography on the topic (see, for example, Fedorov and Leonov, 2013, and the many references therein). Several software packages for optimal design also exist, in particular for applications in pharmacometrics (see Mentré et al., 2007, for a comparison of existing tools).

To use a model in practice, we clearly need modeling and simulation tools, but also a language that allows us to implement it, which is "understood" and can be used by these tools.

1.3.1 Model coding

In this book, we will be working with MLXTRAN, a flexible and powerful declarative language[2] designed for implementing complex hierarchical models.

MLXTRAN allows users to write ordinary differential equation (ODE) based models, implement pharmacokinetic models with complex administration schedules, include inter-individual variability in parameters and define statistical models for different types of data (including continuous, categorical, count and time-to-event data). Another crucial property of MLXTRAN is that it rigorously adopts the model representation formalism proposed in this book. In other words, the model implementation is fully consistent with its mathematical representation.

Furthermore, it is important to note that all of the tools we are going to use, for both modeling and simulation, are based on MLXTRAN. This will allow us to define a complete workflow using the same model implementation, i.e., run several tasks based on the same model.

[2]A declarative language allows variables to be defined using equations and definitions, rather than simply the calculation of their values.

1.3.2 Model exploration

Before using a model to perform modeling and simulation, it may be useful to visualize, i.e., represent graphically, the various functions of time given in the model for several parameter values and run a sensitivity analysis, i.e., "look at" what happens when we change the value of one or several parameters.

Coming back to our usual example, we may want to visualize the growth model $f(t) = a + b(1 - e^{-kt})$ and see how a rat's weight converges to its limiting weight as a function of the parameter k. We may also want to visualize the probability distribution of f when a, b and k are random variables with distributions defined in the model.

Whenever we want to visualize a model, we will use the MLXPLORE software. MLXPLORE allows us to visualize not only the structural model but also the statistical one, for example, visualizing the impact of covariates and inter-individual variability of model parameters on predictions.

1.3.3 Modeling

Modeling is clearly the most difficult and challenging task to perform. It can only be partially automated and requires experience on the modeler's part. Tools for modeling are not designed to build a model automatically, but rather to help a modeler construct a model with the aid of a set of observations.

It is important to differentiate clearly between these distinct concepts: the task to perform, the method to use for this task, the algorithm to implement the method, and the implementation of the algorithm itself. For example, imagine that we want to estimate the population parameters. In this case, the task to perform is estimation and a possible method is maximum likelihood estimation. SAEM (Stochastic Approximation of Expectation-Maximization, Delyon et al., 1999) is an algorithm for computing this estimate and MONOLIX a software in which the algorithm is implemented.

Alternatively, we could choose to perform a Bayesian estimate of the population parameters using an MCMC algorithm implemented, for example, in WinBUGS (Ntzoufras, 2011; Spiegelhalter et al., 2003).

As well as estimating the population parameters, it is important to look at the precision of these estimates. Here again, several methods are available, such as the Fisher information matrix, bootstrapping to obtain standard errors, or posterior distributions.

The estimation of population parameters and their uncertainty supposes that the model is given; we then look for parameter values for this model. Of course, the "best" model is rarely known, so a modeler must progress by trial and error, trying different models, improving and comparing them. We therefore need diagnostic and model selection tools.

Diagnostic tools are used to decide whether a model is acceptable, and if not, to identify which model hypotheses are not valid. We will therefore be able to work in the context of statistical hypothesis testing:

$$H_0: \quad \text{“}\mathcal{M} = \mathcal{M}_0\text{”} \qquad \text{vs} \qquad H_1: \quad \text{“}\mathcal{M} \neq \mathcal{M}_0\text{”}$$

where $\mathcal{M}_0$ is the model the modeler wishes to evaluate. A model remains acceptable if the null hypothesis H_0 is not rejected. The more the diagnostic tools are able to detect model misspecification, the more powerful the test will be. Using this methodology does not imply that we know explicitly the rejection zones of the tests; the approach remains largely empirical, based on graphical outputs and simulation methods.

Methods for model selection that are widely used in our context and that are presented in this book are standard, based on statistical tests such as the likelihood ratio test and Wald test (see Engle 1984; Freedman et al. 2007) and on information criteria such as the Akaike information criterion (Greven and Kneib, 2010) and Bayesian information criterion (Schwarz, 1978). The art of modeling then consists of correctly interpreting and adequately combining all the graphical outputs and statistical criteria in order to improve the model.

We mainly use the software MONOLIX in this book to illustrate the various modeling tasks with which the modeler is faced. MONOLIX has been developed with this in mind: it serves modelers well while fully complying with a coherent mathematical formalism that uses well-known and theoretically justified methods. The algorithms implemented in MONOLIX (SAEM, MCMC, simulated annealing, importance sampling, etc.) are extremely efficient for a wide variety of complex models including count data models (Savic and Lavielle, 2009), categorical data models (Savic et al., 2011), censored data models (Samson et al., 2006), time-to-event data models (Mbogning et al., 2014), mixture models (Lavielle and Mbogning, 2013), hidden Markov models (Delattre and Lavielle, 2012) and SDE-based models (Delattre and Lavielle, 2013; Donnet and Samson, 2008). We also emphasize that the convergence of SAEM and its extensions has been established under quite general hypotheses (Allassonnière et al., 2010; Delyon et al., 1999; Kuhn and Lavielle, 2004).

1.3.4 Simulation

Once a model has been constructed, we may wish to simulate the phenomenon we have been studying by generating data from the model. Here, simulation means simulating both virtual individuals and longitudinal data for them, or simply calculating the values of quantities defined in the model (e.g., the components of a system of ODEs).

We have available to us Simulx, which is both an R and MATLAB function that enables us to compute predictions and sample data from any MLXTRAN model. Simulx combines the flexibility of R and MATLAB scripts with the power of MLXTRAN to easily encode complex models.

1.4 Contents of the book

Part I presents several preliminary concepts that will help the reader to be more comfortable with the methodology that follows. We start in Chapter 2 with linear and nonlinear models, used for modeling a single sequence of longitudinal data. In the population approach, linear and nonlinear mixed models can then be naturally introduced to model continuous longitudinal data and take into account variability in a model's individual parameters. Generalized mixed models allow us to model other data such as categorical data. We will see how these different mixed models can all be also seen as hierarchical ones.

Following this, in Chapter 3 we show how the hierarchical structure of a model leads to a natural decomposition of the joint distribution into a product of conditional and marginal distributions.

Part II focuses on model description, representation and implementation. Models for longitudinal data are described in Chapter 4. In particular, models for continuous, count, categorical and time-to-event data – including joint models which combine several types of outcome – are presented and illustrated in various examples.

Models for individual parameters are described in Chapter 5. We will be particularly interested in Gaussian models, i.e., ones in which there exists some transform (log, logit, probit, etc.) for which the transformed parameters have a Gaussian distribution. Individual covariates may also be introduced into a model in order to explain some of the variability in the individual parameters. This chapter also shows how several levels of variability can be included in a model with the aim of modeling things like *inter-occasion* and *inter-group* variability.

Extensions for mixture models, hidden Markov models and stochastic differential equation-based models are presented in Chapter 6.

Part III is concerned with ways to use models to perform tasks. Chapter 7 presents several methods involved in the practical use of these models for tasks such as parameter estimation, model diagnostics and model selection. We use a classical population pharmacokinetics (PK) example to illustrate these methods.

Chapter 8 illustrates many of the proposed approaches and methods using several examples. The first example describes how to model the growth curves of rats in a toxicity study related to GM corn. The second example involves a classic pharmacokinetics-pharmacodynamics application. We show how to extend a proposed joint model for continuous outcomes to a joint model for continuous and categorical data. The last example then shows that mixed effects models can also be successfully used in quantitative biology for modeling the dynamics of biological networks in cell populations.

Chapter 9 describes several algorithms useful for running tasks that interest us. In particular, the SAEM algorithm, used for estimating population parameters by maximum likelihood, is presented and its implementation described. A simple example then allows us to better understand its excellent theoretical and practical properties.

Appendix A describes how to deal with longitudinal data in the classical context of a unique individual. A PK example accompanied by R code illustrates this approach.

Some prerequisites are required for a good understanding of this book. To help with this, Appendix B recalls some basic probability and statistics results which play fundamental roles in model construction.

This book does not treat only pharmacometric modeling and is not intended for pharmacometricians only. However, many of the illustrative examples do come from pharmacokinetics because it is a domain that frequently uses the population approach and mixed models. For this reason, an overview of PK modeling is proposed in Appendix C to help nonspecialists in this domain better understand the book's examples.

Lastly, Appendix D gives a brief introduction to various modeling tools such as MONOLIX, DATXPLORE, MLXPLORE and Simulx. All of these tools use the same modeling language MLXTRAN. This appendix is not a user guide as such, but its content should be enough to provide the minimal required background knowledge to enable any reader to understand how models are implemented in the book's examples and how to run basic examples.

2

Mixed Effects Models vs Hierarchical Models

This chapter explains why it is necessary 1) to extend linear models, used to describe the variation in a sequence of observations, to nonlinear models, useful to represent numerous biological and physical phenomena, 2) to extend these models to (linear and nonlinear) mixed effects models in order to simultaneously model several sequences of observations coming from different individuals, and 3) to extend these models for continuous data to generalized models for discrete data. We will then consider hierarchical models, which allow us to systematically adopt one standard methodology for the entire population approach, no matter the model or data type.

This chapter is not indispensable for a good understanding of the rest of the book, but it helps to put into context everything that follows.

2.1 From linear models to nonlinear mixed effects models

2.1.1 Linear models

Linear models have an important historical role in statistics when it comes to modeling data series $y_1, y_2, \ldots, y_n$ (Muller and Stewart, 2006; Vonesh and Chinchilli, 1997). Such models by definition assume there is a linear relationship between these observations and d series of variables $(x_j^{(1)}, 1 \le j \le n)$, ..., $(x_j^{(d)}, 1 \le j \le n)$:

$$y_j = a_1 x_j^{(1)} + a_2 x_j^{(2)} + \ldots + a_d x_j^{(d)} + e_j, \qquad 1 \le j \le n, \tag{2.1}$$

where $(e_j, 1 \le j \le n)$ is a sequence of residual errors.

In the case of longitudinal data, measurements are collected at observation times $t_1, t_2, \ldots, t_n$. In this context, y_j is the jth observation measured at time t_j and $x_j^{(1)}, x_j^{(2)}, \ldots, x_j^{(d)}$ are the values of the d explanatory variables – also called regression variables – at time t_j.

The reasons for the success and widespread use of linear models are manifold. The first is the simplicity of methods required for the practical use of such models. These methods come essentially from elementary linear algebra. In particular, estimation of the coefficients $a_1, a_2, \ldots, a_d$ is straightforward. Writing model (2.1) in matrix form

$$y = X\,a + e,$$

where $y = (y_1, \ldots, y_n)'$, $X = (x_j^{(k)}, 1 \leq j \leq n, 1 \leq k \leq d)$, $a = (a_1, \ldots, a_d)'$ and $e = (e_1, \ldots, e_n)'$; the least squares estimator of a is $\hat{a} = (X'X)^{-1}X'y$ as long as the rank of X is d (Rao and Toutenburg, 1999).

A second reason for the popularity of linear models is related to the construction of the model itself: model building is reduced to selecting a collection of explanatory variables $x^{(1)}, \ldots, x^{(d)}$. There is only one way we can add (or remove) a variable in the model: additively. The goal is to find the optimal combination of variables for a given criterion, e.g., how to best explain the variability in the observations with the least possible number of explanatory variables.

For example, we could model our rat weight data by a polynomial function of time: $y_j = a_0 + a_1\,t_j + \ldots + a_d\,t_j^d + e_j$. Figure 2.1 shows that a polynomial of degree 1 (a straight line) provides a very coarse fit. Adding a degree 2 term gives a much better one. The fit can be made almost perfect by adding an additional degree 3 term.

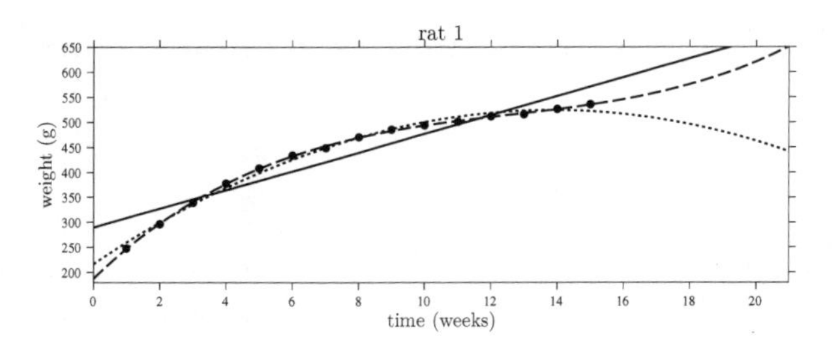

FIGURE 2.1: Weight curve for one rat. The observed weights are displayed with dots, the individual fitted polynomials of degree 1, 2 and 3 with solid, dotted and dashed lines, respectively.

Despite the very good fits of the degree 2 and 3 polynomials, the interest of such models is extremely limited. On the one hand, the polynomials' coefficients have no obvious biological interpretation; for instance, it would be absurd to use a polynomial model to predict the rat weight after 15 weeks since the polynomial of degree 2 is decreasing while that of degree 3 is increasing faster and faster. Using a polynomial model here, we are therefore not seeking to build a structural model f that approximates a physical phenomenon, but merely seeking to capture the variability in the observations due to the explanatory variables $t, t^2, \ldots, t^d$. The underlying biological phenomenon has no place in the construction of such models; we could thus use exactly the same approach to model other data types.

2.1.2 Nonlinear models

We adopt in this book a fundamentally different strategy where we seek to build a structural model that can describe mathematically – even in a rudimentary way – the observed phenomenon. It is in this spirit that we prefer to use a growth model such as shown earlier, $f(t) = a+b(1-e^{-k\,t})$. It is clearly impossible to limit ourselves to linear models and therefore necessary to extend model (2.1) to more general ones, perhaps nonlinear, of the form

$$y_j = f(t_j; \phi) + e_j,$$

where ϕ is a vector of specific parameters for a structural model f. Saying that the model is nonlinear means that f is not a linear function of the components of ϕ.

EXAMPLE 2.1 A rat's weight data can be modeled using the nonlinear model

$$y_j = a + b(1 - e^{-k\,t_j}) + e_j. \tag{2.2}$$

Here, the parameters of the structural model are $\phi = (a, b, k)$.

In many situations, the structural model f is defined as the solution of a system of ordinary differential equations (ODEs). Such solutions do not always have closed-form expressions.

EXAMPLE 2.2 f represents the amount of water in a tank which empties. A is the initial amount of water before opening the plughole at time t_0.

Assume first a linear elimination process. This means that the rate of elimination is proportional to the amount in the tank: $f'(t) = -k\,f(t)$. The solution of this linear ODE is a nonlinear function of k:

$$f(t) = \begin{cases} A & \text{if } t \leq t_0 \\ Ae^{-k\,(t-t_0)} & \text{otherwise.} \end{cases}$$

If we instead assume a saturable elimination process:

$$f'(t) = -\frac{k\,f(t)}{1 + \alpha\,f(t)},$$

there is no analytical solution to the equation. Nevertheless, f "exists" and is defined as the solution of this ODE. It is a nonlinear function of α and k.

Remark: These simple examples show that an extremely elementary physical phenomenon may be modeled using nonlinear models. Many phenomena from many different domains can only be characterized satisfactorily using nonlinear models. In particular, this includes pharmacokinetic (PK) models, compartmental models for which transfers between compartments and elimination are described using ODEs (Bonate, 2011; Gabrielsson and Weiner, 2007). Even the simplest PK models are therefore nonlinear.

2.1.3 Linear mixed effects models

Model (2.1) concerns a single individual. Suppose now that a study is based on N individuals and that we seek to build a global model for all the collected observations for the N individuals. We will denote y_{ij} the jth observation taken of individual i at time t_{ij} and $x_{ij}^{(1)}, \ldots, x_{ij}^{(d)}$ the values of the d explanatory variables for individual i at time t_{ij}. If we assume the parameters of the model can vary from one individual to another, then for any subject i, model (2.1) becomes

$$y_{ij} = a_{i1}x_{ij}^{(1)} + a_{i2}x_{ij}^{(2)} + \ldots + a_{id}x_{ij}^{(d)} + e_{ij}, \quad 1 \leq j \leq n_i. \tag{2.3}$$

Suppose to begin with that each individual parameter a_{ik} can be additively broken down into a *fixed effect* β_k and an *individual effect* η_{ik}, i.e.,

$$a_{ik} = \beta_k + \eta_{ik}.$$

In this model, β_k is the "typical" value of the kth model parameter in the population and η_{ik} the deviation of a_{ik} from this typical value. We can then rewrite (2.3) in matrix form:

$$y_i = X_i\,\beta + X_i\,\eta_i + e_i, \tag{2.4}$$

where X_i is the $n_i \times d$ design matrix formed with the d explanatory variables $x^{(1)}, \ldots, x^{(d)}$, y_i and e_i the $n_i \times 1$ vectors of observations and residual errors, and β and η_i the $d \times 1$ vectors of fixed and individual effects.

EXAMPLE 2.3 Consider the following linear growth model:

$$\begin{aligned} y_{ij} &= a_i + b_i\, t_{ij} + e_{ij} \\ a_i &= a_{\text{pop}} + \eta_{a,i} \\ b_i &= b_{\text{pop}} + \eta_{b,i}. \end{aligned}$$

We can write this model as in (2.4) with $\beta = (a_{\text{pop}}, b_{\text{pop}})'$ and

$$X_i = \begin{pmatrix} 1 & t_{i,1} \\ \vdots & \vdots \\ 1 & t_{i,n_i} \end{pmatrix}.$$

If we place ourselves in a probabilistic framework, the individual parameters (a_{ik}) are going to be considered random variables. Individual effects (η_{ik}) are usually called *random effects* in this context (Verbeke and Molenberghs, 2000). In a linear mixed effects model, η_i and e_i are independent vectors with mean 0. Assuming furthermore that both η_i and e_i are normally distributed with respective variances Ω and Σ_i, we have that y_i is also a Gaussian vector whose mean and variance-covariance matrix are easily computed:

$$y_i \sim \mathcal{N}(X_i\,\beta\ ,\ X_i \Omega X_i' + \Sigma_i).$$

We can extend model (2.4) to models invoking more complicated design matrices that may even differ for fixed and random effects (Laird and Ware, 1982):

$$y_i = X_i\,\beta + Z_i\,\eta_i + e_i. \tag{2.5}$$

We can thus introduce covariates into the model in order to explain part of the variability in the observations.

EXAMPLE 2.4 Consider the same linear growth example but now suppose that the slope b_i is a function of a covariate c_i:

$$b_i = \gamma + \delta\, c_i + \eta_{b,i}.$$

Here, the vector of fixed effects is $\beta = (a_{\text{pop}}, \gamma, \delta)'$ and the design matrices are

$$X_i = \begin{pmatrix} 1 & t_{i,1} & c_i t_{i,1} \\ \vdots & \vdots & \vdots \\ 1 & t_{i,1} & c_i t_{i,n_i} \end{pmatrix}, \qquad Z_i = \begin{pmatrix} 1 & t_{i,1} \\ \vdots & \vdots \\ 1 & t_{i,n_i} \end{pmatrix}.$$

Model (2.4) also includes models for which certain parameters do not exhibit inter-individual variability, as well as models for which variability in the parameters may change over time.

EXAMPLE 2.5 For the sake of simplicity, assume now that $t_{ij} = j$. Suppose that the intercept has no inter-individual variability and the slope changes randomly at time m:

$$y_{ij} = a_{\text{pop}} + b_i\, j + \eta_{2,i}(j - m)^+ + e_{ij},$$

where $b_i = b_{\text{pop}} + \eta_{1,i}$ and $x^+ \stackrel{\text{def}}{=} \max(0, x)$. Then, representation (2.5) holds, with

$$X_i = \begin{pmatrix} 1 & 1 \\ 1 & 2 \\ \vdots & \vdots \\ 1 & n_i \end{pmatrix}, \qquad Z_i = \begin{pmatrix} 1 & 0 \\ 2 & 0 \\ \vdots & \vdots \\ m & 0 \\ m+1 & 1 \\ \vdots & \vdots \\ n & n-m \end{pmatrix}, \qquad \eta_i = \begin{pmatrix} \eta_{1,i} \\ \eta_{2,i} \end{pmatrix}.$$

2.1.4 Nonlinear mixed effects models

Combining these two extensions to the basic linear model (2.1) leads to so-called *nonlinear mixed effects models* (see, for instance, Davidian and Giltinan 1995; Lindstrom and Bates 1990; Pinheiro and Bates 2009):

$$y_{ij} = f(t_{ij}; \beta, \eta_i, c_i) + e_{ij}. \tag{2.6}$$

This mathematical representation of a model therefore considers that the structural model is a function, possibly nonlinear, of fixed and random effects. The linear model (2.5) is a special case of this model when f is a linear function of both the fixed effects β and random effects η. As the model is nonlinear, inclusion of random effects and covariates does not have to be done in a linear way.

EXAMPLE 2.6 We can choose for example to add to growth model (2.2) certain random effects additively and others exponentially:

$$y_{ij} = (a_{\text{pop}} + \eta_{a,i}) + b_{\text{pop}}\, e^{\eta_{b,i}}(1 - e^{-(k_{\text{pop}} + \eta_{k,i})\, t_{ij}}) + e_{ij}.$$

Here, $\beta = (a_{\text{pop}}, b_{\text{pop}}, k_{\text{pop}})$ and $\eta_i = (\eta_{a,i}, \eta_{b,i}, \eta_{k,i})$. There are also several ways to introduce a gender effect into the model. For example, we can set

$c_i = 1$ if rat i is male and $c_i = 0$ if female. One possible model combining covariates and random and fixed effects is then:

$$y_{ij} = (a_{\rm pop} + \gamma\, c_i + \eta_{a,i}) + b_{\rm pop}\, e^{\delta\, c_i + \eta_{b,i}}(1 - e^{-(k_{\rm pop}+\eta_{k,i})\, t_{ij}}) + e_{ij}. \quad (2.7)$$

In this example, the vector of fixed effects includes the coefficients of the covariate c_i: $\beta = (a_{\rm pop}, b_{\rm pop}, k_{\rm pop}, \gamma, \delta)$.

Another form of nonlinearity occurs if we assume that the variability of the residual errors may vary from one individual to another and possibly over time. We can then model the variability of the residual errors by a function g:

$$y_{ij} = f(t_{ij}; \beta, \eta_i, c_i) + g(t_{ij}; \beta, \eta_i, c_i) e_{ij}. \quad (2.8)$$

EXAMPLE 2.7 Suppose that there are random effects that act linearly on the linear structural model $f(t) = a+bt$ and on the variability of the residual errors:

$$y_{ij} = a_{\rm pop} + \eta_{a,i} + (b_{\rm pop} + \eta_{b,i})t_{ij} + (\sigma_{\rm pop} + \eta_{\sigma,i})e_{ij}.$$

Though the structural model f is a linear function and the random effects act additively on the model's parameters, this model is considered to be a nonlinear mixed effects one because it includes products $\eta_{\sigma,i}e_{ij}$ of random effects and residual errors.

2.2 From nonlinear mixed effects models to hierarchical models

The structural models f in which we are going to be interested are all parametric. These are functions of time entirely characterized by a parameter vector ϕ. In the population approach, the same structural model f is used for all individuals, but each has a different set of individual parameters. The mathematical representations of linear models in (2.5) and nonlinear models in (2.6) bring together fixed and random effects and residual errors without explicitly displaying the model's individual parameters.

Another mathematical representation much more frequently used for presenting nonlinear mixed effects models is the *two-stage model* (see Davidian and Giltinan 1995) which both explicitly provides the parameters of the structural model and shows these individual parameters as functions of fixed and random effects and possibly individual covariates:

$$y_{ij} = f(t_{ij}; \phi_i) + e_{ij} \tag{2.9a}$$
$$\phi_i = h(\beta, \eta_i, c_i). \tag{2.9b}$$

Here, having a two-stage model means that the observations for a given individual are described first by a model for the observations that depends on a vector of individual parameters; this is the classic individual approach. The population approach is then a direct extension of this: the second stage adds a component to the model that describes variability in the individual parameters within the population.

EXAMPLE 2.8 The growth model introduced in (2.7) can be rewritten using this two-stage representation:

$$y_{ij} = a_i + b_i(1 - e^{-k_i\, t_{ij}}) + e_{ij} \tag{2.10a}$$

$$\begin{aligned} a_i &= a_{\text{pop}} + \gamma\, c_i + \eta_{a,i} \\ b_i &= b_{\text{pop}}\, e^{\delta\, c_i + \eta_{b,i}} \\ k_i &= k_{\text{pop}} + \eta_{k,i}. \end{aligned} \tag{2.10b}$$

Clearly we still have the same model, but the individual parameters of the model are now explicitly given.

Once the probability distributions for the random effects and residual errors have been defined, model representation (2.9) implicitly defines the joint distribution of the observations (y_i) and individual parameters (ϕ_i). In effect, for each individual, equation (2.9a) defines the conditional distribution of the observations y_i (i.e., conditionally on the individual parameters ϕ_i) while (2.9b) gives the distribution of the individual parameters ϕ_i.

EXAMPLE 2.9 Assume that the random effects and residual errors are mutually independent and normally distributed:

$$e_{ij} \underset{\text{i.i.d.}}{\sim} \mathcal{N}(0, \sigma^2)$$
$$\eta_{a,i} \underset{\text{i.i.d.}}{\sim} \mathcal{N}(0, \omega_a^2), \qquad \eta_{b,i} \underset{\text{i.i.d.}}{\sim} \mathcal{N}(0, \omega_b^2), \qquad \eta_{k,i} \underset{\text{i.i.d.}}{\sim} \mathcal{N}(0, \omega_k^2).$$

Then, the model given in (2.10) implicitly defines the conditional distribution of the observations (y_{ij}) and individual parameters a_i, b_i, and k_i:

$$y_{ij}|a_i, b_i, k_i \sim \mathcal{N}(a_i + b_i(1 - e^{-k_i t_{ij}}), \sigma^2) \tag{2.11a}$$

$$\begin{aligned} a_i \underset{\text{i.i.d.}}{\sim} & \begin{cases} \mathcal{N}(a_{\text{pop}}, \omega_a^2) & \text{if rat } i \text{ is female } (c_i = 0) \\ \mathcal{N}(a_{\text{pop}} + \gamma, \omega_a^2) & \text{if rat } i \text{ is male } (c_i = 1) \end{cases} \\ \log(b_i) \underset{\text{i.i.d.}}{\sim} & \begin{cases} \mathcal{N}(\log(b_{\text{pop}}), \omega_b^2) & \text{if rat } i \text{ is female } (c_i = 0) \\ \mathcal{N}(\log(b_{\text{pop}}) + \delta, \omega_b^2) & \text{if rat } i \text{ is male } (c_i = 1) \end{cases} \\ k_i \underset{\text{i.i.d.}}{\sim} & \mathcal{N}(k_{\text{pop}}, \omega_k^2). \end{aligned} \tag{2.11b}$$

This example shows us that there are several possible representations of the same mixed effects model; here, one in terms of equations involving fixed and random effects, the other in terms of definitions. The choice of representation should be guided by the use we wish to make of the model. Both representations can be used in the simulation context, but when evaluating whether the hypotheses of the statistical model are valid, it is best to use explicit definitions as in (2.11).

The representation using definitions is also often preferable when it comes to describing a model. In effect, it is the distribution of the individual parameters that is pertinent when trying to describe the population model, not the random effect's distribution. For our example, perhaps we would like to describe how the limiting weight is distributed within the population, i.e., to know its median value for males and females, the proportion of males with a limiting weight above 600g, etc. All of these questions have real biological meaning because they involve an actual physiological parameter of interest. On the other hand, the random effects do not "exist." They are virtual probabilistic objects used to represent distributions in the form of equations. We cannot see them or measure them, only calculate them. In other words, (2.10b) does not describe the statistical model; it comes from it.

Furthermore, many distributions cannot be written as equations. For instance, a categorical parameter cannot be represented as an equation involving a random effect; a model can only be defined here using its probability distribution.

EXAMPLE 2.10 Patients may react differently to the same HIV treatment. Let us distinguish between patients that respond and those that do not respond to the treatment. Let G_i be the category of patient i:

- $G_i = r$ if i is a responder
- $G_i = nr$ if i is a nonresponder.

G_i is an individual parameter whose distribution is defined by its probability function, i.e., $\mathbb{P}(G_i = r)$ and $\mathbb{P}(G_i = nr)$. There is no alternative representation of this model in equation form that lets us include continuous random effects; it is the distribution of G_i that is the thing of interest. We may look, for example, to model the probability of treatment response with respect to phenotype and genotype covariates or, estimate the conditional distribution of G_i when observations such as viral charge are available.

Finally, let us note that model (2.9) can be extended to the situation where the standard deviation of the residual error e_{ij} is a parametric function that can depend on ϕ_i and some additional parameter ξ_i:

$$e_{ij} = g(t_{ij}, \phi_i, \xi_i)\varepsilon_{ij}.$$

Here, ε_{ij} is a random variable with mean 0 and variance 1 for identifiability reasons, and the vector of individual parameters is $\psi_i = (\phi_i, \xi_i) = h(\beta, \eta_i, c_i)$.

2.3 From generalized mixed models to hierarchical models

2.3.1 Generalized linear mixed models

Many physical phenomena cannot be characterized using linear or nonlinear Gaussian models. This is why, for example, the exponential distribution is often used to model waiting times (Gross et al., 2013) and the gamma distribution for modeling reaction times in visual search experiments (Palmer et al., 2011). These continuous data models do not involve residual errors and therefore cannot be represented in equation form like (2.8). Models for categorical, count and survival data also cannot be represented in equation form (2.8).

Generalized linear mixed models (GLMM) aim to model the expected value $\mathbb{E}(y_{ij})$ of the observations by way of a link function h and a linear predictor (see, for example, Bolker et al. 2009; Hedeker 2005; McCulloch et al. 2008):

$$h(\mathbb{E}(y_i)) = X_i\beta + Z_i\eta_i.$$

The choice of link function is generally guided by constraints on the values that observations (y_{ij}) can reasonably take. Thus, log functions are frequently used as link functions to model data with Poisson or exponential distributions so as to ensure parameters are positive. The logit function $h(x) = \log(x/(1-x))$ and the probit function $h(x) = \mathbb{P}(\mathcal{N}(0,1) < x)$ can be used to model probabilities and thus be used as link functions for modeling, for example, categorical and binomial data.

EXAMPLE 2.11 We would like to compare certain learning abilities between boys and girls. For example, we might want to model how the probability of succeeding at a particular task evolves over time. Defining $y_{ij}^{(1)} = 1$ if subject i succeeds at the task at time t_{ij} and $y_{ij}^{(1)} = 0$ otherwise, we want to model $\mathbb{E}\left(y_{ij}^{(1)}\right) = \mathbb{P}\left(y_{ij}^{(1)} = 1\right)$. Let $s_i = 0$ if subject i is a girl and $s_i = 1$ if a boy. The following model supposes that girls and boys learn to successfully perform the task at different rates:

$$\text{logit}\left(\mathbb{P}\left(y_{ij}^{(1)} = 1\right)\right) = (a + \eta_{a,i}) + (b + c\, s_i + \eta_{b,i})t_{ij}.$$

Here, the random effects allow us to take into account inter-subject variability at the beginning of the trial and the fact that subjects of different sex learn the task at different rates.

Suppose now that we want to look at the time required to complete a given task. We could model this using an exponential distribution and the log as a link function:

$$\log\left(\mathbb{E}\left(y_{ij}^{(2)}\right)\right) = u + \eta_{u,i} - (v + c\, s_i + \eta_{v,i})\frac{t_{ij}}{1 + t_{ij}}.$$

Here, $y_{ij}^{(2)}$ is the time taken by subject i on day j, and u the "typical" time in the population required to execute the task when the experiment starts; i.e., when $t = 0$, and $u - v$ and $u - v - c$ are the typical limiting times – after an infinite training period – for girls and boys, respectively.

2.3.2 Generalized nonlinear mixed models

In the same way that it was necessary to extend linear models for continuous data to nonlinear ones, generalized linear models for other data types often need to be extended to generalized nonlinear mixed models (Vonesh et al., 1996). For instance, we may wish to use a nonlinear model to model the expectation of the observations or parameters other than the expectation. Take for instance the gamma distribution, defined by two parameters: a shape parameter and a scale parameter; we might want to simultaneously model these two parameters. We may even want to use non-Gaussian distributions to model these parameters.

When we are simultaneously in the longitudinal data and population context, a model for the observations must allow us define a distribution that can both evolve with time and vary from one individual to the next. Therefore, whenever this distribution is *parametric*, we must allow the parameter – or parameter vector – that defines the distribution to vary with time and between individuals. In other words, we suppose that there exists some distribution p and parametric function α such that

$$y_{ij} \sim p(\,\cdot\,; \alpha_{ij}) \tag{2.12a}$$
$$\alpha_{ij} = \alpha(t_{ij}, \psi_i). \tag{2.12b}$$

Once the distribution p has been chosen for observations (y_{ij}), the model is defined by the parameter α_{ij}, i.e., the value of the function α at time t_{ij} and parametrized by ψ_i. In this way, we have clearly defined a hierarchical model; (2.12) defines the conditional distribution of the observations, i.e., the first stage of the hierarchical model. The second stage consists of defining a population distribution for the vector of individual parameters ψ_i.

Defining a model for the observations therefore reverts to choosing the parametric distribution p and defining a model for parameter α of distribution p. Here are some examples of distributions p with their parameters defined as functions of time:

distribution		parameters	functions
Gaussian	$y_{ij} \sim \mathcal{N}(f_{ij}, g_{ij}^2)$	$f_{ij} = f(t_{ij}, \psi_i) = \mathbb{E}\,(y_{ij} \vert \psi_i)$ $g_{ij} = g(t_{ij}, \psi_i) = \mathrm{sd}\,(y_{ij} \vert \psi_i)$	$f(t, \psi_i)$ $g(t, \psi_i)$
Poisson	$y_{ij} \sim \mathcal{P}(\lambda_{ij})$	$\lambda_{ij} = \lambda(t_{ij}, \psi_i) = \mathbb{E}\,(y_{ij} \vert \psi_i)$	$\lambda(t, \psi_i)$
Bernoulli	$y_{ij} \sim \mathcal{B}(\pi_{ij})$	$\pi_{ij} = \pi(t_{ij}, \psi_i) = \mathbb{P}(y_{ij} = 1 \vert \psi_i)$	$\pi(t, \psi_i)$
exponential	$y_{ij} \sim \mathcal{E}(\lambda_{ij})$	$\lambda_{ij} = \lambda(t_{ij}, \psi_i) = 1/\mathbb{E}\,(y_{ij} \vert \psi_i)$	$\lambda(t, \psi_i)$

Remark: In the Gaussian case, the residual error model is the function g which may depend on individual parameters. For uniformity of notation, we have regrouped into a single vector ψ_i the parameter vector ϕ_i of the structural model and the parameter vector ξ_i of the residual error model.

Summary. . .

In the population context, models for longitudinal data are hierarchical models:

1. In the first stage, the model for observations y_{ij} is a parametric distribution that depends on a parameter $\alpha_{ij} = \alpha(t_{ij}, \psi_i)$. The function α is a function of time, parametrized by a vector of individual parameters ψ_i.

2. In the second stage, the model for the individual parameter ψ_i is a probability distribution that describes inter-individual variability in the population. This distribution is the population distribution; it is parametrized by a vector of population parameters θ.

3

What is a Model? A Joint Probability Distribution!

There is no universal definition of what a model is. Defining a model is therefore a relatively arbitrary process that depends on your particular point of view. In this chapter, we are going to show that defining a model as a probability distribution allows us to develop a rigorous and coherent framework.

The contents of this chapter are not indispensable for understanding the rest of the book but are extremely useful for understanding the formal framework for models we use. Essentially, a good understanding of this chapter requires the reader to be comfortable with manipulating conditional probability distributions.

3.1 Introduction and notation

A model built for real-world applications can involve various types of variables such as measurements, individual and population parameters, covariates and design. The model allows us to represent relationships between these variables.

If we consider things from a probabilistic point of view, some of the variables will be random, so the model becomes a probabilistic one, representing the joint distribution of these random variables. Defining a model therefore means defining a joint distribution. The hierarchical structure of the model will then allow it to be decomposed into submodels, i.e., a product of conditional distributions.

Tasks such as estimation, model selection, simulation and optimization can then be expressed as specific ways of using these probability distributions.

- A model is a joint probability distribution.
- A submodel is a conditional distribution derived from this joint distribution.
- A task is a specific use of these distributions.

We will illustrate this approach starting with a very simple example that will gradually become more sophisticated. Then we will see in various situations what can be defined as the model and what its inputs are. We start by introducing some general notations and conventions.

- We will call y_i the set of observations recorded for subject i, and $\boldsymbol{y}$ the combined set of observations for all N individuals: $\boldsymbol{y} = (y_1, \ldots, y_N)$. In general, we will use **bold** text (as for $\boldsymbol{y}$) when a variable regroups several individuals. Thus, we write ψ_i for the parameter vector for individual i and $\boldsymbol{\psi}$ for the parameter vector for a set of individuals: $\boldsymbol{\psi} = (\psi_1, \ldots, \psi_N)$.

- We denote p_y and p_ψ the distributions of $\boldsymbol{y}$ and $\boldsymbol{\psi}$, respectively; $p_{y|\psi}$ the conditional distribution of $\boldsymbol{y}$ given $\boldsymbol{\psi}$; and $p_{y,\psi}$ the joint distribution of $\boldsymbol{y}$ and $\boldsymbol{\psi}$. In these (and other distributions), we have placed the variable described by the distribution in the index.

- We use the same p_x notation for the distribution of a random variable x as for its probability density function (pdf).

- When there is no ambiguity when working with whole equations, to simplify notation we may omit the indices and simply use the symbol p. For instance, $p_y(\boldsymbol{y})$, the pdf of $\boldsymbol{y}$, becomes $\mathrm{p}(\boldsymbol{y})$; both are equivalent. The symbol p has no meaning on its own; it is completely defined by its arguments.

- When the distribution of the individual parameters ψ_i of subject i depends on a vector of individual covariates c_i and a population parameter θ, we may choose to explicitly show this dependence by writing the distribution of ψ_i as $\mathrm{p}(\psi_i; c_i, \theta)$.

- We use a semicolon (;) to separate random variables from nonrandom ones, and we use a comma (,) to separate variables of same type. For instance, $\mathrm{p}(y_i, \psi_i; c_i, \theta)$ is the joint pdf of y_i and ψ_i which depends on c_i and θ.

- We use a vertical bar (|) to define conditional distributions. For instance, $\mathrm{p}(y_i|\psi_i)$ is the conditional distribution of y_i given ψ_i.

- When the conditional distribution $p_{y_i|\psi_i}$ of the observations $y_i = (y_{ij}, 1 \leq j \leq n_i)$ of individual i depends on regression variables

$x_i = (x_{ij}, 1 \le j \le n_i)$ and source terms u_i (i.e., inputs of a dynamical system such as doses in a pharmacokinetic model), we may choose to explicitly show this dependence, writing the conditional distribution as $\mathrm{p}(y_i|\psi_i; x_i, u_i)$.

3.2 An illustrative example

3.2.1 A model for the observations from a single individual

Let $y = (y_j, 1 \le j \le n)$ be a vector of *observations* obtained at times $\underline{t} = (t_j, 1 \le j \le n)$. We consider that the y_j are random variables and denote p_y the distribution (or pdf) of y. If we assume a *parametric model*, then there exists a vector of parameters ψ that completely define p_y.

We can then explicitly represent this dependency with respect to ψ by writing $p_y(\,\cdot\,;\psi)$ for the pdf of y. If we wish to be even more precise, we can make it clear that this distribution is defined for a given design, i.e., a given vector of sampling times $\underline{t}$, and write $p_y(\,\cdot\,;\psi,\underline{t})$ instead.

- In this context, the model is the distribution of the observations $p_y(\,\cdot\,;\psi,\underline{t})$.
- The inputs to the model are the parameters ψ and design $\underline{t}$.

EXAMPLE 3.1 500 mg of a drug is given by intravenous (iv) bolus to a patient at time 0. We assume that the evolution of the plasmatic concentration of the drug over time is described by the pharmacokinetic (PK) model

$$f(t; V, k) = \frac{500}{V} e^{-k\,t},$$

where V is the volume of distribution and k the elimination rate constant. The concentration is measured at times $(t_j, 1 \le j \le n)$ with additive residual errors:

$$y_j = f(t_j; V, k) + e_j, \quad 1 \le j \le n.$$

Assuming that the residual errors (e_j) are independent and normally distributed with constant variance a^2, the observed values (y_j) are also independent random variables and

$$y_j \sim \mathcal{N}\left(f(t_j; V, k), a^2\right), \quad 1 \le j \le n. \tag{3.1}$$

Here, the vector of parameters ψ is (V, k, a). V and k are the PK parameters for the structural PK model and a the residual error parameter. As the y_j

are independent, the joint distribution of y is the product of their marginal distributions:

$$p_y(y; \psi, \underline{t}) = \prod_{j=1}^{n} p_{y_j}(y_j; \psi, t_j),$$

where p_{y_j} is the normal distribution defined in (3.1).

3.2.2 A model for several individuals

Now let us move to N individuals. It is natural to suppose that each is represented by the same basic parametric model but not necessarily the exact same parameter values. Thus, individual i has parameters ψ_i. If we consider that individuals are randomly selected from the population, then we can treat $\boldsymbol{\psi} = (\psi_i, 1 \leq i \leq N)$ as if the ψ_i were random vectors.

If p_ψ is a parametric distribution that depends on a vector θ of *population parameters* and a set of *individual covariates* $\mathbf{c} = (c_i, 1 \leq i \leq N)$, this dependence can be made clear by writing $p_\psi(\,\cdot\,; \theta, \mathbf{c})$ for the pdf of $\boldsymbol{\psi}$.

- In this context, the model is the joint distribution of the observations and the individual parameters:

$$\mathrm{p}(\boldsymbol{y}, \boldsymbol{\psi}; \theta, \mathbf{c}, \underline{\boldsymbol{t}}) = \mathrm{p}(\boldsymbol{y}|\boldsymbol{\psi}; \underline{\boldsymbol{t}})\, \mathrm{p}(\boldsymbol{\psi}; \theta, \mathbf{c}).$$

- The inputs to the model are the population parameters θ, individual covariates $\mathbf{c} = (c_i, 1 \leq i \leq N)$ and measurement times $\underline{\boldsymbol{t}} = (t_{ij},\ 1 \leq i \leq N,\ 1 \leq j \leq n_i)$.

EXAMPLE 3.2 Let us suppose N patients receive the same treatment as the single patient did. We now have the same PK model (3.1) for each patient, except that each has its own individual PK parameters V_i and k_i and potentially its own residual error parameter a_i:

$$y_{ij} \sim \mathcal{N}\left(\frac{500}{V_i} e^{-k_i\, t_{ij}}, a_i^2\right). \tag{3.2}$$

Here, $\psi_i = (V_i, k_i, a_i)$. One possible model is then to assume the same residual error model for all patients and log-normal distributions for V and k:

$$\begin{aligned} a_i &= a \\ \log(V_i) &\underset{\text{i.i.d.}}{\sim} \mathcal{N}\left(\log(V_{\text{pop}}) + \beta \log(w_i/70),\ \omega_V^2\right) \\ \log(k_i) &\underset{\text{i.i.d.}}{\sim} \mathcal{N}\left(\log(k_{\text{pop}}),\ \omega_k^2\right), \end{aligned} \tag{3.3}$$

where the only covariate we choose to consider, w_i, is the weight (in kg) of patient i. The model therefore consists of the conditional distribution of the concentrations defined in (3.2) and the distribution of the individual parameters defined in (3.3). The inputs to the model are the population parameters $\theta = (V_{\rm pop}, k_{\rm pop}, \omega_V, \omega_k, \beta, a)$, covariates (here, the weight) $(w_i, 1 \leq i \leq N)$, and design, i.e., the sampling times $(t_{ij}, 1 \leq i \leq N, 1 \leq j \leq n_i)$.

3.2.3 A model for the population parameters

In some cases, it may turn out that it is useful or important to consider that the population parameter θ is itself random, rather than fixed. There are various reasons for this, such as if we want to model uncertainty in its value, introduce prior information in an estimation context, or model inter-population variability if the model is not considering only one given population.

In such cases, let us denote p_θ the distribution of θ. As the status of θ has changed, the model now becomes the joint distribution of its random variables, i.e., of $\boldsymbol{y}$, $\boldsymbol{\psi}$ and θ.

- In this context, the model is the joint distribution of the observations, the individual parameters and the population parameters:

$$\mathrm{p}(\boldsymbol{y}, \boldsymbol{\psi}, \theta; \boldsymbol{c}, \underline{\boldsymbol{t}}) = \mathrm{p}(\boldsymbol{y}|\boldsymbol{\psi}; \underline{\boldsymbol{t}})\, \mathrm{p}(\boldsymbol{\psi}|\theta; \boldsymbol{c})\, \mathrm{p}(\theta).$$

- The inputs to the model are the individual covariates $\boldsymbol{c} = (c_i, 1 \leq i \leq N)$ and measurement times $\underline{\boldsymbol{t}} = (t_{ij}, 1 \leq i \leq N, 1 \leq j \leq n_i)$.

Remarks:

1. The formula is identical for $\mathrm{p}(\boldsymbol{\psi}; \theta)$ and $\mathrm{p}(\boldsymbol{\psi}|\theta)$. What has changed is the status of θ. It is not random in $\mathrm{p}(\boldsymbol{\psi}; \theta)$, the distribution of $\boldsymbol{\psi}$ in terms of θ, whereas it is random in $\mathrm{p}(\boldsymbol{\psi}|\theta)$, the conditional distribution of $\boldsymbol{\psi}$ given θ.

2. If p_θ is a parametric distribution with parameter φ, this dependency can be made explicit by writing $p_\theta(\,\cdot\,; \varphi)$ for the distribution of θ.

3. Not necessarily all of the components of θ need be random. If it is possible to decompose θ into (θ_F, θ_R) where θ_F is fixed and θ_R random, we get

$$\mathrm{p}(\boldsymbol{y}, \boldsymbol{\psi}, \theta_R; \underline{\boldsymbol{t}}, \theta_F, \boldsymbol{c}) = \mathrm{p}(\boldsymbol{y}|\boldsymbol{\psi}; \underline{\boldsymbol{t}})\, \mathrm{p}(\boldsymbol{\psi}|\theta_R; \theta_F, \boldsymbol{c})\, \mathrm{p}(\theta_R).$$

EXAMPLE 3.3 We can introduce prior distributions in order to model the inter-population variability of the population parameters $V_{\rm pop}$ and $k_{\rm pop}$:

$$\begin{aligned} V_{\rm pop} &\sim \mathcal{N}\left(30, 3^2\right) \\ k_{\rm pop} &\sim \mathcal{N}\left(0.1, 0.01^2\right). \end{aligned} \tag{3.4}$$

As before, the conditional distribution of the concentration is given by (3.2). Now, (3.3) is the *conditional distribution* of the individual PK parameters, given $\theta_R = (V_{\rm pop}, k_{\rm pop})$. The distribution of θ_R is defined in (3.4). Here, the inputs of the model are the fixed population parameters $\theta_F = (\omega_V, \omega_k, \beta, a)$, weights (w_i) and design $\underline{\boldsymbol{t}}$.

3.2.4 A model for the covariates

Another scenario is to suppose that in fact it is the covariates $\boldsymbol{c}$ that are random, not the population parameters. This may be in the context of wanting to simulate individuals, or when modeling and wanting to take into account uncertainty in covariate values. If we note p_c the distribution of the covariates, the joint distribution $p_{\psi,c}$ of the individual parameters and the covariates decomposes naturally as

$$\mathrm{p}(\boldsymbol{\psi}, \boldsymbol{c}; \theta) = \mathrm{p}(\boldsymbol{\psi}|\boldsymbol{c}; \theta)\, \mathrm{p}(\boldsymbol{c}).$$

- In this context, the model is the joint distribution of the observations, the individual parameters and the covariates:

$$\mathrm{p}(\boldsymbol{y}, \boldsymbol{\psi}, \boldsymbol{c}; \theta, \underline{\boldsymbol{t}}) = \mathrm{p}(\boldsymbol{y}|\boldsymbol{\psi}; \underline{\boldsymbol{t}})\, \mathrm{p}(\boldsymbol{\psi}|\boldsymbol{c}; \theta)\, \mathrm{p}(\boldsymbol{c}).$$

- The inputs to the model are the population parameters θ and measurement times $\underline{\boldsymbol{t}}$.

EXAMPLE 3.4 We assume a normal distribution as prior for the weights:

$$w_i \sim_{i.i.d.} \mathcal{N}\left(70, 10^2\right). \tag{3.5}$$

Once more, (3.2) defines the conditional distribution of the concentrations. Now, (3.3) is the *conditional distribution* of the individual PK parameters given the weight $\boldsymbol{w}$, now a random variable whose distribution is defined in (3.5). The inputs to the model are the population parameters $\theta = (V_{\rm pop}, k_{\rm pop}, \omega_V, \omega_k, \beta, a)$ and design $\underline{\boldsymbol{t}}$.

3.2.5 A model for the measurement times

Another scenario is to suppose that there is uncertainty in the measurement times $\underline{t} = (t_{ij})$. If we note $\underline{t}^* = (t^*_{ij},\ 1 \leq i \leq N,\ 1 \leq j \leq n_i)$ the nominal measurement times (i.e., those presented in a data set), then the "true" measurement times $\underline{t}$ at which the measurements were made can be considered random fluctuations around $\underline{t}^*$ following some distribution $p_t(\,\cdot\,; \underline{t}^*)$.

Randomness with respect to time can also appear in the presence of dropout, i.e., individuals that prematurely leave a clinical trial. For an individual i who leaves at the random time T_i, measurement times are the nominal times before T_i: $t_i = (t^*_{ij},\ t^*_{ij} \leq T_i)$. In such situations, measurement times are therefore random and can be thought to come from a distribution $p_t(\,\cdot\,; \underline{t}^*)$.

- In this context, the model is the joint distribution of the observations, the individual parameters and the measurement times:

$$\mathrm{p}(\boldsymbol{y}, \boldsymbol{\psi}, \underline{t}; \theta, \boldsymbol{c}, \underline{t}^*) = \mathrm{p}(\boldsymbol{y}|\boldsymbol{\psi}, \underline{t})\, \mathrm{p}(\boldsymbol{\psi}; \theta, \boldsymbol{c})\, \mathrm{p}(\underline{t}; \underline{t}^*).$$

- The inputs to the model are the population parameters θ, individual covariates $\boldsymbol{c}$ and nominal measurement times $\underline{t}^*$.

EXAMPLE 3.5 Let us assume as prior a normal distribution around the nominal measurement times with standard deviation 3 min = 0.05 h:

$$t_{ij} \sim_{i.i.d.} \mathcal{N}\left(t^*_{ij}, 0.05^2\right). \tag{3.6}$$

Here, (3.6) defines the distribution of the now random variable $\underline{t}$. The other components of the model defined in (3.2) and (3.3) remain unchanged. The inputs of the model are the population parameters θ, weights (w_i) and nominal measurement times $\underline{t}^*$.

Remark: If there are also other regression variables $\boldsymbol{x} = (x_{ij})$, the same approach can be used by considering $\boldsymbol{x}$ to be a random variable fluctuating around $\boldsymbol{x}^*$.

3.2.6 A model for the dose regimen

If the structural model is a dynamical system (e.g., defined by a system of ordinary differential equations (ODEs)), the *source terms* $\boldsymbol{u} = (u_i,\ 1 \leq i \leq N)$, i.e., the inputs of the dynamical system, are usually considered fixed and known. This is the case, for example, with doses administered to patients for a given treatment. Here, the source term u_i is made up of the dose(s) given to patient i, the time(s) of administration, and their type (iv bolus, infusion, oral, etc.).

Here again, there may be differences between the nominal dose regimen stated in the protocol and given in the data set, and the dose regimen that was in reality administered. For example, it might be that the times of administration and/or dose were not exactly respected or recorded. Also, there may have been noncompliance, i.e., certain doses that were not taken by the patient.

If we denote $\boldsymbol{u}^* = (u_i^*, 1 \leq i \leq N)$ the nominal dose regimens (reported in the dataset), then in this context the "real" dose regimen $\boldsymbol{u}$ can be considered to randomly fluctuate around $\boldsymbol{u}^*$ with some distribution $p_u(\,\cdot\,; \boldsymbol{u}^*)$.

- In this context, the model is the joint distribution of the observations, the individual parameters and the dose regimen:

$$\mathrm{p}(\boldsymbol{y}, \boldsymbol{\psi}, \boldsymbol{u}; \theta, \boldsymbol{c}, \underline{\boldsymbol{t}}, \boldsymbol{u}^*) = \mathrm{p}(\boldsymbol{y}|\boldsymbol{\psi}, \boldsymbol{u}; \underline{\boldsymbol{t}})\, \mathrm{p}(\boldsymbol{u}; \boldsymbol{u}^*)\, \mathrm{p}(\boldsymbol{\psi}; \theta, \boldsymbol{c}).$$

- The inputs to the model are the population parameters θ, individual covariates $\boldsymbol{c}$, nominal design $\boldsymbol{\tau}$ and nominal dose regimen $\boldsymbol{u}^*$.

EXAMPLE 3.6 Suppose that instead of the one dose given in the example up to now, there are repeated doses $(d_{ik}, k \geq 1)$ administered to patient i at times $(\tau_{ik}, k \geq 1)$. Then, it is easy to see that

$$y_{ij} \sim \mathcal{N}\left(f(t_{ij}; V_i, k_i), a_i^2\right), \tag{3.7}$$

where

$$f(t; V_i, k_i) = \sum_{k, \tau_{ik} < t} \frac{d_{ik}}{V_i}\, e^{-k_i\,(t - \tau_{ik})}. \tag{3.8}$$

The "real" dose regimen administered to patient i can be written $u_i = (d_{ik}, \tau_{ik}, k \geq 1)$ and the prescribed dose regimen $u_i^* = (d_{ik}^*, \tau_{ik}^*, k \geq 1)$. We can, for example, model the random fluctuations of the administration times τ_{ik} around the nominal times (τ_{ij}^*):

$$\tau_{ik} \sim_{i.i.d.} \mathcal{N}\left(\tau_{ik}^*, 0.02^2\right), \tag{3.9}$$

and noncompliance (here meaning that a dose is not taken):

$$\mathbb{P}(d_{ik} = 0) = 1 - \mathbb{P}(d_{ik} = d_{ik}^*) = 0.10. \tag{3.10}$$

Here, (3.7) and (3.8) define the conditional distributions of the concentrations (y_{ij}), (3.3) the distribution of $\boldsymbol{\psi}$ and (3.9) and (3.10) the distribution of $\boldsymbol{u}$. The inputs are the population parameters θ, weights (w_i), measurement times $\underline{\boldsymbol{t}}$ and nominal dose regimen $\boldsymbol{u}^*$.

3.2.7 A complete model

We have now seen the variety of ways in which the variables in a model play either the role of random variables whose distribution is defined by the model, or that of nonrandom variables or parameters. Any combination is possible, depending on the context. For instance, the population parameters θ and covariates $\boldsymbol{c}$ could be random with parametric probability distributions $p_\theta(\,\cdot\,;\varphi)$ and $p_c(\,\cdot\,;\gamma)$, and the dose regimen $\boldsymbol{u}$ and measurement times $\underline{\boldsymbol{t}}$ could be reported with uncertainty and therefore modeled as random variables with distribution p_u and p_t.

- In this context, the model is the joint distribution of the observations, the individual parameters, the population parameters, the dose regimen, the covariates and the measurement times:

$$\begin{aligned}&\mathrm{p}(\boldsymbol{y},\boldsymbol{\psi},\theta,\boldsymbol{u},\boldsymbol{c},\underline{\boldsymbol{t}};\boldsymbol{u}^*,\underline{\boldsymbol{t}}^*,\varphi,\gamma) =\\ &\quad \mathrm{p}(\boldsymbol{y}|\boldsymbol{\psi},\boldsymbol{u},\underline{\boldsymbol{t}})\,\mathrm{p}(\boldsymbol{\psi}|\theta,\boldsymbol{c})\,\mathrm{p}(\theta;\varphi)\,\mathrm{p}(\boldsymbol{c};\gamma)\,\mathrm{p}(\boldsymbol{u};\boldsymbol{u}^*)\,\mathrm{p}(\underline{\boldsymbol{t}};\underline{\boldsymbol{t}}^*).\end{aligned}$$

- The inputs to the model are the nominal dose regimen $\boldsymbol{u}^*$, nominal measurement times $\underline{\boldsymbol{t}}^*$ and "hyper-parameters" φ and γ.

3.3 Using a model for executing tasks

In a modeling and simulation context, the tasks to execute make specific use of the various probability distributions associated with a model.

3.3.1 Simulation

By definition, simulation makes direct use of the probability distribution that defines the model. Simulation of the global model is straightforward as soon as the joint distribution can be decomposed into a product of easily simulated conditional distributions.

Consider, for example, that the variables involved in the model are those introduced in Section 3.2. Simulation of the complete model then consists of sequentially performing the following steps:

1. The dose regimen $\boldsymbol{u}$ can be either given or sampled from the distribution p_u.
2. The measurement times $\underline{\boldsymbol{t}}$ (respectively regression variables $\boldsymbol{x}$) can be either given or sampled from the distribution p_t (respectively p_x).
3. The individual covariates $\mathbf{c}$ can be either given or sampled from the distribution p_c.
4. The population parameters θ can be either given or sampled from the distribution p_θ.
5. The individual parameters $\boldsymbol{\psi}$ can be sampled from the distribution $p_{\psi|\theta,c}$ using the values of $\mathbf{c}$ and θ obtained in steps 3 and 4.
6. Lastly, observations $\boldsymbol{y}$ can be sampled from the distribution $p_{y|\psi,u,t}$ using the values of $\boldsymbol{u}$, $\underline{\boldsymbol{t}}$ and $\boldsymbol{\psi}$ obtained at steps 1, 2 and 5.

Simulation of a set of variables w using a given set of variables z requires

- a model, i.e., a parametric distribution p_w if the z are treated as nonrandom variables, or a conditional distribution $p_{w|z}$ if they are treated as random variables.
- the input z, i.e., a value of z which allows the parametric distribution $p_w(\,\cdot\,;z)$ or the conditional distribution $p_{w|z}(\,\cdot\,|z)$ to be defined.
- an algorithm which allows us to draw w from p_w or $p_{w|z}$.

EXAMPLE 3.7

1. Imagine now that the population parameter θ and design $(\boldsymbol{u},\underline{\boldsymbol{t}})$ are given, and we want to simulate the individual covariates $\mathbf{c}$, individual parameters $\boldsymbol{\psi}$ and observations $\boldsymbol{y}$. Here, the variables to simulate are $w=(\mathbf{c},\boldsymbol{\psi},\boldsymbol{y})$ and the variables given are $z=(\theta,\boldsymbol{u},\underline{\boldsymbol{t}})$. If the components of z are taken to be nonrandom variables, then:
   - The model is the joint distribution $p_{y,\psi,c}(\,\cdot\,;\theta,\boldsymbol{u},\underline{\boldsymbol{t}})$ of $(\boldsymbol{y},\boldsymbol{\psi},\mathbf{c})$.
   - The inputs required for simulation are the values of $(\theta,\boldsymbol{u},\underline{\boldsymbol{t}})$.

- The algorithm should be able to generate $(\boldsymbol{y}, \boldsymbol{\psi}, \boldsymbol{c})$ from the joint distribution $p_{y,\psi,c}(\,\cdot\,;\theta, \boldsymbol{u}, \underline{\boldsymbol{t}})$. Decomposing the model into three submodels leads to a decomposition of the joint distribution as

$$\mathrm{p}(\boldsymbol{y}, \boldsymbol{\psi}, \boldsymbol{c}; \theta, \boldsymbol{u}, \underline{\boldsymbol{t}}) = \mathrm{p}(\boldsymbol{c})\,\mathrm{p}(\boldsymbol{\psi}|\boldsymbol{c}; \theta)\,\mathrm{p}(\boldsymbol{y}|\boldsymbol{\psi}; \boldsymbol{u}, \underline{\boldsymbol{t}}).$$

The algorithm therefore reduces to successively drawing $\boldsymbol{c}$, $\boldsymbol{\psi}$ and $\boldsymbol{y}$ from p_c, $p_{\psi|c}(\,\cdot\,|\boldsymbol{c}; \theta)$ and $p_{y|\psi}(\,\cdot\,|\boldsymbol{\psi}; \boldsymbol{u}, \underline{\boldsymbol{t}})$.

2. Imagine instead that the individual covariates $\boldsymbol{c}$, observations $\boldsymbol{y}$, design $(\boldsymbol{u}, \underline{\boldsymbol{t}})$ and population parameter θ are given (in a modeling context, for instance, θ may have been estimated), and we want to simulate the individual parameters $\boldsymbol{\psi}$. The only variable to simulate is $w = \boldsymbol{\psi}$ and the variables which are given are $z = (\boldsymbol{y}, \boldsymbol{c}, \theta, \boldsymbol{u}, \underline{\boldsymbol{t}})$. Here, we will treat $\boldsymbol{y}$ as if it were a random variable. The other components of z can be treated as nonrandom variables. Now,

   - The model is the conditional distribution $p_{\psi|y}(\,\cdot\,|\boldsymbol{y}; \boldsymbol{c}, \theta, \boldsymbol{u}, \underline{\boldsymbol{t}})$ of ψ.
   - The inputs required for simulation are the values of $(\boldsymbol{y}, \boldsymbol{c}, \theta, \boldsymbol{u}, \underline{\boldsymbol{t}})$.
   - The algorithm should be able to draw $\boldsymbol{\psi}$ from the conditional distribution $p_{\psi|y}(\,\cdot\,|\boldsymbol{y}; \boldsymbol{c}, \theta, \boldsymbol{u}, \underline{\boldsymbol{t}})$. Markov chain Monte Carlo (MCMC) algorithms can be used for sampling from such complex conditional distributions.

3.3.2 Estimation of the population parameters

In the modeling context, we usually assume that we have data that includes the observations $\boldsymbol{y}$ and measurement times $\underline{\boldsymbol{t}}$. There may also be individual covariates $\boldsymbol{c}$ and in pharmacological applications the dose regimen $\boldsymbol{u}$. For clarity, let us consider the most general case where all are present.

Estimation of the population parameters is one of the most challenging tasks. Any statistical method for estimating the population parameters θ will be based on some specific probability distribution. Let us illustrate this with two common statistical methods: maximum likelihood and Bayesian estimation.

Maximum likelihood estimation consists of maximizing, with respect to θ, the likelihood, defined as

$$\begin{aligned}\mathcal{L}_{\boldsymbol{y}}(\theta) &\stackrel{\text{def}}{=} \mathrm{p}(\boldsymbol{y}; \boldsymbol{c}, \boldsymbol{u}, \underline{\boldsymbol{t}}, \theta) \\ &= \int \mathrm{p}(\boldsymbol{y}, \boldsymbol{\psi}; \boldsymbol{c}, \boldsymbol{u}, \underline{\boldsymbol{t}}, \theta)\, d\boldsymbol{\psi}.\end{aligned}$$

The variance of the estimator $\hat{\theta}$ and therefore confidence intervals can be derived from the observed Fisher information matrix, which itself is calculated using the likelihood (i.e., the pdf of the observations $\boldsymbol{y}$):

$$I_{\boldsymbol{y}}(\hat{\theta}) \stackrel{\text{def}}{=} -\frac{\partial^2}{\partial\theta^2}\log(\mathcal{L}_{\boldsymbol{y}}(\hat{\theta})).$$

Maximum likelihood estimation of the population parameter θ requires

- a model, i.e., a joint distribution $p_{y,\psi}$.
- inputs $\boldsymbol{y}$, $\boldsymbol{c}$, $\boldsymbol{u}$ and $\underline{\boldsymbol{t}}$.
- an algorithm which allows us to maximize $\int \mathrm{p}(\boldsymbol{y},\boldsymbol{\psi};\boldsymbol{c},\boldsymbol{u},\underline{\boldsymbol{t}},\theta)\,d\boldsymbol{\psi}$ with respect to θ and compute $\frac{\partial^2}{\partial\theta^2}\log\int \mathrm{p}(\boldsymbol{y},\boldsymbol{\psi};\boldsymbol{c},\boldsymbol{u},\underline{\boldsymbol{t}},\hat{\theta})\,d\boldsymbol{\psi}$.

Bayesian estimation consists of estimating and/or maximizing the conditional distribution

$$\begin{aligned}
\mathrm{p}(\theta|\boldsymbol{y};\boldsymbol{c},\boldsymbol{u},\underline{\boldsymbol{t}}) &= \frac{\mathrm{p}(\boldsymbol{y},\theta;\boldsymbol{c},\boldsymbol{u},\underline{\boldsymbol{t}})}{\mathrm{p}(\boldsymbol{y};\boldsymbol{c},\boldsymbol{u},\underline{\boldsymbol{t}})} \\
&= \frac{\int \mathrm{p}(\boldsymbol{y},\boldsymbol{\psi},\theta;\boldsymbol{c},\boldsymbol{u},\underline{\boldsymbol{t}})\,d\boldsymbol{\psi}}{\mathrm{p}(\boldsymbol{y};\boldsymbol{c},\boldsymbol{u},\underline{\boldsymbol{t}})}.
\end{aligned}$$

Bayesian estimation of the population parameter θ requires

- a model, i.e., a joint distribution $p_{y,\psi,\theta}(\,\cdot\,;\boldsymbol{c},\boldsymbol{u},\underline{\boldsymbol{t}})$ for $(\boldsymbol{y},\boldsymbol{\psi},\theta)$.
- inputs $\boldsymbol{y}$, $\boldsymbol{c}$, $\boldsymbol{u}$ and $\underline{\boldsymbol{t}}$.
- algorithms able to estimate and maximize $\mathrm{p}(\theta|\boldsymbol{y};\boldsymbol{c},\boldsymbol{u},\underline{\boldsymbol{t}})$. MCMC methods can be used for estimating this conditional distribution. For nonlinear models, optimization tools are required for computing its mode, i.e., finding the maximum of the posterior density.

3.3.3 Estimation of the individual parameters

When θ is given (or estimated), various estimators of the individual parameters $\boldsymbol{\psi}$ are available. They are all based on a conditional distribution of $\boldsymbol{\psi}$.

The *maximum a posteriori* (MAP) estimator is obtained by maximizing, with respect to $\boldsymbol{\psi}$, the *conditional distribution*

$$\mathrm{p}(\boldsymbol{\psi}|\boldsymbol{y};\theta,\boldsymbol{c},\boldsymbol{u},\underline{\boldsymbol{t}}) = \frac{\mathrm{p}(\boldsymbol{y},\boldsymbol{\psi};\theta,\boldsymbol{c},\boldsymbol{u},\underline{\boldsymbol{t}})}{\mathrm{p}(\boldsymbol{y};\theta,\boldsymbol{c},\boldsymbol{u},\underline{\boldsymbol{t}})}.$$

The *conditional mean* of ψ is defined as the mean of the conditional distribution $p_{\psi|y}$ of ψ and denoted as $\mathbb{E}(\boldsymbol{\psi}|\boldsymbol{y};\theta,\boldsymbol{c},\boldsymbol{u},\underline{\boldsymbol{t}})$.

Estimation of the individual parameters $\boldsymbol{\psi}$ requires

- a model, i.e., a joint distribution $p_{y,\psi}(\,\cdot\,;\theta,\boldsymbol{c},\boldsymbol{u},\underline{\boldsymbol{t}})$ for $(\boldsymbol{y},\boldsymbol{\psi})$.
- inputs $\boldsymbol{y}$, θ, $\boldsymbol{c}$, $\boldsymbol{u}$ and $\underline{\boldsymbol{t}}$.
- algorithms able to estimate and maximize $\mathrm{p}(\boldsymbol{\psi}|\boldsymbol{y};\theta,\boldsymbol{c},\boldsymbol{u},\underline{\boldsymbol{t}})$. MCMC methods can be used for estimating this conditional distribution. For nonlinear models, optimization tools are required for computing its mode (i.e., the MAP estimator).

3.3.4 Model selection

Likelihood ratio tests and statistical information criteria (Bayesian information criterion, Akaike information criteria) compare likelihoods computed under different models, i.e., the probability distribution functions $\mathrm{p}^{(1)}(\boldsymbol{y};\boldsymbol{c},\boldsymbol{u},\underline{\boldsymbol{t}},\hat{\theta}_1)$, $\mathrm{p}^{(2)}(\boldsymbol{y};\boldsymbol{c},\boldsymbol{u},\underline{\boldsymbol{t}},\hat{\theta}_2)$,..., $\mathrm{p}^{(K)}(\boldsymbol{y};\boldsymbol{c},\boldsymbol{u},\underline{\boldsymbol{t}},\hat{\theta}_K)$ computed under models $\mathcal{M}_1,\mathcal{M}_2,\ldots,\mathcal{M}_K$, where $\hat{\theta}_k$ is the maximum likelihood estimate of θ under model $\mathcal{M}_k$, i.e., the value of θ which maximizes $\mathrm{p}^{(k)}(\boldsymbol{y};\boldsymbol{c},\boldsymbol{u},\underline{\boldsymbol{t}},\theta)$.

Computing the likelihood and information criteria requires

- a model, i.e., a joint distribution $p_{y,\psi}(\,\cdot\,;\theta,\boldsymbol{c},\boldsymbol{u},\underline{\boldsymbol{t}})$ for $(\boldsymbol{y},\boldsymbol{\psi})$.
- inputs $\boldsymbol{y}$, θ, $\boldsymbol{c}$, $\boldsymbol{u}$ and $\underline{\boldsymbol{t}}$.
- an algorithm able to compute $\int \mathrm{p}(\boldsymbol{y},\boldsymbol{\psi};\theta,\boldsymbol{c},\boldsymbol{u},\underline{\boldsymbol{t}})\,d\boldsymbol{\psi}$. For nonlinear models, linearization or Monte Carlo methods can be used.

3.3.5 Optimal design

In designing experiments for estimating statistical models, optimal design methods allow parameters to be estimated with minimum variance by optimizing some statistical criterion. Common optimality criteria are functionals of the eigenvalues of the expected Fisher information matrix

$$I^*(\theta;\boldsymbol{u},\underline{\boldsymbol{t}}) \stackrel{\text{def}}{=} -\mathbb{E}_y\left(\frac{\partial^2}{\partial\theta^2}\log\mathrm{p}(\boldsymbol{y};\boldsymbol{u},\underline{\boldsymbol{t}},\theta)\right).$$

Optimal design for minimum variance estimation requires

- a model, i.e., a joint distribution $p_{y,\psi}(\,\cdot\,;\theta,\boldsymbol{u},\underline{\boldsymbol{t}})$ for $(\boldsymbol{y},\boldsymbol{\psi})$.
- a vector of population parameters θ.
- a criterion $\mathcal{D}(\boldsymbol{u},\underline{\boldsymbol{t}},\theta)$ derived from the expected Fisher information matrix $I^*(\theta;\boldsymbol{u},\underline{\boldsymbol{t}})$.
- an algorithm able to compute $I^*(\theta;\boldsymbol{u},\underline{\boldsymbol{t}})$ for any design $(\boldsymbol{u},\underline{\boldsymbol{t}})$ and maximize $\mathcal{D}(\boldsymbol{u},\underline{\boldsymbol{t}},\theta)$ with respect to $\boldsymbol{u}$ and $\underline{\boldsymbol{t}}$.

Remark: In a clinical trial context, studies are designed to optimize the probability of reaching some predefined target $\mathcal{A}$, i.e., $\mathbb{P}((\boldsymbol{y},\boldsymbol{\psi})\in\mathcal{A};\boldsymbol{u},\underline{\boldsymbol{t}},\theta)$. This may include maximizing some utility function for safety and efficacy and such things as the probability of reaching sustained virologic response, etc.

3.4 Implementing hierarchical models with MLXTRAN

MLXTRAN takes advantage of the hierarchical structure of a joint probability distribution by decomposing the joint model into several submodels. Then, each component of the model is implemented in a different section:

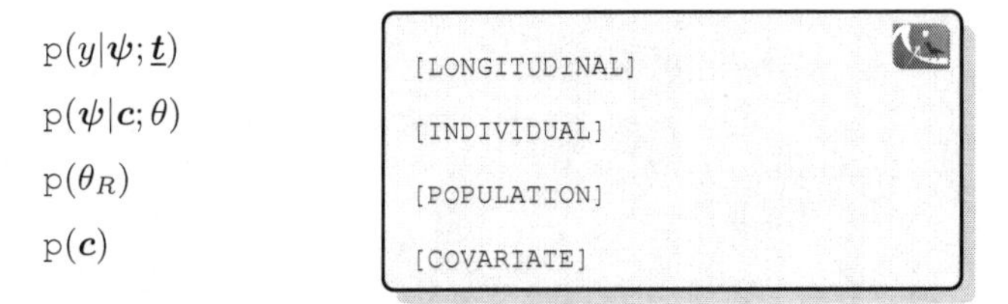

Consider first the model defined by the joint distribution

$$\mathrm{p}(\boldsymbol{y},\boldsymbol{\psi};\theta,\underline{\boldsymbol{t}})=\mathrm{p}(\boldsymbol{y}|\boldsymbol{\psi};\underline{\boldsymbol{t}})\mathrm{p}(\boldsymbol{\psi};\theta),$$

where, as in our running example introduced in (3.2) and (3.3),

- $\boldsymbol{y}=(y_{ij},\,1\leq i\leq N, 1\leq j\leq n_i)$ are concentrations;
- $\boldsymbol{\psi}=(\psi_i,\,1\leq i\leq N)$ are individual PK parameters, here $\psi_i=(V_i,k_i,a_i)$;

- $\theta = (V_{\text{pop}}, k_{\text{pop}}, \omega_V, \omega_k, a)$ are population parameters;
- $\underline{t} = (t_{ij}, 1 \leq i \leq N, 1 \leq j \leq n_i)$ are the measurement times.

We aim to define a joint model for $\boldsymbol{y}$ and $\boldsymbol{\psi}$. To do this, we will define each model component and show how to implement it with MLXTRAN.

1) $\mathrm{p}(y|\boldsymbol{\psi};\underline{t})$

$$f(t; V_i, k_i) = \frac{500}{V_i} e^{-k_i\,t}$$

$$y_{ij} \sim \mathcal{N}\left(f(t_{ij}; V_i, k_i), a^2\right)$$

2) $\mathrm{p}(\boldsymbol{\psi}|\boldsymbol{c};\theta)$

$$\ell_i = \log(w_i/70)$$

$$\log(V_i) \sim \mathcal{N}\left(\log(V_{\text{pop}}) + \beta\ell_i, \omega_V^2\right)$$

$$\log(k_i) \sim \mathcal{N}\left(\log(k_{\text{pop}}), \omega_k^2\right)$$

distribution1_model.txt

```
[LONGITUDINAL]
input={V,k,a}

EQUATION:
f = 500/V*exp(-k*t)

DEFINITION:
y={distribution=normal,prediction=f,sd=a}


[INDIVIDUAL]
input={V_pop,k_pop,omega_V,omega_k,beta,w}

EQUATION:
l = log(w/70)

DEFINITION[model=linear]:
V={distribution=lognormal,reference=V_pop,
  covariate=l,coefficient=beta,sd=omega_V}
k={distribution=lognormal,reference=k_pop,
   sd=omega_k}
```

Remark: In this example, a_i is fixed. Thus, only the distributions of V_i and k_i need to be defined.

We can then use different tools on this model for executing different tasks: MLXPLORE for model exploration, MONOLIX for modeling, Simulx for simulation, etc.

It is important to remember that MLXTRAN is not a "function" that calculates an output. It is a declarative – not imperative – language which allows us to describe a model. It is then the tasks we choose to run which use MLXTRAN like a function, "asking" it to give predictions, draw random variables, compute a pdf, maximize a likelihood, etc.

Imagine now that we also want to introduce a statistical model for the covariates and population parameters. We need to add to the overall distribution only a distribution for the covariates and one for the population parameters, i.e., add `[COVARIATE]` and `[POPULATION]` blocks to the MLXTRAN model file.

3) $\mathrm{p}(\boldsymbol{c})$

$$w_i \sim \mathcal{N}\left(70, 10^2\right)$$

4) $\mathrm{p}(\theta_R)$

$$V_{\text{pop}} \sim \mathcal{N}\left(30, 3^2\right)$$
$$k_{\text{pop}} \sim \mathcal{N}\left(0.1, 0.01^2\right)$$

```
[COVARIATE]

DEFINITION:
weight = {distribution=normal, mean=70, sd=10}


[POPULATION]

DEFINITION:
V_pop = {distribution=normal, mean=30, sd=3}
k_pop = {distribution=normal, mean=0.1,sd=0.01}
```

Remark: A model that incorporates a [COVARIATE] block for the covariates and a [POPULATION] one for the population parameters can be used for simulation by the function Simulx (see Appendix D.2) and to explore models using MLXPLORE (see Appendix D.1). The [POPULATION] block can be used for estimation in MONOLIX in the Bayesian estimation case. However, the [COVARIATE] block cannot be used with MONOLIX because it supposes that the covariates are known (see Appendix D.4).

Part II

Defining Models

Models are attempts to describe observations in a logical, simple way and involve the relationship between measurements, parameters, covariates and so on. If working in a probabilistic framework – as we are here – there will be randomness in the model involving random variables, probability distributions, errors, etc.

Because of this, and in accordance with the formal point of view described in Chapter 3, we are going to make the following definition of a model: **a model is a joint probability distribution**.

Therefore, defining a model means defining a joint probability distribution, which can then be decomposed into a product of conditional distributions on which we can perform tasks: visualization, estimation, model selection, simulation, etc. This part of the book is therefore about defining appropriate probability distributions. In what follows, we will use the notation introduced in Section 3.1.

There are two important pieces to the puzzle: the longitudinal data $\boldsymbol{y}$ whose distribution p_y depends on the individual parameters, and the individual parameters $\boldsymbol{\psi}$ themselves with distribution p_ψ. In the population approach, the base distribution is the joint distribution $p_{y,\psi}$ of the data and the individual parameters:

$$\mathrm{p}(\boldsymbol{y}, \boldsymbol{\psi}) = \mathrm{p}(\boldsymbol{y}|\boldsymbol{\psi})\mathrm{p}(\boldsymbol{\psi}).$$

In this part of the book, we concentrate essentially on these two components: the conditional distribution $p_{y|\psi}$ of the observations, and the distribution p_ψ of the individual parameters.

Depending on the required complexity of the model, its other components such as covariates, population parameters and design can also be modeled as random variables, but we will not go into much detail about that here.

For each model we will deal with, we will aim to precisely identify the minimal amount of information needed to represent it mathematically so that it remains possible to implement and analyze.

4

Modeling the Observations

4.1 Introduction

We focus in this chapter on models for the longitudinal data $\boldsymbol{y} = (y_i,\ 1 \leq i \leq N)$, i.e., the conditional probability distributions $(p_{y_i|\psi_i},\ 1 \leq i \leq N)$ when the individual parameters $\boldsymbol{\psi} = (\psi_i,\ 1 \leq i \leq N)$ are given and where

- N is the number of subjects.
- $y_i = (y_{ij},\ 1 \leq j \leq n_i)$ are the n_i observations for individual i. Here, y_{ij} is the measurement made on individual i at time t_{ij}.
- ψ_i is the vector of individual parameters for subject i.

Remarks:

- We suppose that the model we will use to describe the observations is a function of regression variables $x_i = (x_{ij},\ 1 \leq j \leq n_i)$. Each x_{ij} is made up of the time t_{ij} and perhaps other variables that vary with time. For example, a pharmacokinetic model can depend on time and weight: $x_{ij} = (t_{ij}, w_{ij})$ where w_{ij} is the weight of individual i at time t_{ij}, whereas a pharmacodynamic model can depend on time and concentration: $x_{ij} = (t_{ij}, c_{ij})$.
- The model for observations from individual i can also depend on *input terms* u_i. For example, a pharmacokinetic model can include the dose regimen administered to patients: u_i is made up of the dose(s) given to patient i, the time(s) of administration and its type (iv bolus, infusion, oral, etc.). If the structural model is a dynamical system (e.g., defined by a system of ordinary differential equations), the input terms (u_i) are also called *source terms*.

In our framework, observations $\boldsymbol{y}$ are longitudinal. So, for a given individual i, the model has to describe the change in $y_i = (y_{ij})$ over time. To do this, we suppose that each observation y_{ij} comes from a probability distribution, one that evolves with time. As we have decided to work with parametric models, we suppose that there exists a function α such that the distribution of y_{ij} depends on $\alpha(t_{ij}, \psi_i)$. Implicitly, this includes the time-varying variables x_{ij} mentioned above.

The time-dependence in α helps us to describe the change with time of each y_{ij}, while the fact it depends on the vector of individual parameters ψ_i helps us to describe the inter-individual variability in y_i.

We will distinguish in the following between continuous data models, discrete data models (including categorical and count data) and time-to-event (or survival) data models. Here are some examples of these types of data:

- Continuous data with a normal distribution:

$$y_{ij} \sim \mathcal{N}\left(f(t_{ij}, \psi_i),\, g^2(t_{ij}, \psi_i)\right).$$

Here, $\alpha(t_{ij}, \psi_i) = (f(t_{ij}, \psi_i),\, g(t_{ij}, \psi_i))$, where $f(t_{ij}, \psi_i)$ is the mean and $g(t_{ij}, \psi_i)$ the standard deviation of y_{ij}.

- Categorical data with a Bernoulli distribution:

$$y_{ij} \sim \mathcal{B}\left(\pi(t_{ij}, \psi_i)\right).$$

Here, $\alpha(t_{ij}, \psi_i) = \pi(t_{ij}, \psi_i)$ is the probability that y_{ij} takes the value 1.

- Count data with a Poisson distribution:

$$y_{ij} \sim \mathcal{P}\left(\lambda(t_{ij}, \psi_i)\right).$$

Here, $\alpha(t_{ij}, \psi_i) = \lambda(t_{ij}, \psi_i)$ is the Poisson parameter, i.e., the expected value of y_{ij}.

- Time-to-event data:

$$\begin{aligned} \mathbb{P}(y_i > t) &= S(t, \psi_i) \\ -\tfrac{d}{dt} \log S(t, \psi_i) &= h(t, \psi_i). \end{aligned}$$

Here, $\alpha(t, \psi_i) = h(t, \psi_i)$ is known as the hazard function.

In summary, defining a parametric model for the observations means choosing a parametric distribution. Then, a structural model must be chosen for the parameters of this distribution. This structural model is itself a parametric function of time: $\alpha(t, \psi)$.

4.2 Models for continuous data

4.2.1 The data

Continuous data is data that can take any real value within a given range. For instance, a concentration takes its values in $\mathbb{R}^+$, the log of the viral load takes values in $\mathbb{R}$, an effect expressed as a percentage takes values in $[0, 100]$.

The data can be stored in a table and represented graphically. Table 4.1 contains some simple pharmacokinetics (PK) data involving four individuals after a single intravenous (iv) bolus administration at time 0:

TABLE 4.1: Raw PK data for four patients.

id	time	concentration
1	1.0	9.84
1	2.0	8.19
1	4.0	6.91
1	8.0	3.71
1	12.0	1.25
2	1.0	17.23
2	3.0	11.14
2	5.0	4.35
2	10.0	2.92
3	2.0	9.78
3	3.0	10.40
3	4.0	7.67
3	6.0	6.84
3	11.0	1.10
4	4.0	8.78
4	6.0	3.87
4	12.0	1.85

A common plot for representing continuous data is a scatter plot. Figure 4.1 gives scatter plots of the data for each individual.

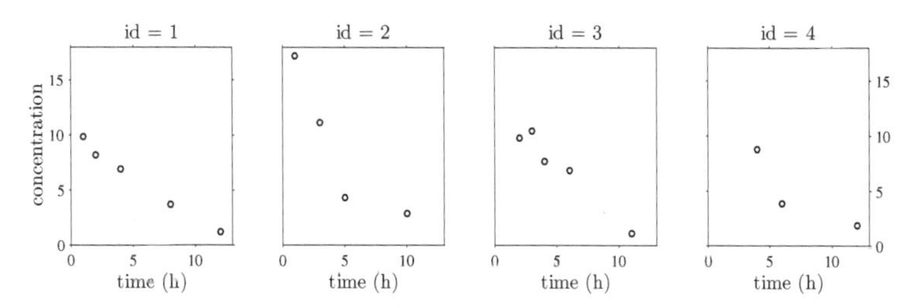

FIGURE 4.1: Scatter plots of the data for each individual.

Instead of individual plots, we can plot them all together and connect the points of the same individual with line segments (Figure 4.2). Such plots are usually called *spaghetti plots*.

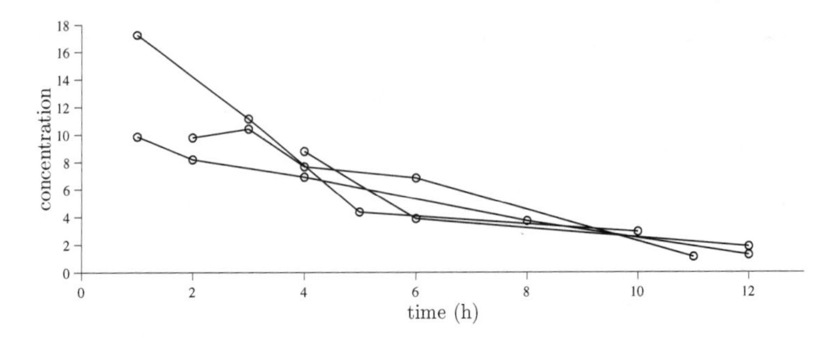

FIGURE 4.2: Spaghetti plot of the data.

4.2.2 The model

For continuous data, we are going to consider scalar outcomes ($y_{ij} \in \mathcal{Y} \subset \mathbb{R}$) and assume the following general model:

$$y_{ij} = f(t_{ij}, \phi_i) + g(t_{ij}, \phi_i, \xi_i)\varepsilon_{ij}, \quad 1 \leq i \leq N, \ 1 \leq j \leq n_i, \tag{4.1}$$

where ϕ_i is the parameter vector of the structural model f for individual i. The residual error model is defined by the function g which may depend on some additional vector of parameters ξ_i. For the sake of simplicity in the notation, we can group together all the individual parameters of subject i into one vector $\psi_i = (\phi_i, \xi_i)$ and rewrite model (4.1) as

$$y_{ij} = f(t_{ij}, \psi_i) + g(t_{ij}, \psi_i)\varepsilon_{ij}, \quad 1 \leq i \leq N, \ 1 \leq j \leq n_i. \tag{4.2}$$

We will use representations (4.1) and (4.2) interchangeably in the following.

The residual errors (ε_{ij}) are standardized random variables (mean 0 and standard deviation 1). In this case, it is clear that $f(t_{ij}, \phi_i)$ and $g(t_{ij}, \phi_i, \xi_i)$ are the conditional mean and standard deviation of y_{ij}, i.e.,

$$\mathbb{E}\left(y_{ij}|\psi_i\right) = f(t_{ij}, \phi_i)$$
$$\text{sd}\left(y_{ij}|\psi_i\right) = g(t_{ij}, \phi_i, \xi_i).$$

4.2.3 The structural model

f is known as the *structural model* and aims to describe the time evolution of the phenomena being studied. For a given subject i and vector of individual parameters $\psi_i = (\phi_i, \xi_i)$, $f(t_{ij}, \phi_i)$ is the prediction of the observed variable at time t_{ij}. In other words, it is the value that would be measured at time t_{ij} if there were no error ($\varepsilon_{ij} = 0$).

In the current example, the structural model is used for predicting the drug concentration as a function of time. We can use for example a model of the form $f(t) = C_0 \exp(-k\,t)$ to represent the exponential decay of the concentration. Figure 4.3 displays examples of curves obtained with various combinations of C_0 and k.

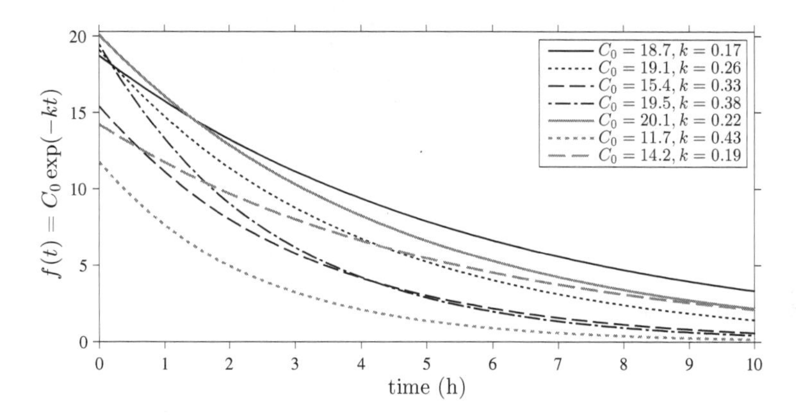

FIGURE 4.3: Examples of exponential decay curves.

We can see that different values of the parameters C_0 and k let us generate curves that behave like the data points in Figure 4.2. In other words, this structural model provides a set of curves that is rich enough to predict the concentrations for the four subjects.

There may exist several mathematical representations of the same structural model. Consider for instance the following PK model for iv bolus administration (Gabrielsson and Weiner, 2007):

$$\dot{A}_c(t) = -k\,A_c(t), \tag{4.3}$$

where A_c is the drug quantity in the central compartment (see Appendix C for a short introduction to PK modeling). Assume now that a single dose D was administered at time 0. The solution of (4.3) can be computed in closed form:

$$A_c(t) = D\,e^{-k\,t}. \tag{4.4}$$

If our observations are plasmatic concentrations, then $C_c(t) = A_c(t)/V$ (where V is the volume of distribution) can be used for predicting the plasmatic concentration at time t. The constant $C_0 = D/V$ can then be interpreted as the initial concentration at time $t = 0$ and k as the elimination rate constant.

Implementing this model using representation (4.4) will be much more efficient in terms of computational complexity than (4.3) which requires numerically solving a system of ordinary differential equations (ODEs). On the other hand, representing a PK model in terms of ODEs as in (4.3) provides a much better description of the PK model in that the elimination process is presented explicitly. In any case, both representations define the same structural model.

If instead of the linear elimination represented in (4.3) we assume a saturable elimination process (Gabrielsson and Weiner, 2007):

$$\dot{A}_c(t) = -\frac{V_m \, A_c(t)}{V \, K_m + A_c(t)}, \tag{4.5}$$

it turns out that there is no analytic solution (see Appendix C for more on this model). Nevertheless, the amount A_c is still a function of time and defined as the solution of the ODE. Thus, the concentration predicted by the model is mathematically well-defined as $C_c(t) = A_c(t)/V$. This model can be implemented and C_c calculated by numerically solving ODE (4.5).

Other models involving more complicated dynamical systems can be imagined, such as those defined as solutions of complex systems of ordinary or partial differential equations. Real-life examples are found in the study of viral kinetics (Snoeck et al., 2010), pharmacokinetics (Gabrielsson and Weiner, 2007), diabetes (Mari, 2002), tumor growth (Ribba et al., 2012) and system biology (Gonzalez et al., 2013).

4.2.4 The residual error model

For a given structural model f, the conditional probability distribution of the observations (y_{ij}) is completely defined by the residual error model, i.e., the probability distribution of the residual errors (ε_{ij}) and the standard deviation $g(t_{ij}, \phi_i, \xi_i)$.

4.2.4.1 Examples of residual error models

A residual error model can take many forms (Buonaccorsi, 2010; Carroll et al., 2010; Davidian and Giltinan, 1995). For example,

- Constant error models assume that $g(t_{ij}, \phi_i, \xi_i) = a_i$. Then, $\xi_i = a_i$ and model (4.1) becomes

$$y_{ij} = f(t_{ij}, \phi_i) + a_i \varepsilon_{ij}.$$

- Proportional error models assume that the standard error of the residual error is proportional to the prediction, i.e., $g(t_{ij}, \phi_i, \xi_i) =$

$b_i f(t_{ij}, \phi_i)$. Then $\xi_i = b_i$ and model (4.1) becomes

$$y_{ij} = f(t_{ij}, \phi_i)(1 + b_i \varepsilon_{ij}).$$

- A possible combined error model additively combines a constant and a proportional error model by assuming $g(t_{ij}, \phi_i, \xi_i) = a_i + b_i f(t_{ij}, \phi_i)$. Here, $\xi_i = (a_i, b_i)$ and

$$y_{ij} = f(t_{ij}, \phi_i) + (a_i + b_i f(t_{ij}, \phi_i))\varepsilon_{ij}. \tag{4.6}$$

- Another combined error model combines two residual errors:

$$y_{ij} = f(t_{ij}, \phi_i) + a_i \varepsilon_{ij}^{(1)} + b_i f(t_{ij}, \phi_i)\varepsilon_{ij}^{(2)}, \tag{4.7}$$

  where $(\varepsilon_{ij}^{(1)})$ and $(\varepsilon_{ij}^{(2)})$ are sequences of standardized random variables. If we furthermore assume that these two sequences are uncorrelated, the mean and variance of $a_i \varepsilon_{ij}^{(1)} + b_i f(t_{ij}, \phi_i)\varepsilon_{ij}^{(2)}$ are, respectively, 0 and $a_i^2 + b_i^2 f^2(t_{ij}, \phi_i)$. We can therefore rewrite model (4.7) using the general representation (4.1) with $g(t_{ij}, \phi_i, \xi_i) = \sqrt{a_i^2 + b_i^2 f^2(t_{ij}, \phi_i)}$, where $\xi_i = (a_i, b_i)$.

Figure 4.4 shows four simulated sequences of observations (y_{ij}, $1 \leq i \leq 4$, $1 \leq j \leq 10$) with their respective structural models $f(t, \phi_i)$. The same constant error model has been used for all four individuals with $a_i = 0.5$. Thus, $a_i = 0.5$ is the standard deviation of the conditional distribution of y_{ij} for all $j = 1, 2, \ldots, n_i$.

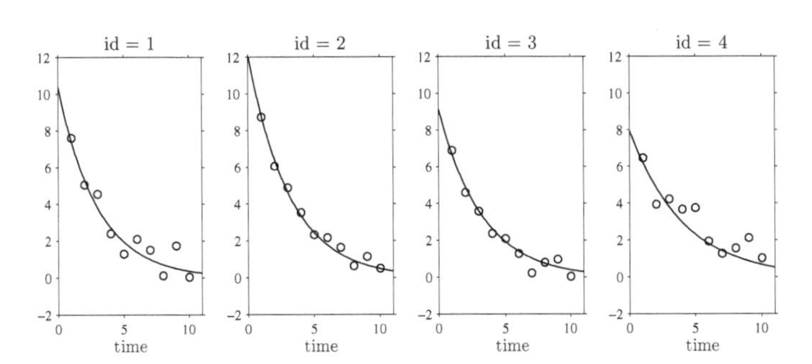

FIGURE 4.4: Four simulated sequences of observations using a constant error model. The structural model is shown as a solid line.

These graphs let us visualize the structural model f and get a general idea of the quality of the model fit, but do not help when it comes to the residual error model g. Let us therefore define by $(\tilde{y}_{ij})$ the predictions provided by model (4.1), where $\tilde{y}_{ij} = f(t_{ij}, \phi_i)$ is the predicted value of y_{ij}, and also define the prediction errors (e_{ij}) as the difference between the predictions and the observations:

$$\begin{aligned} e_{ij} &= y_{ij} - \tilde{y}_{ij} \\ &= y_{ij} - f(t_{ij}, \phi_i) \\ &= g(t_{ij}, \phi_i, \xi_i)\varepsilon_{ij}. \end{aligned}$$

If we want to try to visualize the link between the error model g and structural model f, we can plot the prediction errors (e_{ij}) against the predictions $(\tilde{y}_{ij})$. We can also plot the observations (y_{ij}) against the predictions $(\tilde{y}_{ij})$. Let us take a look at these types of plots for some basic error models.

Our first example is shown in Figure 4.5. Here, the same constant error model with $a_i = a = 0.5$ has been used for 50 individuals, followed by the calculation $e_{ij} = a\varepsilon_{ij}$. We thus obtain figures which are typical for constant error models: the standard deviation of the prediction errors does not depend on the value of the predictions $(\tilde{y}_{ij})$ since $\mathrm{sd}\,(e_{ij}) = a = 0.5$, so both intervals have constant amplitude.

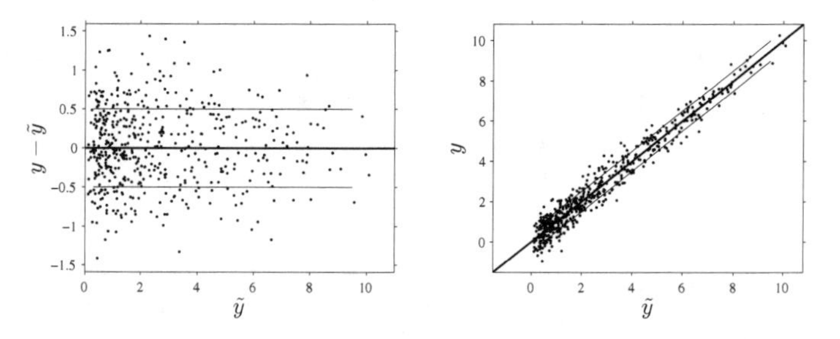

FIGURE 4.5: Constant error model. Left: prediction errors (e_{ij}) vs predictions $(\tilde{y}_{ij})$. Horizontal lines are the theoretical mean $\mathbb{E}\,(e_{ij}) = 0$ and $\pm$ 1 standard deviations: $\mathrm{sd}\,(e_{ij}) = a_i = 0.5$. Right: observations (y_{ij}) vs predictions $(\tilde{y}_{ij})$. The solid lines are $y = \tilde{y}$ and ± 1 standard deviations around $\tilde{y}_{ij}$: $[\tilde{y}_{ij} - \mathrm{sd}\,(e_{ij})\,, \tilde{y}_{ij} + \mathrm{sd}\,(e_{ij})]$.

The same plots are shown in Figure 4.6, but this time the same proportional error model is used for all 50 individuals with $b_i = b = 0.4$. Here, $e_{ij} = bf(t_{ij}, \phi_i)\varepsilon_{ij}$. The standard deviation of the prediction error e_{ij} is then proportional to the prediction $\tilde{y}_{ij}$, and hence we can see that the amplitude of the ± 1 standard deviation intervals increases linearly with f.

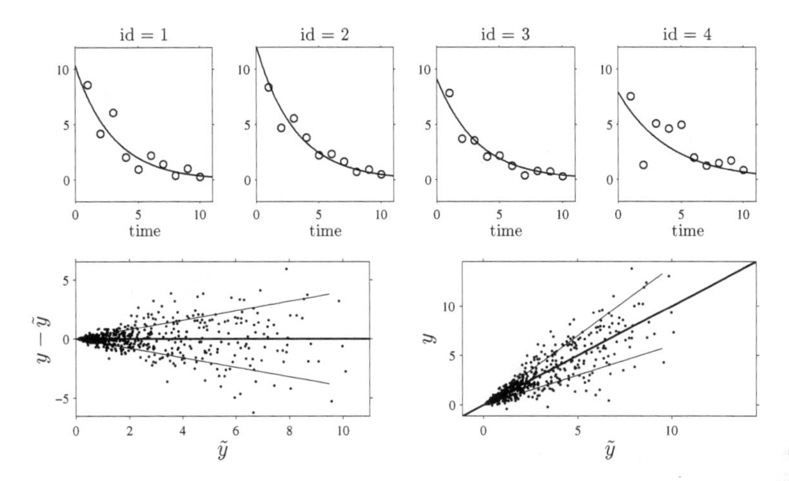

FIGURE 4.6: Proportional error model. Top: four simulated sequences of observations; bottom left: prediction errors (e_{ij}) vs predictions ($\tilde{y}_{ij}$); bottom right: observations (y_{ij}) vs predictions ($\tilde{y}_{ij}$).

The combined error model defined in (4.6) is used in Figure 4.7 with $a_i = 0.5$ and $b_i = 0.3$ for the 50 individuals. Here, $e_{ij} = (a+bf(t_{ij}, \phi_i))\varepsilon_{ij}$ and its standard deviation is $a + bf(t_{ij}, \phi_i)$. The standard deviation of the prediction error e_{ij} and thus the amplitude of the intervals are now affine[1] functions of the prediction $\tilde{y}_{ij}$.

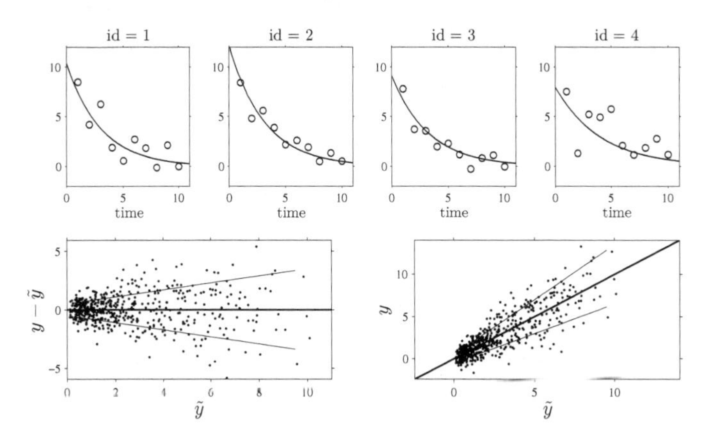

FIGURE 4.7: Combined error model $g(t_{ij}, \phi_i, \xi_i) = a_i + b_i f(t_{ij}, \phi_i)$. Top: four simulated sequences of observations; bottom left: prediction errors (e_{ij}) vs predictions ($\tilde{y}_{ij}$); bottom right: observations (y_{ij}) vs predictions ($\tilde{y}_{ij}$).

[1] An affine function of t has the form $f(t) = a + b\,t$ while a linear one has the form $f(t) = b\,t$.

We can then see in Figure 4.8 that using the combined error model defined in (4.7) gives intervals that look fairly similar to the previous ones, though they are no longer linear since the standard deviation of e_{ij} is $\sqrt{a_i^2 + b_i^2 f^2(t_{ij}, \phi_i)}$.

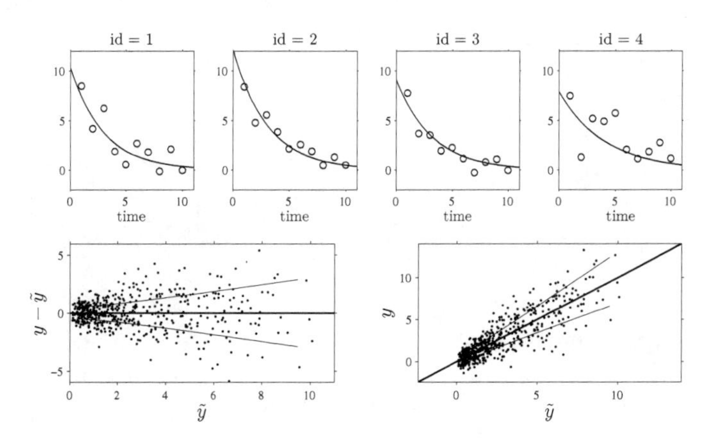

FIGURE 4.8: Combined error model $g(t_{ij}, \phi_i, \xi_i) = \sqrt{a_i^2 + b_i^2 f^2(t_{ij}, \phi_i)}$. Top: four simulated sequences of observations; bottom left: prediction errors (e_{ij}) vs predictions $(\tilde{y}_{ij})$; bottom right: observations (y_{ij}) vs predictions $(\tilde{y}_{ij})$.

Remark: We assumed in these examples the same residual error parameter ξ_i for all individuals. In the population context, if ξ_i is an individual parameter, things become a little more complicated when we pool all prediction errors.

Assume that the residual error parameters (ξ_i) are independent and identically distributed (i.i.d.) random variables, and that for all i, ξ_i and the structural model parameter ϕ_i are independent.

- If the error model is constant, then $e_{ij} = a_i \varepsilon_{ij}$ and $\text{sd}\,(e_{ij}) = \sqrt{\mathbb{E}\,(a_i^2)}$. We see therefore that mixing constant error models does not alter the basic form of the plots in Figure 4.5; the amplitude remains constant.

- For a proportional error model where $e_{ij} = b_i f(t_{ij}, \phi_i)\varepsilon_{ij}$, we have $\text{sd}\,(e_{ij}) = \sqrt{\mathbb{E}\,(b_i^2)} f(t_{ij}, \phi_i)$. Here again, mixing proportional error models does not alter the basic form of the plots in Figure 4.6; the amplitude of the intervals remains a linear function of $f(t_{ij}, \phi_i)$.

- In the case of combined error models as defined in (4.6), the look of the plots in Figure 4.7 will change slightly. Indeed, the standard deviation of e_{ij} is no longer an affine function of $f(t_{ij}, \phi_i)$ since $\mathrm{sd}(e_{ij}) = \sqrt{\mathbb{E}(a_i^2) + \mathbb{E}(b_i^2) f^2(t_{ij}, \phi_i)}$. Nevertheless, the global behavior remains the same since we can detect the presence of an intercept ($\mathrm{sd}(e_{ij}) = \sqrt{\mathbb{E}(a_i^2)}$ when $f = 0$) and $\mathrm{sd}(e_{ij})$ increases with $f(t_{ij}, \phi_i)$.

Things can get much more complicated if ξ_i and ϕ_i are not independent, essentially due to identifiability concerns in the error model. Consider for example the simple model:

$$y_{ij} = \phi_i + a_i \varepsilon_{ij}, \tag{4.8}$$

where ϕ_i and a_i are Gaussian random variables. If ϕ_i and a_i are correlated, there exists a coefficient b and Gaussian random variable u_i independent of ϕ_i such that $a_i = b\phi_i + u_i$. We can therefore rewrite the additive error model (4.8) as a combined error model:

$$y_{ij} = \phi_i + (u_i + b\phi_i)\varepsilon_{ij}.$$

For identifiability reasons, we will therefore always assume that the parameters of the residual error model ξ_i and those of the structural model ϕ_i are independent.

4.2.4.2 Extensions to autocorrelated errors

For any subject i, the residual errors $(\varepsilon_{ij}, 1 \leq j \leq n_i)$ are usually assumed to be independent random variables. The extension to autocorrelated errors is possible by assuming, for instance, that (ε_{ij}) is a stationary ARMA (autoregressive moving average) process (Box et al., 2008). For example, an autoregressive process of order 1, AR(1), assumes that autocorrelation decreases exponentially:

$$\mathrm{corr}(\varepsilon_{ij}, \varepsilon_{i,j+1}) = \rho_i^{(t_{i,j+1} - t_{ij})},$$

where $0 \leq \rho_i < 1$ for each individual i. If we assume that $t_{ij} = j$ for any (i, j), then $t_{i,j+1} - t_{i,j} = 1$ and the autocorrelation function γ_i for individual i is given by

$$\begin{aligned} \gamma_i(\tau) &= \mathrm{corr}(\varepsilon_{ij}, \varepsilon_{i,j+\tau}) \\ &= \rho_i^{\tau}. \end{aligned}$$

The residual errors are uncorrelated when $\rho_i = 0$. Figure 4.9 displays three different sequences of normally distributed residual errors simulated with three different autocorrelations, $\rho_1 = 0.1$, $\rho_2 = 0.7$ and $\rho_3 = 0.9$. The autocorrelation functions $(\gamma_i, 1 \leq i \leq 3)$ are also displayed.

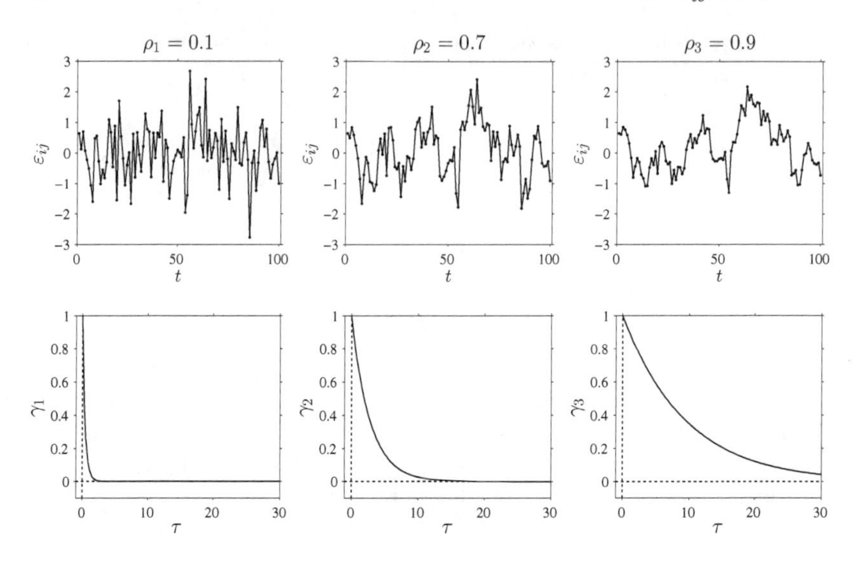

FIGURE 4.9: Examples of correlated residual errors (ε_{ij}) (top) and the associated autocorrelation functions (bottom).

4.2.4.3 Distribution of the standardized residual errors

The distribution of the standardized residual errors (ε_{ij}) is usually assumed to be the same for each individual i and any observation time t_{ij}. Furthermore, for identifiability reasons it is also assumed to be symmetrical around 0, i.e., $\mathbb{P}(\varepsilon_{ij} < -u) = \mathbb{P}(\varepsilon_{ij} > u)$ for all $u \in \mathbb{R}$. Thus, for any (i, j) the distribution of the observation y_{ij} is also symmetrical around its prediction $f(t_{ij}, \phi_i)$. This $f(t_{ij}, \phi_i)$ is therefore both the mean and median of the conditional distribution of y_{ij}: $\mathbb{E}(y_{ij}|\psi_i) = f(t_{ij}, \phi_i)$ and $\mathbb{P}(y_{ij} > f(t_{ij}, \phi_i)|\psi_i) = \mathbb{P}(y_{ij} < f(t_{ij}, \phi_i)|\psi_i) = 1/2$. If we make the additional hypothesis that 0 is the mode of the distribution of ε_{ij}, then $f(t_{ij}, \phi_i)$ is also the mode of the distribution of y_{ij}.

A widely used bell-shaped distribution for modeling residual errors is the normal distribution. If we assume that $\varepsilon_{ij} \sim \mathcal{N}(0, 1)$, then y_{ij} is also normally distributed: $y_{ij} \sim \mathcal{N}(f(t_{ij}, \phi_i), g(t_{ij}, \phi_i, \xi_i))$.

Other distributions can be used, such as Student's t-distribution (also known simply as the t-distribution) which is also symmetric and bell-shaped but with heavier tails, as shown in Figure 4.10, meaning that it is more prone to producing values that fall far from its mean (Pinheiro et al., 2001).

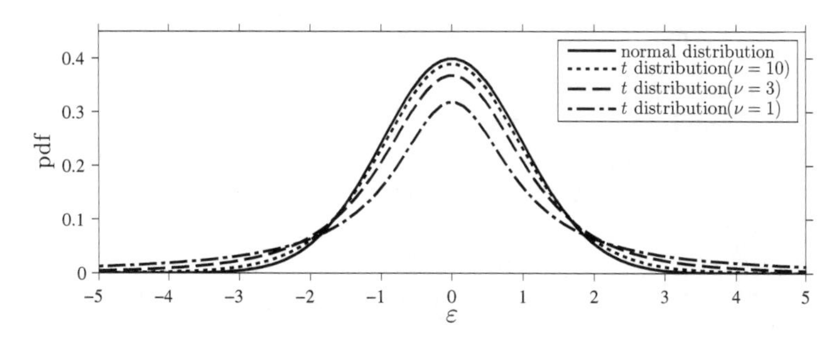

FIGURE 4.10: The pdf of the normal distribution and several t-distributions with different degrees of freedom ν.

A t-distribution with ν *degrees of freedom* has a finite variance $\nu/(\nu-2)$ if and only if $\nu > 2$. If we assume that the standardized residual errors (ε_{ij}) are such that $\sqrt{\nu/(\nu-2)}\varepsilon_{ij} \sim t(\nu)$, with $\nu > 2$, then the y_{ij} defined in (4.1) have nonstandardized Student's t-distributions with finite variance.

4.2.5 The conditional density function

When the individual parameters $\boldsymbol{\psi}$ are given and assuming that the residual errors $(\varepsilon_{ij},\ 1 \leq i \leq N,\ 1 \leq j \leq n_i)$ are i.i.d., the conditional density function of the observations $\boldsymbol{y}$ is straightforward to compute:

$$\begin{aligned}
\mathrm{p}(\boldsymbol{y}|\boldsymbol{\psi}) &= \prod_{i=1}^{N} \mathrm{p}(y_i|\psi_i) \\
&= \prod_{i=1}^{N}\prod_{j=1}^{n_i} \mathrm{p}(y_{ij}|\psi_i) \\
&= \prod_{i=1}^{N}\prod_{j=1}^{n_i} \frac{1}{g(t_{ij},\psi_i)}\, p_\varepsilon\left(\frac{y_{ij}-f(t_{ij},\psi_i)}{g(t_{ij},\psi_i)}\right),
\end{aligned}$$

where p_ε is the pdf of the i.i.d. residual errors (ε_{ij}). For example, if we assume that the residual errors (ε_{ij}) are Gaussian random variables with mean 0 and variance 1, then $p_\varepsilon(x) = e^{-x^2/2}/\sqrt{2\pi}$, and

$$\mathrm{p}(\boldsymbol{y}|\boldsymbol{\psi}) = \prod_{i=1}^{N}\prod_{j=1}^{n_i} \frac{1}{\sqrt{2\pi}g(t_{ij},\psi_i)} \exp\left\{-\frac{1}{2}\left(\frac{y_{ij}-f(t_{ij},\psi_i)}{g(t_{ij},\psi_i)}\right)^2\right\}.$$

4.2.6 Transforming the data

The assumption that the distribution of any observation y_{ij} is symmetrical around its predicted value is a very strong one. If this assumption does not hold, we may want to transform the data to make it more symmetric around its (transformed) predicted value (Oberg and Davidian, 2000). In other cases, constraints on the values that observations can take may also lead us to transform the data.

Model (4.1) can be extended to include a transformation of the data:

$$u(y_{ij}) = u(f(t_{ij}, \phi_i)) + g(t_{ij}, \phi_i, \xi_i)\varepsilon_{ij}, \tag{4.9}$$

where u is a monotonic transformation (a strictly increasing or decreasing function). As we can see, both the data y_{ij} and the structural model f are transformed by the function u so that $f(t_{ij}, \phi_i)$ remains the prediction of y_{ij}. Let us see now some examples of basic transformations:

- If y takes nonnegative values, a log transformation can be used: $u(y) = \log(y)$. We can then write the model with one of two equivalent representations:

$$\begin{aligned} \log(y_{ij}) &= \log(f(t_{ij}, \phi_i)) + g(t_{ij}, \phi_i, \xi_i)\varepsilon_{ij} \\ y_{ij} &= f(t_{ij}, \phi_i)\, e^{g(t_{ij}, \phi_i, \xi_i)\varepsilon_{ij}}. \end{aligned}$$

  Figure 4.11 shows three simulated sequences with the following model:

$$y_{ij} = A_i e^{-\alpha_i t_{ij}}\, e^{a\varepsilon_{ij}},$$

  where $a = 0.5$ and $\varepsilon_{ij} \sim \mathcal{N}(0, 1)$. Plotting the log-transformed data helps us to better visualize both the structural and error models because we now have a function that is linear with time and has a constant error model:

$$\log(y_{ij}) = \log(A_i) - \alpha_i t_{ij} + a\,\varepsilon_{ij}.$$

- If y takes its values between 0 and 1, a logit transformation can be used:

$$\begin{aligned} \text{logit}(y_{ij}) &= \text{logit}(f(t_{ij}, \phi_i)) + g(t_{ij}, \phi_i, \xi_i)\varepsilon_{ij} \\ y_{ij} &= \frac{f(t_{ij}, \phi_i)}{f(t_{ij}, \phi_i) + (1 - f(t_{ij}, \phi_i))\, e^{-g(t_{ij}, \phi_i, \xi_i)\varepsilon_{ij}}}. \end{aligned}$$

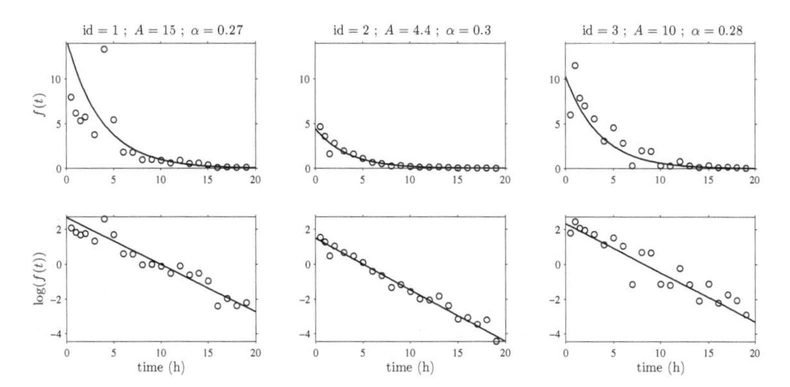

FIGURE 4.11: Top: original data (y_{ij}) and model $f(t) = A_i\, e^{-\alpha_i\, t}$ for three subjects; bottom: log-transformation of the data and the model.

Figure 4.12 displays three simulated series under this model, where $f(t_{ij}, \phi_i) = e^{-\alpha_i t_{ij}}$ and $g(t_{ij}, \phi_i, \xi_i) = 0.8$. Here, the data (y_{ij}) are constrained to take values between 0 and 1 due to the logit transformation.

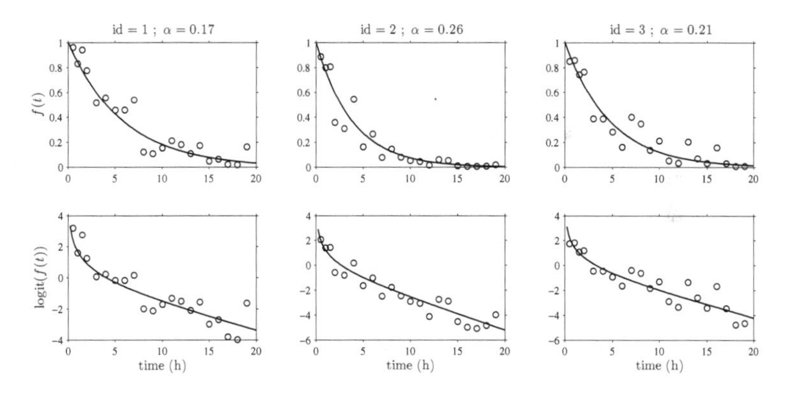

FIGURE 4.12: Top: original data (y_{ij}) and model $f(t) = e^{-\alpha_i\, t}$ for three subjects; bottom: logit transformation of the data and the model.

- The logit model can be extended if the y_{ij} are known to take their values in an interval (A, B):

$$u(y_{ij}) = \log((y_{ij} - A)/(B - y_{ij})),$$

$$y_{ij} = A + (B - A)\frac{f(t_{ij}, \phi_i) - A}{f(t_{ij}, \phi_i) - A + (B - f(t_{ij}, \phi_i))e^{-g(t_{ij},\phi_i,\xi_i)\varepsilon_{ij}}}.$$

Using the transformation proposed in (4.9), the conditional density

$p_{y|\psi}$ of the observations becomes

$$\begin{aligned}
\mathrm{p}(\boldsymbol{y}|\boldsymbol{\psi}) &= \prod_{i=1}^{N} \prod_{j=1}^{n_i} \mathrm{p}(y_{ij}|\psi_i) \\
&= \prod_{i=1}^{N} \prod_{j=1}^{n_i} u'(y_{ij})\, \mathrm{p}(u(y_{ij})|\psi_i) \\
&= \prod_{i=1}^{N} \prod_{j=1}^{n_i} \frac{u'(y_{ij})}{g(t_{ij}, \phi_i, \xi_i)}\, p_\varepsilon \left(\frac{u(y_{ij}) - u(f(t_{ij}, \phi_i))}{g(t_{ij}, \phi_i, \xi_i)} \right).
\end{aligned}$$

For example, if the observations are log-normally distributed given the individual parameters ($u(y) = \log(y)$) with a constant error model ($g(t; \psi_i) = a$), then $\psi_i = (\phi_i, a)$ and

$$\mathrm{p}(\boldsymbol{y}|\boldsymbol{\psi}) = \prod_{i=1}^{N} \prod_{j=1}^{n_i} \frac{1}{\sqrt{2\pi a^2}\, y_{ij}} \exp\left\{ -\frac{1}{2\,a^2} \left(\log(y_{ij}) - \log(f(t_{ij}, \phi_i))\right)^2 \right\}.$$

4.2.7 Censored data

Censoring occurs when the value of a measurement or observation is only partially known. For continuous data measurements in the longitudinal context, censoring refers to the values of the measurements, not the times at which they were taken (Schluchter, 1992; Van der Laan and Robins, 2003; Vock et al., 2012).

For example, in analytical chemistry, the lower limit of detection (LLOD) is the lowest quantity of a substance that can be distinguished from its absence (Armbruster et al., 1994). Therefore, any time the quantity is below the LLOD, the "observation" is not a measurement but the information that the measured quantity is less than the LLOD.

Similarly, in longitudinal studies of viral kinetics, measurements of the viral load below a certain limit, referred to as the lower limit of quantification (LLOQ), are so low that their reliability is considered suspect (Jacqmin-Gadda et al., 2000; Lavielle et al., 2011; Snoeck et al., 2010). A measuring device can also have an upper limit of quantification (ULOQ) such that any value above this limit cannot be measured and reported.

As hinted above, censored values are not typically reported as a number, but their existence is known, as well as the type of censoring. Thus, the observation $y_{ij}^{(r)}$ (i.e., what is reported) is the measurement y_{ij} if not censored, and the type of censoring otherwise. We usually distinguish between three types of censoring: left, right and interval. We now introduce these, along with some illustrative data sets.

- *Left censoring*: A data point is below a certain value L but it is not known by how much:

$$y_{ij}^{(r)} = \begin{cases} y_{ij} & \text{if } y_{ij} \geq L \\ \text{"}y_{ij} < L\text{"} & \text{otherwise.} \end{cases}$$

In Figure 4.13, the "data" below the limit $L = -0.30$ and shown in grey are left censored. These values should therefore not be reported in the dataset, but the information that they are below the limit should be. MONOLIX uses an additional column `cens` to indicate if an observation is left censored (`cens=1`) or not (`cens=0`). The column of observations `logVL` displays the observed log-viral load when it is above the limit $L = -0.30$, and the limit $L = -0.30$ otherwise. The data for the first individual are

id	time	logVL	cens
1	1.0	0.26	0
1	2.0	0.02	0
1	3.0	-0.13	0
1	4.0	-0.13	0
1	5.0	-0.30	1
1	6.0	-0.30	1
1	7.0	-0.25	0
1	8.0	-0.30	1
1	9.0	-0.29	0
1	10.0	-0.30	1

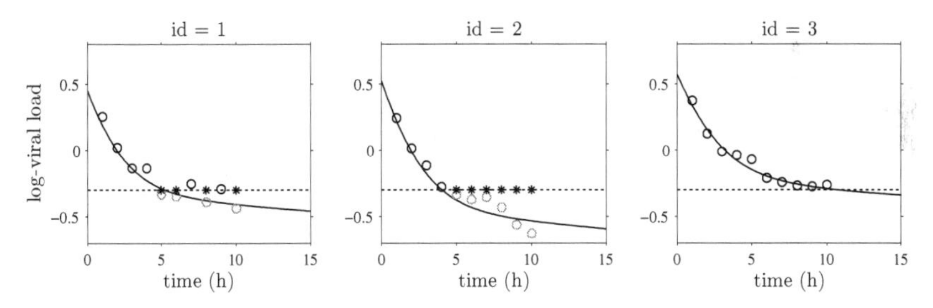

FIGURE 4.13: Observed and left censored data for three individuals. The limit L is shown with a dotted line, the data below the limit with grey circles and the reported data with stars.

- *Interval censoring*: A data point is in interval I but its exact value is not known:

$$y_{ij}^{(r)} = \begin{cases} y_{ij} & \text{if } y_{ij} \notin I \\ \text{"}y_{ij} \in I\text{"} & \text{otherwise.} \end{cases}$$

For example, suppose we are measuring a concentration which naturally takes only nonnegative values, but again we cannot measure it below the level $L = 1$. Then, any data point y_{ij} below 1 will be recorded only as "$y_{ij} \in [0, 1)$". Figure 4.14 displays observed and interval censored data for three individuals. In the table, an additional column `llimit` is required to indicate the lower bound of the censoring interval. Here, the data for the first individual are

id	time	concentration	llimit	cens
1	0.3	1.20	.	0
1	0.5	1.93	.	0
1	1.0	3.38	.	0
1	2.0	3.88	.	0
1	4.0	3.24	.	0
1	6.0	1.82	.	0
1	8.0	1.07	.	0
1	12.0	1.00	0	1
1	16.0	1.00	0	1
1	20.0	1.00	0	1

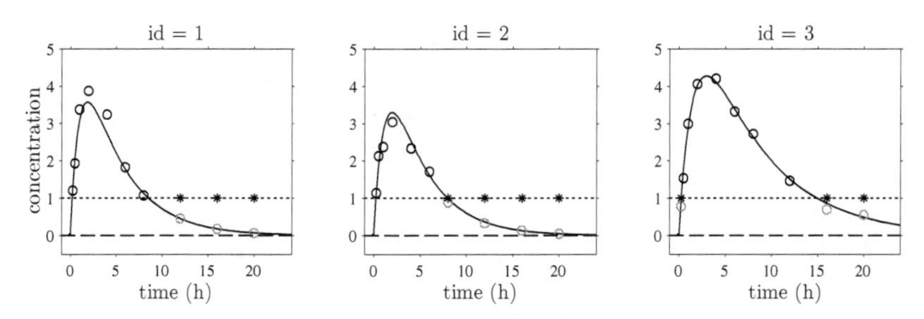

FIGURE 4.14: Observed and interval censored data for three individuals. The upper limit of the censoring interval is shown with a dotted line and the lower limit with a dashed line; data within the censoring interval are shown as grey circles and the reported data as asterisks.

- *Right censoring*: A data point is above a certain value U but it is not known by how much:

$$y_{ij}^{(r)} = \begin{cases} y_{ij} & \text{if } y_{ij} \leq U \\ \text{"}y_{ij} > U\text{"} & \text{otherwise.} \end{cases}$$

Figure 4.15 displays observed and right censored data for three individuals, where the limit is $U = 3.80$. Column `cens` is used to indicate if an observation is right censored (`cens=-1`) or not (`cens=0`). Data for the first individual are

id	time	volume	cens
1	2.0	1.85	0
1	7.0	2.40	0
1	12.0	3.27	0
1	17.0	3.28	0
1	22.0	3.62	0
1	27.0	3.02	0
1	32.0	3.80	-1
1	37.0	3.80	-1
1	42.0	3.80	-1
1	47.0	3.80	-1

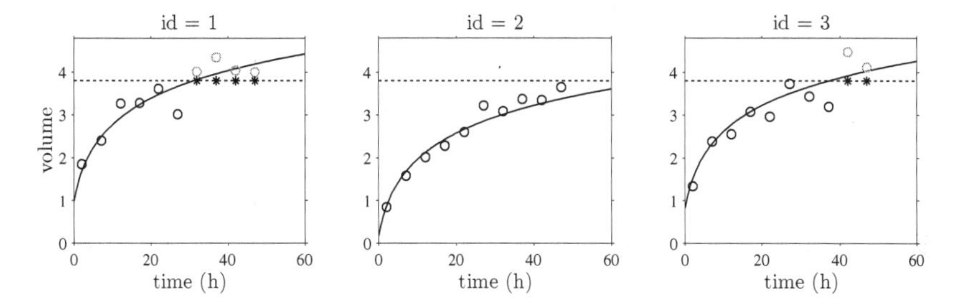

FIGURE 4.15: Observed and right censored data for three individuals. The limit U is shown with a dotted line, the data above it as grey circles and the reported data as stars.

Remarks:

- Different censoring limits and intervals can be in play at different times and for different individuals.
- Interval censoring covers any type of censoring, i.e., we can set $I = (-\infty, L]$ for left censoring and $I = [U, +\infty)$ for right censoring.

The conditional density function needs to be computed carefully in the presence of censored data. To cover all three types of censoring in one go, let I_{ij} be the (finite or infinite) censoring interval existing for individual i at time t_{ij}. Then,

$$\mathrm{p}(\boldsymbol{y}^{(r)}|\boldsymbol{\psi}) = \prod_{i=1}^{N}\prod_{j=1}^{n_i} \mathrm{p}(y_{ij}|\psi_i)^{\mathbb{1}_{y_{ij}\notin I_{ij}}}\, \mathbb{P}(y_{ij} \in I_{ij}|\psi_i)^{\mathbb{1}_{y_{ij}\in I_{ij}}} ,$$

where

$$\mathbb{P}(y_{ij} \in I_{ij}|\psi_i) = \int_{I_{ij}} p_{y_{ij}|\psi_i}(u|\psi_i)\, du.$$

We see that if y_{ij} is not censored (i.e., $\mathbb{1}_{y_{ij}\notin I_{ij}} = 1$), its contribution to the likelihood is the usual $\mathrm{p}(y_{ij}|\psi_i)$, whereas if it is censored, the contribution is $\mathbb{P}(y_{ij} \in I_{ij}|\psi_i)$.

4.2.8 Extensions to multidimensional continuous observations

- The extension to multidimensional observations is straightforward. If d outcomes are simultaneously measured at t_{ij}, then y_{ij} is a now a vector in $\mathbb{R}^d$ and we can suppose that equation (4.1) still holds for each component of y_{ij}. Thus, for $1 \leq m \leq d$,

  $$y_{ij}^{(m)} = f_m(t_{ij}, \phi_i) + g_m(t_{ij}, \phi_i, \xi_i)\varepsilon_{ij}^{(m)}, \quad 1 \leq i \leq N, \quad 1 \leq j \leq n_i.$$

  It is then possible to introduce correlation between the components of each observation by assuming that $\varepsilon_{ij} = (\varepsilon_{ij}^{(m)}, 1 \leq m \leq d)$ is a random vector with mean 0 and correlation matrix Σ_{ij}.

- Suppose instead that K replicates of the same measurement are taken at time t_{ij}. Then, a straightforward extension of model (4.1) gives, for $1 \leq k \leq K$,

  $$y_{ijk} = f(t_{ij}, \phi_i) + g(t_{ij}, \phi_i, \xi_i)\varepsilon_{ijk}, \quad 1 \leq i \leq N, \quad 1 \leq j \leq n_i.$$

  This model assumes the same model for the inter-replicate variability (between the K replicates at a given observation time) and the inter-measurement variability (between different observation times for a given replicate).

  It is possible to extend this model and distinguish between these two sources of variability by decomposing the residual error into inter-measurement (IM) and inter-replicate (IR) components:

  $$y_{ijk} = f(t_{ij}, \phi_i) + g_{IM}(t_{ij}, \phi_i, \xi_i^{IM})\varepsilon_{ij}^{(IM)} + g_{IR}(x_{ij}, \phi_i, \xi_i^{IR})\varepsilon_{ijk}^{(IR)}.$$

  In this model, residual error models g_{IM} and g_{IR} may depend on two different vectors of parameters ξ_i^{IM} and ξ_i^{IR}.

  We will use the same approach in Section 5.5 for decomposing random effects into inter-individual and inter-occasion components.

4.2.9 Mlxtran for continuous data models

Model 1: Basic continuous data model.
Mlxtran allows us to combine equations and definitions of continuous random variables. In this first example, the structural model f is defined in the `EQUATION` block and used for prediction in the `DEFINITION` block.

$$\phi_i = (A_i, \alpha_i, B_i, \beta_i)$$
$$\psi_i = (\phi_i, a)$$

$$f(t, \phi_i) = A_i \, e^{-\alpha_i \, t} + B_i \, e^{-\beta_i \, t}$$

$$y_{ij} = f(t_{ij}, \phi_i) + a \, \varepsilon_{ij}$$

```
continuous1_model.txt

[LONGITUDINAL]
INPUT:
parameter = {A, alpha, B, beta, a}

EQUATION:
f = A*exp(-alpha*t) + B*exp(-beta*t)

DEFINITION:
y = {type=continuous,distribution=normal,
     prediction=f, sd=a}
```

Model 2: Viral kinetics model.
The structural model can be defined as the solution of a system of ODEs. Initial conditions and derivatives are defined in the `EQUATION` block.

$$\phi_i = (\delta_i, c_i, \beta_i, p_i, s_i, d_i, \nu_i, \rho_i)$$
$$\psi_i = (\phi_i, a_1, a_2)$$

if $t < 0$

$$N(t) = \delta_i \, c_i / (\beta_i \, p_i)$$
$$I(t) = (s_i - d_i \, N)/\delta_i$$
$$V(t) = p_i \, I/c_i$$

else

$$\dot{N}(t) = s_i - \beta_i(1-\nu_i)N(t)V(t) - d_i N(t)$$
$$\dot{I}(t) = \beta_i(1-\nu_i)N(t)V(t) - \delta_i \, I(t)$$
$$\dot{V}(t) = p_i(1-\rho_i) \, I(t) - c_i \, V(t)$$

$$f_1(t, \phi) = V(t)$$
$$f_2(t, \phi) = N(t) + I(t)$$

$$\log(y_{ij}^{(1)})|\psi_i \sim \mathcal{N}(\log(f_1(t_{ij}, \phi_i), a_1^2)$$

$$\log(y_{ij}^{(2)})|\psi_i \sim \mathcal{N}(\log(f_2(t_{ij}, \phi_i), a_2^2)$$

```
continuous2_model.txt

[LONGITUDINAL]
INPUT:
parameter = {delta,c,beta,p,s,
             d,nu,rho,a1,a2}


EQUATION:
t0=0

N_0 = delta*c/(beta*p)
I_0 = (s - d*N_0)/delta
V_0 =  p*I_0/c

ddt_N = s - beta*(1-nu)*N*V - d*N
ddt_I = beta*(1-nu)*N*V - delta*I
ddt_V = p*(1-rho)*I - c*V

f1 = V
f2 = N+I


DEFINITION:
y1={type=continuous,
    distribution=lognormal,
    prediction=f1,sd=a1}
y2={type=continuous,
    distribution=lognormal,
    prediction=f2,sd=a2}
```

4.3 Models for count data

Longitudinal count data is a special type of longitudinal data that can take only nonnegative integer values $\{0, 1, 2, \ldots\}$ that come from counting something, e.g., the number of seizures, hemorrhages or lesions in each given time period (Sutradhar, 2011; Thall and Vail, 1990; Winkelmann, 2008; Zeileis et al., 2008). In this context, data from individual i is the sequence $y_i = (y_{ij}, 1 \leq j \leq n_i)$ where y_{ij} is the number of events observed in the jth time interval I_{ij}.

Count data models can also be used for modeling other types of data such as the number of trials required for completing a given task or the number of successes (or failures) during some exercise. Here, y_{ij} is either the number of trials or successes (or failures) for subject i at time t_{ij}.

For any of these data types we will then model $y_i = (y_{ij}, 1 \leq j \leq n_i)$ as a sequence of random variables that take their values in $\{0, 1, 2, \ldots\}$. If we assume that they are independent, then the model is completely defined by the probability mass functions $\mathbb{P}(y_{ij} = k)$ for $k \geq 0$ and $1 \leq j \leq n_i$. Here, we will consider only parametric distributions; in this context, building a model for longitudinal count data means defining:

1. the probability mass function $\mathbb{P}(y_{ij} = k; \alpha_{ij})$ which is assumed to depend on a parameter α_{ij}.

2. a parameter function α that depends on individual parameters ψ_i and possibly the time t_{ij} such that $\alpha_{ij} = \alpha(t_{ij}, \psi_i)$ for any individual i.

The conditional distribution of the observations is therefore written as

$$\mathbb{P}(y_{ij} = k | \psi_i) = \mathbb{P}(y_{ij} = k; \alpha(t_{ij}, \psi_i)) .$$

Let us now look at a few examples of distributions for modeling either the number of successes or failures at a given time t_{ij} or the number of events during a given time period I_{ij}.

4.3.1 Modeling success and failure numbers

The choice of distribution essentially depends on the type of data we want to model. We limit ourselves here to looking at two types of distribution that are particularly well suited to the two specific data types:

- *The binomial distribution.* The probability mass function of a binomial distribution (B) with parameters (n, p) is

$$\mathbb{P}(y = k; n, p) = \binom{n}{k} (1 - p)^{n-k} p^k, \quad 0 \leq k \leq n,$$

with $0 \leq p \leq 1$ and $n > 0$. The binomial distribution $B(n,p)$ is the probability distribution of the number of successes in a sequence of n independent Bernoulli trials with probability of success p.

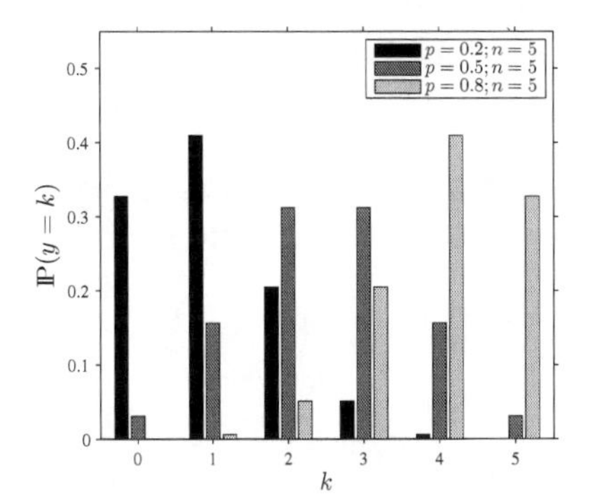

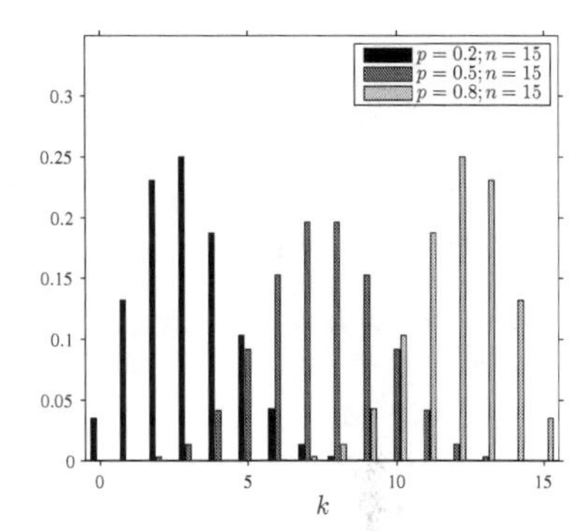

FIGURE 4.16: The binomial distribution $B(n,p)$ for different values of n and p.

EXAMPLE 4.1 Imagine that an archer has for each arrow a probability p of hitting a target with his bow and that he shoots n of them. Then, the number of arrows that reach the target is a binomial random variable with parameters (n,p). Figure 4.16 shows the distribution of this number of successfully shot arrows when $p = 0.2, 0.5$ and 0.8, and $n = 5$ or 15.

In the population context with longitudinal data, y_{ij} represents the number of times archer i hits the target at time t_{ij}. This number can be characterized using a binomial distribution $B(n, p_{ij})$. We then look to model p_{ij} as a function of time (in order to model how this probability increases with practice) and also as a variable that varies among individuals.

As we are looking to model a probability that is increasing, we have to construct a function of time that is increasing and takes values in $(0,1)$. It is therefore better to model $\text{logit}(p_{ij})$ rather than p_{ij}. For example, we could use the function:

$$\pi(t\,,\,\psi_i) = d_i + (e_i - d_i)(1 - e^{-k_i\,t}),$$

where $\psi_i = (d_i, e_i, k_i)$, and define

$$\begin{aligned}\text{logit}(p_{ij}) &= \frac{\log(p_{ij})}{1 - \log(p_{ij})} \\ &= \pi(t_{ij}\,,\,\psi_i).\end{aligned}$$

Then,

$$p_{ij} = \frac{1}{1 + e^{-\pi(t_{ij}\,,\,\psi_i)}}.$$

Here, d_i defines the level of individual i at the start of training ($p_{i,0} = 1/(1+e^{-d_i})$), and e_i the level he can hope to reach after an "infinite" training period ($p_{i,\infty} = 1/(1+e^{-e_i})$). The speed at which he progresses is represented by k_i. In Chapter 5 we will see how to model the inter-individual variability of the individual parameter vector ψ_i, i.e., the variation in competence at a certain activity in a given population.

- *The negative binomial distribution.* The probability mass function of the negative binomial (NB) distribution with parameters (r, p) is

$$\mathbb{P}(y = k; r, p) = \frac{\Gamma(k+r)}{k!\,\Gamma(r)}(1-p)^r p^k,$$

with $r > 0$ and $0 \leq p \leq 1$. If r is an integer, then $NB(r, p)$ is the probability distribution of the number of failures in a sequence of independent Bernoulli trials with probability of success p before r successes occur, and

$$\mathbb{P}(y = k; r, p) = \binom{k+r-1}{k}(1-p)^r p^k.$$

Remark: $NB(1, p)$ is known as the *geometric distribution*: it is the probability distribution of the number of failures before the first success.

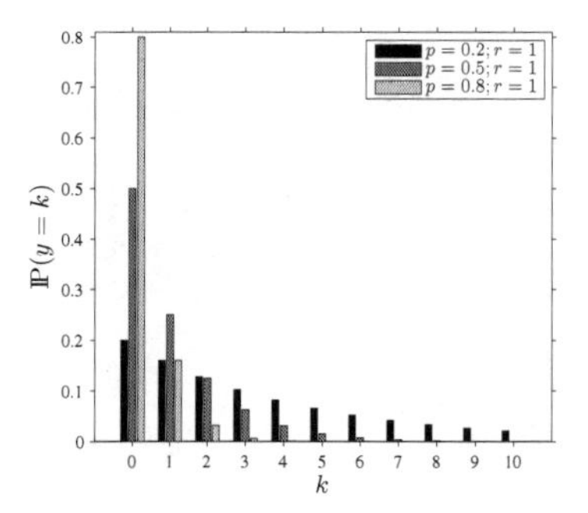

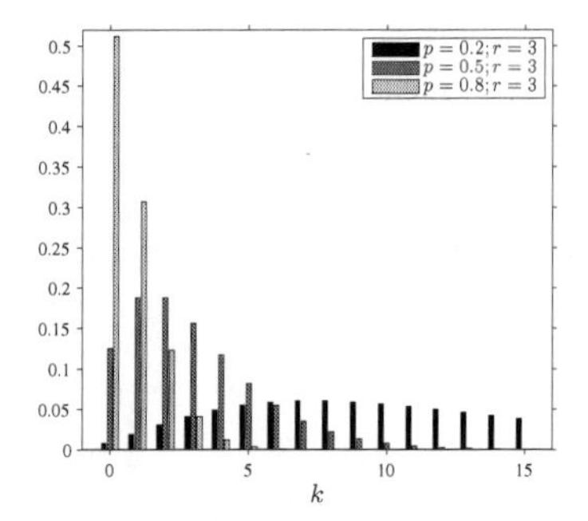

FIGURE 4.17: The geometric distribution $NB(1, p)$ (left) and negative binomial distribution $NB(3, p)$ (right) for different values of p.

EXAMPLE 4.2 Imagine that we are now interested in the number of misses the archer makes before he hits the target r times. This number is a random variable with a negative binomial distribution $NB(r, p)$. Figure 4.17 shows the distribution of this number of misses when $p = 0.2, 0.5$ and 0.8, when $r = 1, 2$ or 3.

In the population context with longitudinal data, y_{ij} now represents the number of misses archer i makes before he has 1, 2 or 3 successes, when shooting at time t_{ij}. This number is characterized by a negative binomial distribution $NB(r, p_{ij})$ where $\text{logit}(p_{ij}) = \pi(t_{ij}, \psi_i)$ as defined in the previous example.

4.3.2 Modeling the number of events

Let us now consider that the data is the number of events of a certain type that occurred in a given time interval. For the moment, let us assume that all intervals have the same length. This is the case, for instance, if data are daily seizure counts: I_{ij} is the jth day after the start of the experiment and y_{ij} the number of seizures observed during that day for patient i.

First, let us look at some possible distributions for this type of data.

- *The Poisson distribution.* The probability mass function of a Poisson distribution with parameter λ is

$$\mathbb{P}(y = k; \lambda) = \frac{\lambda^k e^{-\lambda}}{k!}.$$

One of the main properties of the Poisson distribution is that λ is both its mean and its variance:

$$\mathbb{E}(y) = \text{Var}(y) = \lambda.$$

Another important property is the link between the Poisson and exponential[2] distributions. Indeed, if we assume that the time between consecutive events has an exponential distribution with parameter λ, then the number of events in an interval of length τ has a Poisson distribution with parameter $\lambda\tau$. Figure 4.18 shows several Poisson distributions with different parameters λ.

[2]The probability density function of an exponential distribution is $p(t; \lambda) = \lambda e^{-\lambda t}$ for any $t \geq 0$.

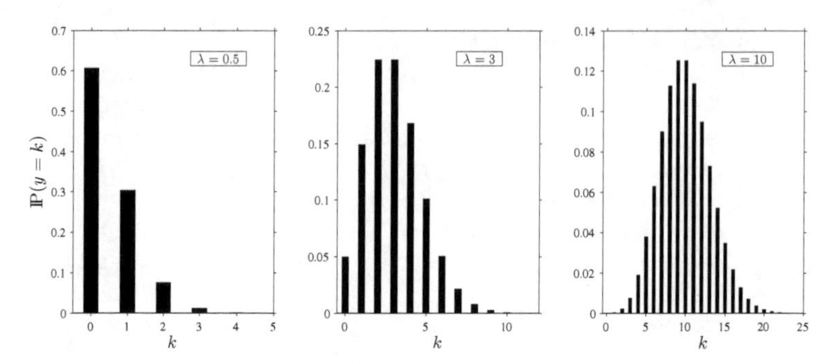

FIGURE 4.18: The Poisson distribution for different parameters λ.

- *The inflated Poisson distribution.* This distribution can be useful when data seem to follow a Poisson distribution except for having an overly large quantity of cases when $k = 0$:

$$\mathbb{P}(y = k; \lambda, p_0) = \begin{cases} p_0 + (1 - p_0)e^{-\lambda} & \text{if } k = 0 \\ (1 - p_0)\frac{e^{-\lambda}\lambda^k}{k!} & \text{if } k > 0, \end{cases}$$

where $0 \leq p_0 < 1$. Figure 4.19 displays several inflated Poisson distributions with different parameters (λ, p_0).

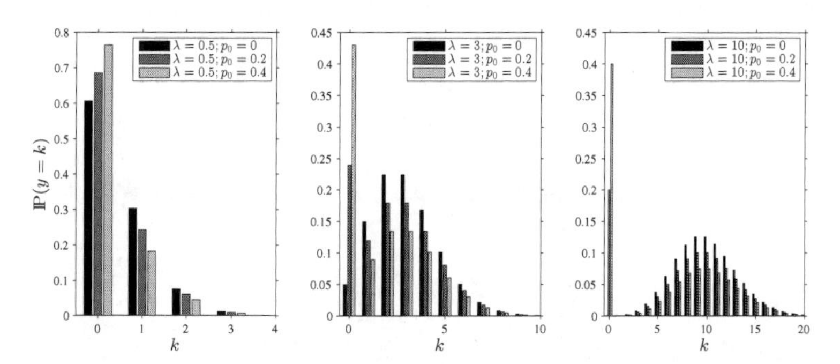

FIGURE 4.19: The inflated Poisson distribution for different parameters (λ, p_0).

- *The generalized Poisson distribution.* The probability mass function of the generalized Poisson (GP) distribution with parameters (λ, δ) is

$$\mathbb{P}(y = k; \lambda, \delta) = \frac{\lambda(\lambda + k\delta)^{k-1}e^{-\lambda - k\delta}}{k!},$$

with $\lambda > 0$ and $0 \leq \delta < 1$. The generalized Poisson distribution includes the Poisson distribution as a special case ($\delta = 0$) and is overdispersed relative to the Poisson. Indeed, the variance to mean ratio exceeds 1:

$$\mathbb{E}(y) = \frac{\lambda}{1-\delta}$$
$$\text{Var}(y) = \frac{\lambda}{1-\delta^3}.$$

Figure 4.20 shows several generalized Poisson distributions with different parameters (λ, δ).

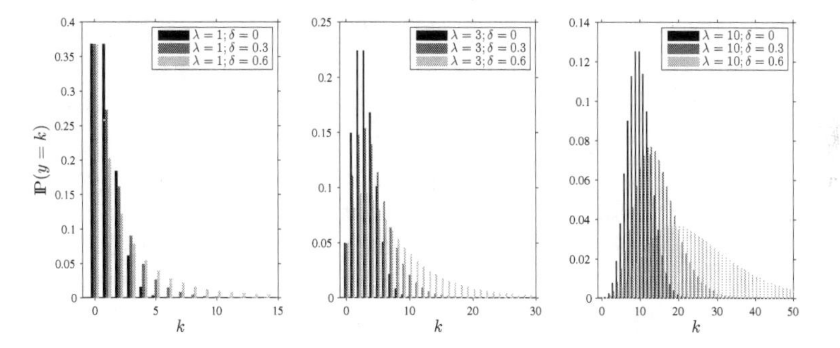

FIGURE 4.20: The generalized Poisson distribution for different parameters (λ, δ).

In the population context, if we assume that model parameters are constant over time for each individual, then the model is reduced to describing the inter-individual variability of these parameters.

> EXAMPLE 4.3 Assume that daily seizure counts for individual i are independent and follow a Poisson distribution with parameter λ_i. Then $\psi_i = \lambda_i$ and
>
> $$y_{ij} \,|\, \psi_i \underset{\text{i.i.d.}}{\sim} \text{Poisson}(\lambda_i).$$
>
> Here, λ_i is the expected number of seizures per day for individual i. This is assumed to remain constant over time.

On the other hand, if model parameters for the longitudinal data are not constant over time, we can make the approximation that they are constant over each time interval I_{ij}. We can then construct a model to characterize the value of these parameters in each interval.

EXAMPLE 4.4 Suppose that we believe that a disease-related event has a linearly increasing frequency. We can model this by defining a continuous function of time $\lambda(t, \psi_i) = \alpha_i + \beta_i t$, where $\psi_i = (\alpha_i, \beta_i)$, setting $\lambda_{ij} = \lambda(t_{ij}, \psi_i)$.

Assume furthermore that taking a certain drug tends to reduce the number of events. We can then link the time-varying drug concentration C to the value of λ at any time using for instance an *inhibition Imax model* (Gabrielsson and Weiner, 2007):

$$\lambda(t, \psi_i) = (\alpha_i + \beta_i\, t) \left(1 - Imax_i \frac{C_i(t)}{IC_{50,i} + C_i(t)}\right),$$

where $0 \leq Imax_i \leq 1$. Here, $\psi_i = (\alpha_i, \beta_i, Imax_i, IC_{50,i})$. As before, we suppose that the conditional distribution of y_{ij} given ψ_i is Poisson with parameter $\lambda(t_{ij}, \psi_i)$.

A more realistic framework consists of supposing that there exists an underlying *continuous* process and that the data we observe in each time interval issue from this process. The construction of such a framework is only possible for certain special distributions such as the Poisson; we will see in effect in Section 4.5 that there exists a direct link between the intensity of a Poisson process and the hazard function associated with time-to-event data.

EXAMPLE 4.5 If y_{ij} is the number of a given type of event (seizures, hemorrhages, etc.) in time interval I_{ij}, and if $h_i(t) = h(t, \psi_i)$ is the hazard function associated with this sequence of events for individual i, then y_{ij} is a nonhomogeneous Poisson process with Poisson intensity

$$\lambda_{ij} = \int_{I_{ij}} h(t, \psi_i) dt \qquad (4.10)$$

in interval I_{ij}. It is thus immediately clear from (4.10) that we can consider intervals with different lengths. In particular, if we assume a *homogeneous Poisson process*, i.e., with intensity λ_i constant over time, then the expected number of events in interval I_{ij} of length τ_{ij} is $\lambda_i \tau_{ij}$.

Such extensions are not possible for the inflated and generalized Poisson distributions. For example, there is no obvious way to define p_0 for the inflated Poisson when dealing with intervals of different lengths.

4.3.3 MLXTRAN for count data models

Model 1: Poisson model with time varying intensity.
Using MLXTRAN we can easily define the observations (y_{ij}) as random

variables where, for example, the distribution of y_{ij} is Poisson with parameter $\lambda(t_{ij}, \psi_i)$.

$$\psi_i = (\alpha_i, \beta_i)$$

$$\lambda(t, \psi_i) = \alpha_i + \beta_i \, t$$

$$y_{ij} \mid \psi_i \sim \text{Poisson}(\lambda(t_{ij}, \psi_i))$$

```
count1_model.txt

[LONGITUDINAL]
INPUT:
parameter = {alpha, beta}

EQUATION:
lambda = alpha + beta*t

DEFINITION:
y ~ poisson(lambda)
```

Example 2: Generalized Poisson model.
With MLXTRAN it is possible to use a library of predefined distributions (including Poisson and binomial). It is also possible for users to explicitly define the data's distribution by giving the probability mass function of y_{ij}. Here, the generalized Poisson distribution is used for defining the distribution of y_{ij}.

$$\psi_i = (\lambda_i, \delta_i)$$

$$\log\left(\mathbb{P}(y_{ij} = k \mid \psi_i)\right) = \log(\lambda_i) - k\delta_i \\ -\lambda_i + (k-1)\log(\lambda_i + k\delta_i) - \log(k!)$$

```
count2_model.txt

[LONGITUDINAL]
INPUT:
parameter = {lbd, dlt}

DEFINITION:
Y = {type = count,
  log(P(Y=k)) = log(lbd)-lbd-k*dlt
  +(k-1)*log(lbd+k*dlt) -factln(k)
    }
```

4.4 Models for categorical data

Assume now that the observed data takes its values in a fixed and finite set of nominal categories $\{c_1, c_2, \ldots, c_K\}$ (Agresti, 2007; Molenberghs and Verbeke, 2005; Powers and Xie, 2008). Considering the observations $(y_{ij}, 1 \leq j \leq n_i)$ for any individual i as a sequence of conditionally independent random variables, the model is completely defined by the probability mass functions $\mathbb{P}(y_{ij} = c_k | \psi_i)$ for $k = 1, \ldots, K$ and $1 \leq j \leq n_i$.

For a given (i, j), the sum of the K probabilities is 1, so in fact only $K-1$ of them need to be defined. In the most general way possible, any model can be considered so long as it defines a probability distribution, i.e., for each k, $\mathbb{P}(y_{ij} = c_k|\psi_i) \in [0, 1]$, and $\sum_{k=1}^{K} \mathbb{P}(y_{ij} = c_k|\psi_i) = 1$.

For instance, we could define K time-dependent parametric functions a_1, a_2, …,a_K and set for any individual i, time t_{ij} and $k \in \{1, \ldots, K\}$,

$$\mathbb{P}(y_{ij} = c_k|\psi_i) = \frac{e^{a_k(t_{ij},\psi_i)}}{\sum_{m=1}^{K} e^{a_m(t_{ij},\psi_i)}}. \tag{4.11}$$

Odds may sometimes be more convenient than probabilities. The odds in favor of a given event are the ratio of the probability that the event will happen to the probability it will not. Thus, the odds for y_{ij} in favor of category c_k are

$$\text{odds}_{ij}(c_k) = \frac{\mathbb{P}(y_{ij} = c_k|\psi_i)}{\mathbb{P}(y_{ij} \neq c_k|\psi_i)}, \tag{4.12}$$

and the associated log-odds are

$$\text{log-odds}_{ij}(c_k) = \text{logit}(\mathbb{P}(y_{ij} = c_k|\psi_i) .$$

EXAMPLE 4.6 Suppose we want to model binary data, i.e., data where $y_{ij} \in \{0, 1\}$ (Lee et al., 2009; Meza et al., 2009). Let $\psi_i = (\alpha_i, \beta_i)$ and let $a_0(t, \psi_i) = 0$ and $a_1(t, \psi_i) = \alpha_i + \beta_i\, t$. Then, (4.11) gives a probability distribution for binary outcomes:

$$\mathbb{P}(y_{ij} = 0|\psi_i) = \frac{1}{1 + e^{\alpha_i+\beta_i\, t_{ij}}} \quad \text{and} \quad \mathbb{P}(y_{ij} = 1|\psi_i) = \frac{e^{\alpha_i+\beta_i\, t_{ij}}}{1 + e^{\alpha_i+\beta_i\, t_{ij}}}.$$

Such a parameterization is extremely flexible and easy to interpret in this example since $\mathbb{P}(y_{ij} = 1|\psi_i)$ and $a_1(t_{ij}, \psi_i)$ move in the same direction as time increases. Indeed,

$$\begin{aligned}\text{odds}_{ij}(1) &= \frac{\mathbb{P}(y_{ij} = 1|\psi_i)}{\mathbb{P}(y_{ij} = 0|\psi_i)} \\ &= e^{\alpha_i+\beta_i\, t_{ij}}\end{aligned}$$

and

$$\begin{aligned}\text{log-odds}_{ij}(1) &= \text{logit}(\mathbb{P}(y_{ij} = 1|\psi_i) \\ &= \alpha_i + \beta_i\, t_{ij}.\end{aligned}$$

4.4.1 Ordinal data

Ordinal data further assume that the categories are ordered (Agresti, 2010; Molenberghs and Verbeke, 2005), i.e., there exists an order $\prec$ such that

$$c_1 \prec c_2, \prec \ldots \prec c_K.$$

We can think, for instance, of levels of pain (low $\prec$ moderate $\prec$ severe) or scores on a discrete scale, e.g., from 1 to 10.

Instead of defining the probabilities of each category, it may be convenient to define the cumulative probabilities $\mathbb{P}(y_{ij} \preceq c_k|\psi_i)$ for $k = 1, \ldots, K-1$, or in the other direction: $\mathbb{P}(y_{ij} \succeq c_k|\psi_i)$ for $k = 2, \ldots, K$. Any model is possible as long as it defines a probability distribution, i.e., it satisfies

$$0 \leq \mathbb{P}(y_{ij} \preceq c_1|\psi_i) \leq \mathbb{P}(y_{ij} \preceq c_2|\psi_i) \leq \ldots \leq \mathbb{P}(y_{ij} \preceq c_K|\psi_i) = 1.$$

We can then extend the definition of odds given in (4.12) for categorical data to cumulative odds for ordinal data:

$$\text{cumulative-odds}_{ij}(c_k) = \frac{\mathbb{P}(y_{ij} \preceq c_k|\psi_i)}{\mathbb{P}(y_{ij} \succ c_k|\psi_i)}$$

and

$$\text{log-cumulative-odds}_{ij}(c_k) = \text{logit}(\mathbb{P}(y_{ij} \preceq c_k|\psi_i)\,. \tag{4.13}$$

Without loss of generality, we will consider numerical categories in what follows. The order $\prec$ then reduces to the usual order ($<$) on $\mathbb{R}$.

Currently, the most popular model for ordinal data is the proportional odds model (Molenberghs and Verbeke, 2005; Williams, 2006; Zeng et al., 2005) which uses *logits* of these cumulative probabilities, also called *cumulative logits*, as defined in (4.13). We assume that there exist $\alpha_{i,1} \geq 0$, $\alpha_{i,2} \geq 0$, $\ldots$, $\alpha_{i,K-1} \geq 0$ such that for $k = 1, 2, \ldots, K-1$,

$$\text{logit}\left(\mathbb{P}(y_{ij} \leq c_k|\psi_i)\right) = \sum_{m=1}^{k} \alpha_{im} \; + \beta_i \cdot x(t_{ij}), \tag{4.14}$$

where $x(t_{ij})$ is a vector of regression variables and β_i a vector of coefficients.[3] Here, $\psi_i = (\alpha_{i,1}, \alpha_{i,2}, \ldots, \alpha_{i,K-1}, \beta_i)$.

Recall that $\text{logit}(p) = \log\left(p/(1-p)\right)$. The probability defined in (4.14) can therefore also be expressed as

$$\mathbb{P}(y_{ij} \leq c_k|\psi_i) = \frac{1}{1 + \exp\left\{-\sum_{m=1}^{k} \alpha_{im} \; - \beta_i \cdot x(t_{ij})\right\}}.$$

[3]Here, $a \cdot b = \sum_k a_k b_k$ is the *dot product* of vectors a and b.

Example 4.7 We give to patients a drug which is supposed to decrease the level of a given type of pain. The level of pain y_{ij} for patient i at time t_{ij} is measured on a scale from 1 to 3: 1=low, 2=moderate, 3=high. We consider the following model for y_{ij}:

$$\begin{aligned}\text{logit}\left(\mathbb{P}(y_{ij} \leq 1|\psi_i)\right) &= \alpha_{i,1} + \beta_{i,1}\, t_{ij} + \beta_{i,2}\, C_{ij} \\ \text{logit}\left(\mathbb{P}(y_{ij} \leq 2|\psi_i)\right) &= \alpha_{i,1} + \alpha_{i,2} + \beta_{i,1}\, t_{ij} + \beta_{i,2}\, C_{ij},\end{aligned}$$

where C_{ij} is the drug concentration at time t_{ij}. This model defines a probability distribution for y_{ij} if furthermore $\mathbb{P}(y_{ij} \leq 3|\psi_i) = 1$ and $\alpha_{i,2} \geq 0$. The model parameters are quite easy to explain:

- $\beta_{i,1} = 0$ means that without treatment, the level of pain tends to remain stable over time.
- $\beta_{i,1} < 0$ ($\beta_{i1} > 0$) means that without treatment, pain tends to increase (decrease) over time.
- $\beta_{i,2} = 0$ means that the drug has no effect on pain.
- $\beta_{i,2} > 0$ means that the level of pain tends to decrease when the drug concentration increases, whereas $\beta_{i2} < 0$ means that pain is an adverse drug effect.

Remark: The exclusive use of linear models (or generalized linear models) has no real justification today since very efficient algorithms and tools are available for nonlinear models. Model (4.14) can be easily extended to a model that is nonlinear in the regression variables:

$$\text{logit}\left(\mathbb{P}(y_{ij} \leq k|\psi_i)\right) = \sum_{m=1}^{k} \alpha_{im} + \beta(x(t_{ij})),$$

where β is any (linear or nonlinear) function of $x(t_{ij})$. More generally, we can use any nonlinear function for the cumulative logits so long as they define a probability distribution. Let γ_1, γ_2, ...,γ_{K-1} be $K-1$ parametric functions of time such that for parameter vector ψ and any time t,

$$\gamma_1(t, \psi) \leq \gamma_2(t, \psi) \leq \ldots \leq \gamma_{K-1}(t, \psi).$$

We can then define the conditional distribution of the data by setting for each individual i, each $1 \leq j \leq n_i$ and $1 \leq k \leq K-1$,

$$\text{logit}\left(\mathbb{P}(y_{ij} \leq k|\psi_i)\right) = \gamma_k(t_{ij}, \psi_i).$$

4.4.2 Markovian dependence

For the sake of simplicity, we will assume here that the observations (y_{ij}) take their values in $\{1, 2, \ldots, K\}$.

We have so far assumed that the categorical observations $(y_{ij}, j = 1, 2, \ldots, n_i)$ for individual i are independent. It is however possible to introduce dependence between observations from the same individual by assuming that $(y_{ij}, j = 1, 2, \ldots, n_i)$ forms a Markov chain. For instance, a Markov chain with memory 1 assumes that all that is required from the past to determine the distribution of y_{ij} is the value of the previous observation $y_{i,j-1}$, i.e., for all $k = 1, 2, \ldots, K$,

$$\mathbb{P}(y_{ij} = k \mid y_{i,j-1}, y_{i,j-2}, y_{i,j-3}, \ldots, \psi_i) = \mathbb{P}(y_{ij} = k | y_{i,j-1}, \psi_i) .$$

4.4.2.1 Discrete-time Markov chains

If observation times are regularly spaced (constant length of time between successive observations), we can consider the observations $(y_{ij}, j = 1, 2, \ldots, n_i)$ to be a discrete-time Markov chain (Durrett, 2010; Meyn and Tweedie, 2009). Here, for each individual i, the probability distribution of the sequence (y_{ij}) is defined by

- The distribution $\pi_i = (\pi_i^k, k = 1, 2, \ldots, K)$ of the first observation $y_{i,1}$:
$$\pi_i^k = \mathbb{P}(y_{i,1} = k | \psi_i) .$$
- The sequence of *transition matrices* $(Q_{ij}, j = 2, 3, \ldots)$ where for each j, $Q_{ij} = (q_{ij}^{\ell,k}, 1 \leq \ell, k \leq K)$ is a matrix of size $K \times K$ such that
$$q_{ij}^{\ell,k} = \mathbb{P}(y_{ij} = k | \, y_{i,j-1} = \ell, \psi_i) \qquad \text{for all } \ 1 \leq \ell, k \leq K,$$
$$\sum_{k=1}^{K} q_{ij}^{\ell,k} = 1 \quad \text{ for all } \ 1 \leq \ell \leq K.$$

The conditional distribution of $y_i = (y_{ij}, j = 1, 2, \ldots, n_i)$ is then well defined as

$$\mathrm{p}(y_i | \psi_i) = \mathrm{p}(y_{i,1} | \psi_i) \prod_{j=2}^{n_i} \mathrm{p}(y_{ij} | y_{i,j-1}, \psi_i).$$

For a given individual i, Q_{ij} defines the transition probabilities between states at a given time t_{ij}. Figure 4.21 shows the transitions of a 3-state Markov chain for individual i at time t_{ij}.

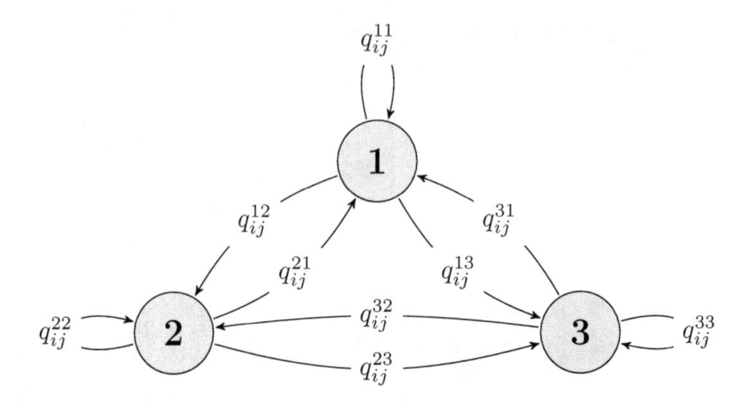

FIGURE 4.21: Transitions of a 3-state Markov chain for individual i at time t_{ij}.

Our model must therefore give for each individual i the distribution of the first observation $(y_{i,1})$ and a description of how the transition probabilities evolve with time.

EXAMPLE 4.8 Figure 4.22 shows several examples of simulated sequences coming from a 2-state Markov model defined for any individual i by

$$\begin{aligned}\mathbb{P}(y_{i,1} = 1) &= 0.5 \\ q_{ij}^{12} &= \alpha_1(t_j) \\ q_{ij}^{21} &= \alpha_2(t_j),\end{aligned}$$

where $t_j = j$ and

$$\begin{aligned}\text{logit}\,(\alpha_1(t)) &= a + bt \\ \text{logit}\,(\alpha_2(t)) &= c + dt.\end{aligned}$$

In the first example (left), the logits of the transitions between states are constant ($b = d = 0$). Transition probabilities are therefore constant over time. Here, $q^{12} = 1/(1+\exp(2.5)) = 0.076$ and $q^{21} = 1/(1+\exp(2)) = 0.119$. As q^{12} and q^{21} are small with $q^{12} < q^{21}$, transitions between the two states are rare, and a larger amount of time (on average) is spent in state 1. Indeed, the stationary distribution is the eigenvector of the transition matrix P': $\mathbb{P}(y_{ij} = 1) = 0.611$ and $\mathbb{P}(y_{ij} = 2) = 0.389$. The figure (left) displays the transition rates q^{12} and q^{21} as functions of the time (top left) and one simulated sequences of states (bottom left).

In the second example (center), b and d are negative. This means that as time progresses, transitions from state 1 to 2 become rarer, and the same is true from 2 to 1.

In the third example (right), b and d are now positive. This means that as time progresses, transitions from state 1 to 2 become more and more frequent, and also more frequent from 2 to 1.

Note that the value of a (resp. c) can be seen as the transition probability from state 1 to 2 (resp. 2 to 1) at time $t = 0$.

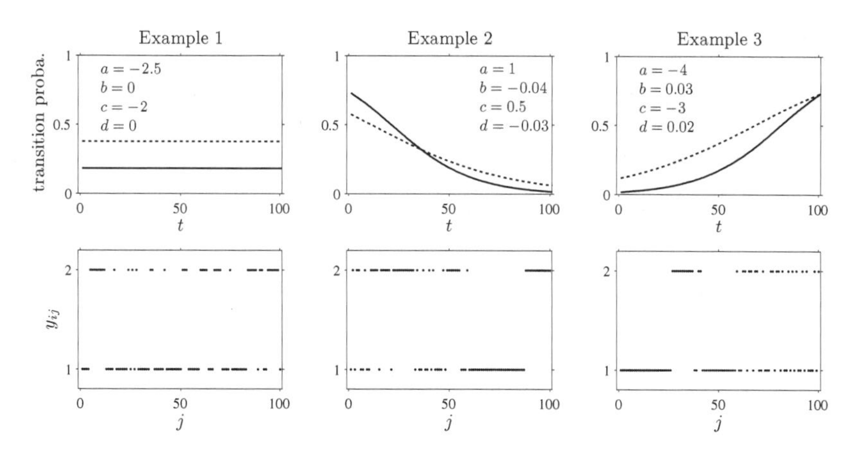

FIGURE 4.22: Three examples of Markov models for categorical data. Top: $\alpha_1(t) = 1/(1 + e^{-a-b\,t})$ as a solid line and $\alpha_2(t) = 1/(1 + e^{-c-d\,t})$ as a dotted line; bottom: three sequences $(y_{1,j})$ sampled with three Markov models defined by transition probabilities $q_{ij}^{12} = \alpha_1(t_j)$ and $q_{ij}^{21} = \alpha_2(t_j)$.

Various choices can be made for defining an initial distribution π_i:

- The initial state can be defined arbitrarily: $y_{i,1} = k_0$. This means that $\pi_i^{k_0} = 1$ and $\pi_i^k = 0$ for $k \neq k_0$.
- More generally, any simple probability distribution can be used for choosing the initial state, e.g., the uniform distribution $\pi_i^k = 1/K$ for $k = 1, 2, \ldots, K$.
- If a transition matrix $Q_{i,1}$ has been defined at time t_1, we can consider using its stationary distribution, i.e., taking for π_i the solution to

$$\pi_i = \pi_i Q_{i,1}.$$

4.4.2.2 Continuous-time Markov chains

The previous situation can be extended to the case where time intervals between observations are irregular by modeling the sequence of states as a continuous-time Markov process (Gardiner, 1996). The difference is that rather than transitioning to a new (possibly the same) state at each time step, the system remains in the current state for some random amount of time before transitioning. This process is now characterized by *transition rates* instead of transition probabilities:

$$\mathbb{P}(y_i(t+h) = k \,|\, y_i(t) = \ell, \psi_i) = h\, \rho_{\ell k}(t, \psi_i) + o(h), \qquad k \neq \ell.$$

The probability that no transition happens between t and $t+h$ is

$$\mathbb{P}(y_i(s) = \ell, \forall s \in (t, t+h) \mid y_i(t) = \ell, \psi_i) = e^{h\, \rho_{\ell\ell}(t, \psi_i)}.$$

Furthermore, for any individual i and time t, the transition rates $(\rho_{\ell,k}(t, \psi_i))$ satisfy for any $1 \leq \ell \leq K$,

$$\sum_{k=1}^{K} \rho_{\ell k}(t, \psi_i) = 0.$$

Constructing a model therefore means defining parametric functions of time $(\rho_{\ell,k})$ that satisfy this condition. Defining $(\rho_{\ell,k})$ as a function of time allows one to take into account variation in transition rates over time, and dependence of the transition rates on a vector of individual parameters ψ_i allows us to take into account inter-individual variability.

4.4.3 MLXTRAN for categorical data models

Model 1: $y_{ij} \in \{0, 1\}$.

$$\psi_i = \pi_i$$

$$\mathbb{P}(y_{ij} = 1 \,|\, \psi_i) = \pi_i$$
$$\mathbb{P}(y_{ij} = 0 \,|\, \psi_i) = 1 - \pi_i$$

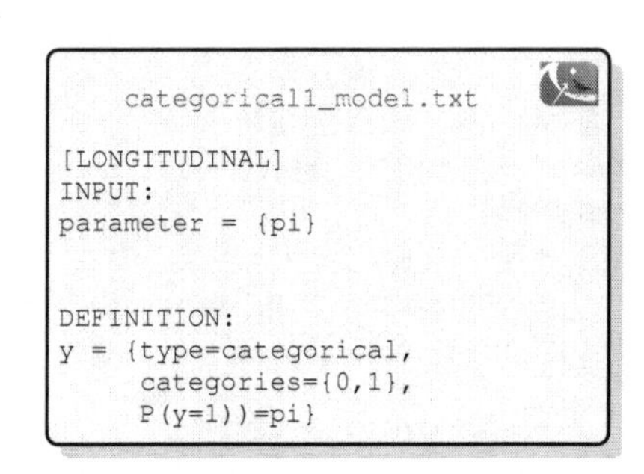

```
categorical1_model.txt

[LONGITUDINAL]
INPUT:
parameter = {pi}

DEFINITION:
y = {type=categorical,
     categories={0,1},
     P(y=1))=pi}
```

Model 2: $y_{ij} \in \{0, 1, 2\}$.

$$\psi_i = (V_i, k_i, \alpha_i, \beta_i, \gamma_i)$$

$$D = 100$$
$$C(t, \psi_i) = D/V_i \, e^{-k_i \, t}$$
$$l_0(t, \psi_i) = \alpha_i + \gamma \, C(t, \psi_i)$$
$$l_1(t, \psi_i) = \alpha_i + \beta_i + \gamma_i \, C(t, \psi_i)$$

$$\text{logit}(\mathbb{P}(y_{ij} \le 0 | \psi_i)) = l_0(t_{ij}, \psi_i)$$
$$\text{logit}(\mathbb{P}(y_{ij} \le 1 | \psi_i)) = l_1(t_{ij}, \psi_i)$$
$$\mathbb{P}(y_{ij} \le 2 | \psi_i) = 1$$

categorical2_model.txt

```
[LONGITUDINAL]
INPUT:
parameter={V,k,alpha,beta,gamma}


EQUATION:
D = 100
C = D/V*exp(-k*t)
l0 = alpha + gamma*C
l1 = alpha + beta + gamma*C


DEFINITION:
y = {type=categorical,
     categories={0,1,2},
     logit(P(y<=0))=l0,
     logit(P(y<=1))=l1}
```

Model 3: 2-state discrete-time Markov chain.

$$\psi_i = (a_i, b_i, c_i, d_i)$$

$$\mathbb{P}(y_{i,1} = 1) = 0.5$$
$$\text{logit}(\mathbb{P}(y_{ij} = 2 | y_{i,j-1} = 1, \psi_i)) = a_i + b_i t_{ij}$$
$$\text{logit}(\mathbb{P}(y_{ij} = 1 | y_{i,j-1} = 2, \psi_i)) = c_i + d_i t_{ij}$$

markov1_model.txt

```
[LONGITUDINAL]
INPUT:
parameter = {a, b, c, d}

DEFINITION:
Y={type = categorical,
   categories = {1, 2},
   dependence = Markov
   P(Y_1=1) = 0.5
   logit(P(Y=2 |Y_p=1))=a+b*t
   logit(P(Y=1 |Y_p=2))=c+d*t}
```

Model 4: 2-state continuous-time Markov chain.

$$\psi_i = (a_i, b_i, c_i, d_i, \pi_i)$$

$$\mathbb{P}(y_{i,1} = 1 | \psi_i) = \pi_i$$
$$\rho_{1,2}(t, \psi_i) = e^{a_i + b_i t}$$
$$\rho_{2,1}(t, \psi_i) = e^{c_i + d_i t}$$

markov2_model.txt

```
[LONGITUDINAL]
INPUT:
parameter = {a, b, c, d, pi}

DEFINITION:
Y = {type = categorical,
     categories = {1, 2},
     dependence = Markov
     P(Y_1=1) = pi
     transitionRate(1,2)=exp(a+b*t)
     transitionRate(2,1)=exp(c+d*t)
     }
```

4.5 Models for time-to-event data

Here, observations are the "times at which events occur." An event may be one-off (e.g., death, hardware failure) or repeated (e.g., epileptic seizures, mechanical incidents, strikes).

4.5.1 Single events

To begin with, we will consider a one-off event. Depending on the application, the length of time to this event may be called the *survival* time (until death, for instance, see Andersen, 2006; Klein et al., 2013; Kleinbaum, 2011; Miller, 2011), *failure* time (until hardware fails, see, for example, Kalbfleisch and Prentice, 2011), and so on. In general, we simply say *time-to-event.*

4.5.1.1 Different possible situations

The random variable representing the time-to-event for subject i is typically written T_i. There are then several ways to define observations, depending on the situation:

1. The event time is exactly observed at time t_i. Here, observation y_i for individual i is "$T_i = t_i$" which can equally be written $y_i = t_i$.

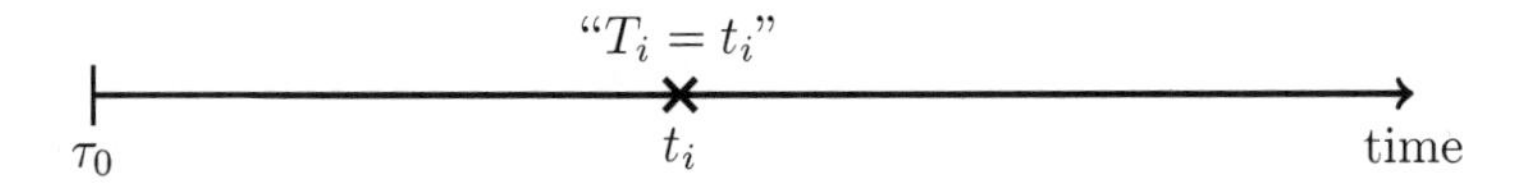

2. We may know the event has happened in an interval I_i but not know the exact time t_i. This is *interval censoring.* For example, at a routine check-up, cancer recurrence may be detected and we only know that it has occurred at some point in time since the last check-up. Here, observation y_i is the event: "$a_i < T_i \leq b_i$".

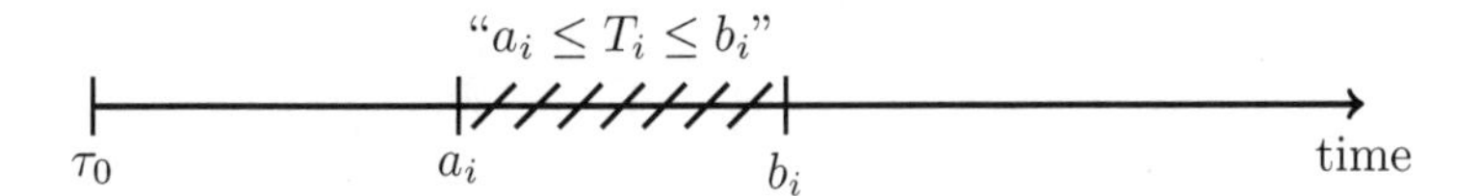

3. If we assume that the trial ends at time τ_{end}, the event may happen after the end. This is *right censoring.* Here, observation y_i is the event: "$T_i > \tau_{\text{end}}$".

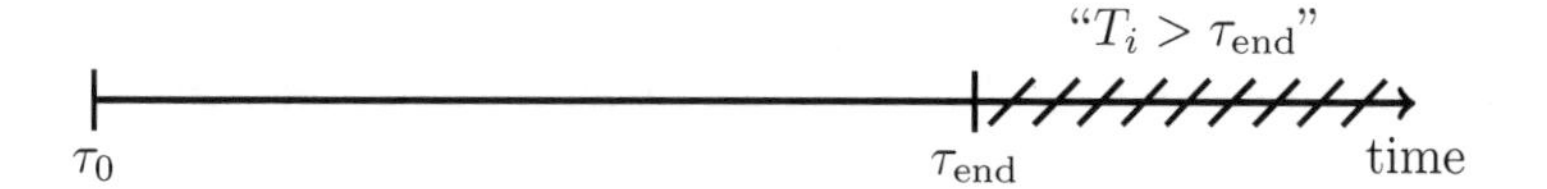

4.5.1.2 Probability distributions

Several functions play key roles in time-to-event analysis: the survival, hazard and cumulative hazard functions. We are still working under a population approach here so these functions, detailed below, are thus individual functions, i.e., each subject has its own. As we are using parametric models, this means that these functions depend on individual parameters (ψ_i).

- The *survival function* $S(t, \psi_i)$ gives the probability that the event happens to individual i after time $t > \tau_0$:

$$S(t, \psi_i) \stackrel{\text{def}}{=} \mathbb{P}(T_i > t; \psi_i)\,.$$

- The *hazard function* $h(t, \psi_i)$ is defined for individual i as the instantaneous rate of the event at time t, given that the event has not already occurred:

$$h(t, \psi_i) \stackrel{\text{def}}{=} \lim_{dt \to 0} \frac{S(t, \psi_i) - S(t + dt, \psi_i)}{S(t, \psi_i)\, dt}.$$

  This is equivalent to

$$h(t, \psi_i) = -\frac{d}{dt} \log S(t, \psi_i). \tag{4.15}$$

- Another useful quantity is the *cumulative hazard function* $H(a, b; \psi_i)$, defined for individual i as

$$H(a, b; \psi_i) \stackrel{\text{def}}{=} \int_a^b h(t, \psi_i)\, dt.$$

  Note that (4.15) implies:

$$S(t, \psi_i) = e^{-H(\tau_0, t; \psi_i)}. \tag{4.16}$$

Equation (4.15) shows that the hazard function $h(t, \psi_i)$ characterizes the problem, because knowing it is the same as knowing the survival function $S(t, \psi_i)$. The probability distribution of survival data is therefore completely defined by the hazard function. The conditional distribution $p_{y_i|\psi_i}$ can be easily computed for the various censoring situations discussed above.

1. If the event is exactly observed with $y_i = t_i$, the pdf is the derivative of the cumulative distribution function (cdf), i.e., the derivative of $1 - S(t_i; \psi_i)$:

$$\begin{aligned} \mathrm{p}(y_i|\psi_i) &= \frac{d}{dt_i}\left(1 - e^{-H(\tau_0, t_i; \psi_i)}\right) \\ &= h(t_i; \psi_i) e^{-H(\tau_0, t_i; \psi_i)}. \end{aligned}$$

2. If the event is interval-censored with $y_i =$"$a_i < T_i \leq b_i$",

$$\begin{aligned} \mathrm{p}(y_i|\psi_i) &= \mathbb{P}(T_i \in (a_i, b_i] \mid \psi_i) \\ &= \mathbb{P}(T_i > a_i|\psi_i)\, \mathbb{P}(T_i \leq b_i|T_i > a_i, \psi_i) \\ &= e^{-H(\tau_0, a_i; \psi_i)}(1 - e^{-H(a_i, b_i; \psi_i)}). \end{aligned} \tag{4.17}$$

3. If the event is right-censored with $y_i =$"$T_i > \tau_{\text{end}}$",

$$\begin{aligned} \mathrm{p}(y_i|\psi_i) &= \mathbb{P}(T_i > \tau_{\text{end}}|\psi_i) \\ &= S(\tau_{\text{end}}, \psi_i) \\ &= e^{-H(\tau_0, \tau_{\text{end}}; \psi_i)}. \end{aligned}$$

4.5.1.3 Applications

There are several possible ways to define observations in real-world situations:

- If events (before τ_{end}) are precisely observed, then for $i = 1, 2, \ldots, N$,

$$y_i = \begin{cases} t_i & \text{if } t_i \leq \tau_{\text{end}} \\ \text{"}T_i > \tau_{\text{end}}\text{"} & \text{otherwise.} \end{cases}$$

EXAMPLE 4.9 Assume that a trial starts at $\tau_0 = 0$ and ends at $\tau_{\text{end}} = 5$, and that we obtain the following observations from four individuals: $y_1 = 3.2$, $y_2 =$"$T_2 > 5$", $y_3 = 2.7$, $y_4 =$"$T_4 > 5$". These observations can be stored in a data file, as shown to the left.

id	time	event
1	0	0
1	3.2	1
2	0	0
2	5	0
3	0	0
3	2.7	1
4	0	0
4	5	0

pdf
1
$h(3.2; \psi_1) \exp(-H(0, 3.2; \psi_1))$
1
$\exp(-H(0, 5; \psi_2))$
1
$h(2.7; \psi_3) \exp(-H(0, 2.7; \psi_3))$
1
$\exp(-H(0, 5; \psi_4))$

Here, "event=0" at time t means that the event happened after t and "event=1" means that the event happened at time t. The rows with $t = 0$ are included to show the trial start time $\tau_0 = 0$. In the table on the right, we display the contributions of each observation to the conditional pdf of $\boldsymbol{y}$.

- If events before τ_{end} are interval censored, then for $i = 1, 2, \ldots, N$,

$$y_i = \begin{cases} \text{“}a_i < T_i \leq b_i\text{”} & \text{if } t_i \leq \tau_{\text{end}} \\ \text{“}T_i > \tau_{\text{end}}\text{”} & \text{otherwise.} \end{cases}$$

EXAMPLE 4.10 Assume that we have intervals of length 1: $(0, 1], (1, 2], \ldots, (4, 5]$. For the same four individuals as the previous example, we now have the following observations: y_1 =“$3 < T_1 \leq 4$”, y_2 =“$T_2 > 5$”, y_3 =“$2 < T_3 \leq 3$”, y_4 =“$T_4 > 5$”. The table below shows how the data can be stored in a data file and how to compute the contributions of each observation to the conditional pdf of $\boldsymbol{y}$.

id	time	event
1	0	0
1	3	0
1	4	1
2	0	0
2	5	0
3	0	0
1	2	0
1	3	1
4	0	0
4	5	0

pdf
1
$\exp(-H(0, 3; \psi_1))$
$1 - \exp(-H(3, 4; \psi_1))$
1
$\exp(-H(0, 5; \psi_2))$
1
$\exp(-H(0, 2; \psi_3))$
$1 - \exp(-H(2, 3; \psi_3))$
1
$\exp(-H(0, 5; \psi_4))$

Here, "event=0" at time t means that the event happened after t and "event=1" means that the event happened before time t.

4.5.2 Repeated events

Sometimes, an event can potentially happen again and again, e.g., epileptic seizures, heart attacks (Huang and Liu, 2007; Kelly and Jim, 2000). For any given hazard function h, the survival function S for individual i now represents the survival since the previous event at $t_{i,j-1}$, given here in terms of the cumulative hazard from $t_{i,j-1}$ to $t_{i,j}$:

$$\begin{aligned} S(t_{i,j}|t_{i,j-1};\psi_i) &= \mathbb{P}(T_{i,j} > t_{i,j} \,|\, T_{i,j-1} = t_{i,j-1};\psi_i) \\ &= \exp(-H(t_{i,j-1},t_{i,j};\psi_i)) \\ &= \exp\left(-\int_{t_{i,j-1}}^{t_{i,j}} h(t,\psi_i)\,dt\right). \end{aligned}$$

4.5.3 Censoring and probability distributions

Taking into account censoring for repeated events is slightly more complicated than for one-off events. First, let us assume that a trial starts at time τ_0 and ends at time τ_{end}. Let $(T_{i1}, T_{i2}, \ldots)$ be random event times after τ_0 for individual i. Then, we can distinguish between the following two situations:

- *Exactly observed events*: A sequence of n_i event times is precisely observed before τ_{end}, i.e., $y_i = (t_{i,1}, t_{i,2}, \ldots, t_{i,n_i}, \text{"}T_{i,n_i+1} > \tau_{\text{end}}\text{"})$. The conditional pdf of y_i is given by

$$\mathrm{p}(y_i|\psi_i) = \left(\prod_{j=1}^{n_i} h(t_{ij};\psi_i)e^{-H(t_{i,j-1},t_{i,j};\psi_i)}\right) e^{-H(t_{n_i},\tau_{\text{end}};\psi_i)}, \quad (4.18)$$

where $t_{i0} = \tau_0$. For example, suppose that for individual $i = 1$ we know there were at least 7 events but only 6 of them occurred before $\tau_{\text{end}} = 15$. Here is a graphic showing the events that were exactly observed:

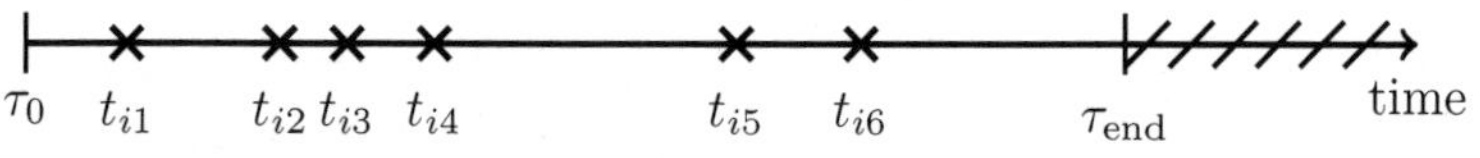

τ_0 t_{i1} t_{i2} t_{i3} t_{i4} t_{i5} t_{i6} τ_{end} time

This data is then stored in a datafile as shown below. We see that the 7th event is noted "event = 0" with time $\tau_{\text{end}} = 15$, indicating that the event was not observed at the end of the time period τ_{end}. In the table on the right, we show the contributions of each observation to the conditional pdf of y_1. Equation (4.18) implies that the pdf of $y_1 = (y_{1,1}, \ldots, y_{1,8})$ is the product of the conditional pdfs given in this table.

id	time	event
1	0.0	0
1	1.4	1
1	3.5	1
1	4.4	1
1	5.6	1
1	9.7	1
1	11.4	1
1	15.0	0

pdf
1
$h(1.4;\psi_1)e^{-H(0,1.4;\psi_1)}$
$h(3.5;\psi_1)e^{-H(1.4,3.5;\psi_1)}$
$h(4.4;\psi_1)e^{-H(3.5,4.4;\psi_1)}$
$h(5.6;\psi_1)e^{-H(4.4,5.6;\psi_1)}$
$h(9.7;\psi_1)e^{-H(5.6,9.7;\psi_1)}$
$h(11.4;\psi_1)e^{-H(9.7,11.4;\psi_1)}$
$e^{-H(11.4,15;\psi_1)}$

- *Interval-censored events*: Let $(b_0, b_1], (b_1, b_2], \ldots, (b_{K-1}, b_K]$ be a sequence of successive intervals with

$$\tau_0 = b_0 < b_1 < b_2 < \ldots < b_K = \tau_{\text{end}}.$$

We do not know the exact event times, but a sequence $(m_{ik}; 1 \leq k \leq K)$ is observed where m_{ik} is the number of events that occurred for individual i in interval $(b_{k-1}, b_k]$. We can show that the conditional pdf of y_i is given by

$$\mathrm{p}(y_i|\psi_i) = \prod_{k=1}^{K} e^{-H(b_{k-1},b_k;\psi_i)} \frac{(H(b_{k-1}, b_k; \psi_i))^{m_{ik}}}{m_{ik}!}. \tag{4.19}$$

In other words, the number of events per interval for individual i is a (possibly nonhomogenous) Poisson process with intensity $H(b_{k-1}, b_k; \psi_i)$ in interval $(b_{k-1}, b_k]$.

Here is a graphic that shows an example of the interval boundaries and the number of events that occurred in each interval for individual $i = 1$:

$m_{i1}=1$ $m_{i2}=3$ $m_{i3}=0$ $m_{i4}=2$ $m_{i5}=0$

$b_0=\tau_0$ b_1 b_2 b_3 b_4 $b_5=\tau_{\text{end}}$ time

The table below shows the same data. Using (4.19) we see that the conditional pdf of $y_1 = (y_{1,1}, \ldots, y_{1,6})$ is the product of the conditional pdfs given in the table on the right.

id	time	event
1	0	0
1	3	1
1	6	3
1	9	0
1	12	2
1	15	0

pdf
1
$\exp(-H(0,3;\psi_1))H(0,3;\psi_1)$
$\exp(-H(3,6;\psi_1))H^3(3,6;\psi_1)/6$
$\exp(-H(6,9;\psi_1))$
$\exp(-H(9,12;\psi_1))H^2(9,12;\psi_1)/2$
$\exp(-H(12,15;\psi_1))$

Remark: If the total number n_i of (observed and unobserved) events for individual i is known to be finite, then formula (4.19) changes slightly when the last event occurs before τ_{end} ($t_{n_i} < \tau_{\text{end}}$). Assume that the last event for individual i occurs in the K_i-th interval. Let $s_i = \sum_{i=1}^{K_i-1} m_{ik}$ be the number of events that occurred before this interval. Then, we can show that

$$\mathrm{p}(y_i|\psi_i) = \prod_{k=1}^{K_i-1}\left(\frac{(H(b_{k-1},b_k;\psi_i))^{m_{ik}}}{m_{ik}!}e^{-H(b_{k-1},b_k;\psi_i)}\right) \times\left(1-\sum_{\ell=0}^{n_i-s_i}\frac{(H(b_{k-1},b_k;\psi_i))^{\ell}}{\ell!}e^{-H(b_{K_i-1},b_{K_i};\psi_i)}\right).$$

This means in particular that we cannot generalize the formulas obtained for repeated events to single events. Indeed, if an event occurs in interval $(a_i, b_i]$ and if we know that it is a unique event, then according to (4.17) the correct formula for computing the pdf is $\exp(-H(\tau_0, a_i; \psi_i))(1 - \exp(-H(a_i, b_i; \psi_i)))$. On the other hand, if this event is not unique and will reoccur in the future, then according to (4.19) the contribution of what was observed between τ_0 and b_i to the pdf is $\exp(-H(\tau_0, a_i; \psi_i)) \exp(-H(a_i, b_i; \psi_i))H(a_i, b_i; \psi_i)$.

4.5.4 Examples of survival models

4.5.4.1 Some classical survival distributions

Let us now take a look at some classical survival distributions, starting with the hazard and survival functions of three widely used distributions in survival analysis (see Andersen, 2006; Kleinbaum, 2011; Miller, 2011).

- The simplest distribution is the *exponential distribution*, derived from a constant hazard function. Here, $\psi_i = \lambda_i$ and

$$h(t, \psi_i) = \lambda_i, \qquad S(t, \psi_i) = e^{-\lambda_i t},$$

  where $\lambda_i > 0$. Figure 4.23 shows the hazard and survival functions of several exponential distributions.

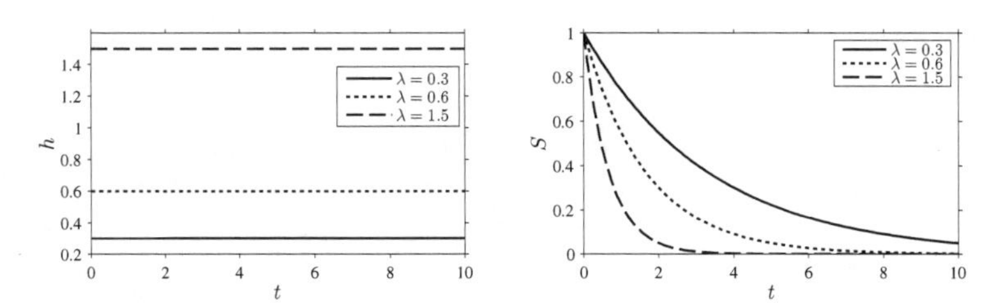

FIGURE 4.23: Exponential distributions: hazard function (left) and survival function (right).

- The *Gompertz distribution* was originally used to describe the distribution of adult lifespans. Here, $\psi_i = (b_i, \eta_i)$ and

$$h(t, \psi_i) = b_i \, \eta_i \, e^{b_i \, t}, \qquad S(t, \psi_i) = \exp(-\eta_i(e^{b_i \, t} - 1)),$$

where $b_i > 0$ and $\eta_i > 0$. Examples of Gompertz distributions are displayed Figure 4.24.

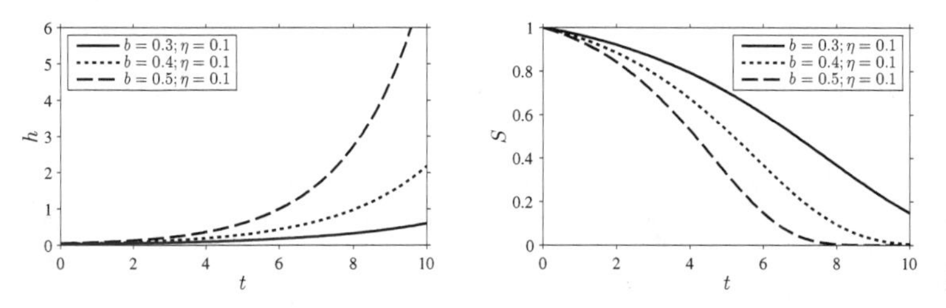

FIGURE 4.24: Gompertz distributions: hazard function (left) and survival function (right).

- The *Weibull distribution* gives a distribution for which the failure rate is proportional to some power of the time. Here, $\psi_i = (k_i, \lambda_i)$ and

$$h(t, \psi_i) = \frac{k_i}{\lambda_i} \left(\frac{t}{\lambda_i} \right)^{k_i - 1}, \qquad S(t, \psi_i) = e^{-(t/\lambda_i)^{k_i}},$$

where $k_i > 0$ is the shape parameter and $\lambda_i > 0$ the scale parameter. Figure 4.25 displays several examples of Weibull distributions.

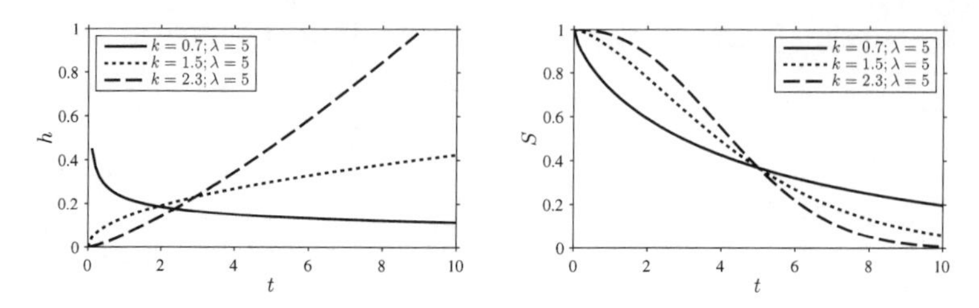

FIGURE 4.25: Weibull distributions: hazard function (left) and survival function (right).

4.5.4.2 Proportional hazards models

These have hazard functions of the form:

$$h(t, \psi_i) = h_0(t, \alpha_i)\, e^{\beta \cdot c_i}.$$

The hazard has two terms: a baseline function h_0 of t and an "individual" term, a function of some individual covariates c_i. Note that this individual term is linear in the covariates: $\beta \cdot c_i = \sum_{\ell=1}^{L} \beta_\ell c_{i\ell}$.

In proportional hazards models, a unit increase in the value of a covariate has a multiplicative effect on the hazard.

The *Cox model* is a *semi-parametric* proportional hazards model where the baseline is a nonparametric function of time (Kalbfleisch and Prentice, 2011; Therneau, 2000). We consider here a parametric extension of the Cox model where the baseline h_0 depends on a vector of individual parameters α_i. In the usual proportional hazards model, α_i is a population constant ($\alpha_i = \alpha$). Then, ψ_i can be decomposed into a set of population parameters α and an individual term $\beta \cdot c_i$. A straightforward extension consists of assuming that α_i is also an individual parameter.

4.5.4.3 Extended proportional hazards models

Another possible extension assumes that the hazard function is a (possibly nonlinear) function u of a regression variable x_i:

$$h(t, \psi_i) = h_0(t, \alpha_i)\, e^{u(\beta_i, x_i(t))}.$$

Consider for example that $x_i(t)$ is the plasmatic concentration of a drug at time t for individual i. Then, $u(\beta_i, x_i(t))$ is the term that represents (i.e., models) the effect of the drug on the hazard, while $h_0(t, \alpha_i)$ might model the effect of disease progression on the hazard.

In this example, $x_i(t)$ is the "true" plasmatic concentration for subject i at time t and is a continuous function of time. However, in practice it is only measured at specific times, so a longitudinal model for plasmatic concentration is needed to give a concentration value for each t. Thus, in practice we need to develop *joint models* in order to simultaneously model time-to-event and longitudinal data. This type of approach is introduced in Section 4.6.

Frailty models are an extension in which the random effect (the frailty) has a multiplicative effect on the hazard (Duchateau and Janssen, 2008; Huang and Liu, 2007; Rondeau et al., 2007; Wienke, 2010). Frailty models can therefore be used to describe the influence of unobserved covariates in a proportional hazards model for univariate (independent) failure times, and for multivariate (dependent) failure times when modeling repeated events.

4.5.4.4 Accelerated failure time models

Unlike proportional hazards models, the accelerated failure time (AFT) model supposes that a change in a covariate has a multiplicative effect not on the hazard but on the *predicted event time* (Kalbfleisch and Prentice, 2011). This can be written as

$$\log(T_i) = \psi_i \cdot c_i + \zeta_i,$$

where ζ_i is a zero-mean random variable, e.g., a centered normal distribution. Usually, parameters are fixed effects: $\psi_i = \psi$ for each subject i.

To calculate the hazard function, let us first denote p_{ζ_i} the density and F_{ζ_i} the cdf of ζ_i, and to simplify, write $\mu_i = \psi_i \cdot c_i$ for the mean of $\log(T_i)$. We begin by calculating the survival function:

$$\begin{aligned} S(t, \psi_i) &= \mathbb{P}(\log T_i > \log t\,;\, \psi_i) \\ &= \int_{\log t - \mu_i}^{\infty} p_{\zeta_i}(u\,;\, \psi_i)\, du \\ &= 1 - F_{\zeta_i}(\log t - \mu_i\,;\, \psi_i). \end{aligned}$$

Calculating (4.15) then gives the hazard function:

$$h(t, \psi_i) = \frac{p_{\zeta_i}(\log t - \mu_i\,;\, \psi_i)}{t(1 - F_{\zeta_i}(\log t - \mu_i\,;\, \psi_i))}.$$

4.5.5 MLXTRAN for time-to-event data models

Model 1: Constant hazard model for a single event.

$$\psi_i = \lambda_i$$

$$y_i|\psi_i \sim \text{TTE}(\text{hazard} = \lambda_i)$$

```
event1_model.txt

[LONGITUDINAL]
INPUT:
parameter = {lambda}

DEFINITION:
y = {type=event,
     maxNumberEvent=1,
     hazard=lambda}
```

Model 2: Constant hazard model for repeated interval-censored events. The survival model is the same but the design is different. Repeated events are observed between $\tau_0 = 0$ and $\tau_{\text{end}} = 200$. Furthermore, events are interval-censored and the intervals are of length 5.

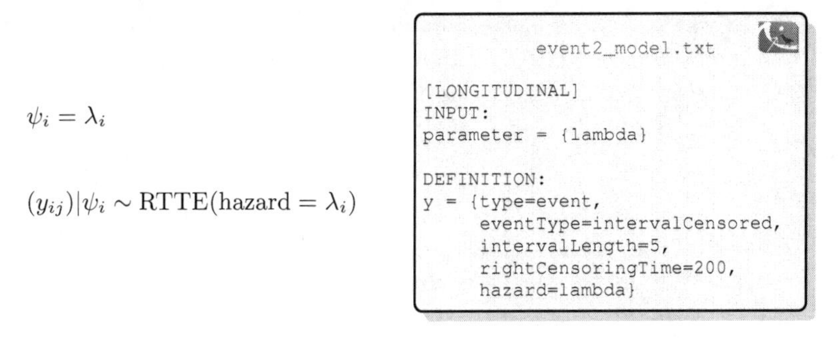

$$\psi_i = \lambda_i$$

$$(y_{ij})|\psi_i \sim \text{RTTE}(\text{hazard} = \lambda_i)$$

```
event2_model.txt

[LONGITUDINAL]
INPUT:
parameter = {lambda}

DEFINITION:
y = {type=event,
     eventType=intervalCensored,
     intervalLength=5,
     rightCensoringTime=200,
     hazard=lambda}
```

Model 3: Weibull baseline model combined with a drug-effect model.

$$\psi_i = (V_i, Cl_i, k_i, \lambda_i, \beta_i)$$

$$D = 100$$

$$C(t, \psi_i) = \frac{D}{V_i} e^{-(Cl_i/V_i)\,t}$$

$$h(t, \psi_i) = \frac{k_i}{\lambda_i}\left(\frac{t}{\lambda_i}\right)^{k_i - 1} e^{-\beta_i C(t,\psi_i)}$$

$$(y_{ij})|\psi_i \sim \text{RTTE}(\text{hazard}{=}h(\cdot, \psi_i))$$

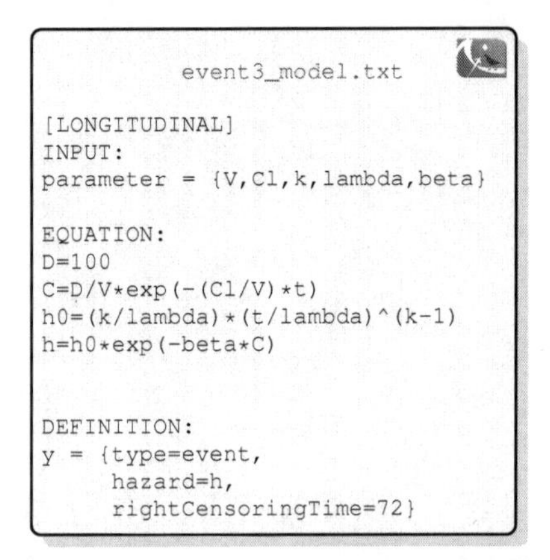

```
event3_model.txt

[LONGITUDINAL]
INPUT:
parameter = {V,Cl,k,lambda,beta}

EQUATION:
D=100
C=D/V*exp(-(Cl/V)*t)
h0=(k/lambda)*(t/lambda)^(k-1)
h=h0*exp(-beta*C)

DEFINITION:
y = {type=event,
     hazard=h,
     rightCensoringTime=72}
```

4.6 Joint models

4.6.1 Introduction

An important goal of longitudinal studies is to characterize relationships between different types of response data.

For instance, in a population PKPD study, we may be interested in the relationship between certain pharmacokinetics (absorption, distribution, metabolism and excretion) and pharmacodynamics (biochemical and physiological effects) of a drug (Bonate, 2011; Gabrielsson and Weiner, 2007). To do this, we need to measure some of both types of response data for several individuals from the same population, then try and characterize their relationship.

Alternatively, many clinical trials and reliability studies generate both longitudinal and survival (time-to-event) data. For example, in HIV clinical trials the viral load and concentration of CD4 cells are widely used as biomarkers for progression to AIDS when studying the efficacy of drugs to treat HIV-infected patients (De Gruttola and Tu, 1994). We might interest ourselves in the relationship between these variables and events such as seroconversion or death.

Therefore, in general, a *joint model* is one that allows us to simultaneously describe the distribution of different types of observations made on the same individual (Elashoff et al., 2008; Ibrahim et al., 2010; Rizopoulos, 2012; Tsiatis and Davidian, 2004). We consider this, as usual, in the population context.

Suppose that we have L different types of observation for individual i: $y_i^{(1)} = (y_{ij}^{(1)}, 1 \le j \le n_{i1})$, $y_i^{(2)} = (y_{ij}^{(2)}, 1 \le j \le n_{i2})$, …, $y_i^{(L)} = (y_{ij}^{(L)}, 1 \le j \le n_{i,L})$, where $n_{i,\ell}$ is the number of observations of type ℓ made on individual i. Note that the numbers of observations $(n_{i,\ell})$ and the observation times $(t_{ij}^{(\ell)})$ may be different for the same individual.

Let us denote y_i the set of observations for individual i: $y_i = (y_i^{(1)}, y_i^{(2)}, \ldots, y_i^{(L)})$. For each individual, the joint probability distribution of the observations y_i and the individual parameters ψ_i can be decomposed as follows:

$$\begin{aligned} \mathrm{p}(y_i, \psi_i; \theta) &= \mathrm{p}(y_i|\psi_i)\, \mathrm{p}(\psi_i; \theta) \\ &= \mathrm{p}(y_i^{(1)}, y_i^{(2)}, \ldots, y_i^{(L)}|\psi_i)\, \mathrm{p}(\psi_i; \theta). \end{aligned}$$

We can then distinguish between different types of dependency between observations: independence, conditional independence and conditional dependence.

4.6.2 Independent observations

Suppose first that the vector of individual parameters ψ_i can be decomposed into L independent subvectors $\psi_i^{(1)}$, $\psi_i^{(2)}$, ..., $\psi_i^{(L)}$ such that $y_i^{(\ell)}$ depends only on $\psi_i^{(\ell)}$:

$$\begin{aligned}
\mathrm{p}(y_i, \psi_i; \theta) &= \mathrm{p}\left(y_i^{(1)}, y_i^{(2)}, \ldots, y_i^{(L)}, \psi_i^{(1)}, \psi_i^{(2)}, \ldots, \psi_i^{(L)}; \theta\right) \\
&= \prod_{\ell=1}^{L} \mathrm{p}\left(y_i^{(\ell)}, \psi_i^{(\ell)}; \theta\right) \\
&= \prod_{\ell=1}^{L} \mathrm{p}\left(y_i^{(\ell)} | \psi_i^{(\ell)}\right) \mathrm{p}\left(\psi_i^{(\ell)}; \theta\right).
\end{aligned}$$

Here, joint modeling does not bring anything new to the picture because all information on $\psi_i^{(\ell)}$ is contained in the related set of observations $y_i^{(\ell)}$. We can therefore model separately each set of observations.

A joint model for two types of longitudinal data might have, for instance, the form:

$$y_{ij}^{(1)} = f_1(t_{ij}^{(1)}, \phi_i^{(1)}) + g_1(t_{ij}^{(1)}, \phi_i^{(1)}, \xi_i^{(1)})\varepsilon_{ij}^{(1)}, \tag{4.20}$$

$$y_{ij}^{(2)} = f_2(t_{ij}^{(2)}, \phi_i^{(2)}) + g_2(t_{ij}^{(2)}, \phi_i^{(2)}, \xi_i^{(2)})\varepsilon_{ij}^{(2)}. \tag{4.21}$$

If the individual parameters $\psi_i^{(1)} = (\phi_i^{(1)}, \xi_i^{(1)})$ and $\psi_i^{(2)} = (\phi_i^{(2)}, \xi_i^{(2)})$ are independent, we can simply use model (4.20) to fit data $(y_{ij}^{(1)})$ and model (4.21) to fit $(y_{ij}^{(2)})$.

EXAMPLE 4.11 32 healthy volunteers received a 1.5 mg/kg single oral dose of warfarin, an anticoagulant normally used in the prevention of thrombosis. We then measured at different times the warfarin plasmatic concentration and the prothrombin complex activity (PCA) for these patients. Figure 4.26 shows the PK and the PD data.

First, we consider two entirely independent parametric models for each of the PK and PD data sets: a simple one-compartment model for the predicted concentration C and a rebound model for the predicted PCA R. For any $t > 0$,

$$C(t, \phi^{(1)}) = \frac{D\, k_a}{V(k_a - k_e)}\left(e^{-k_e t} - e^{-k_a t}\right) \tag{4.22}$$

$$R(t, \phi^{(2)}) = 100\left(\frac{\beta}{1+\beta} e^{-\alpha t} + \frac{1}{1 + \beta\, e^{-\gamma t}}\right), \tag{4.23}$$

where $\phi^{(1)} = (k_a, V, k_e)$ and $\phi^{(2)} = (\alpha, \beta, \gamma)$. Figure 4.27 shows the observed data for four patients and the predictions given by (4.22) and (4.23) for certain values of the individual parameters. We clearly see that it is possible to find parameter values $\phi^{(1)}$ and $\phi^{(2)}$ that allow us to fit quite well curves to the observed data for these four patients.

Nevertheless, even though the PD model fits the data well, it has no biological interpretation and thus little practical interest. Indeed, it is not linked to the PK profile despite the main goal of joint PKPD models being to describe a relationship between a drug's concentration and effect.

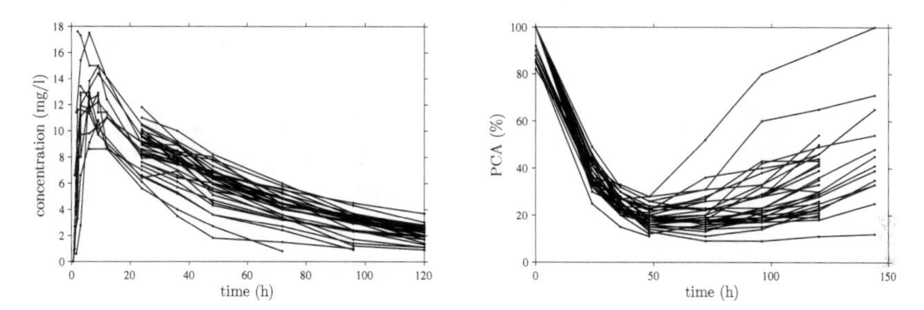

FIGURE 4.26: warfarin PK data (left) and PD data (right).

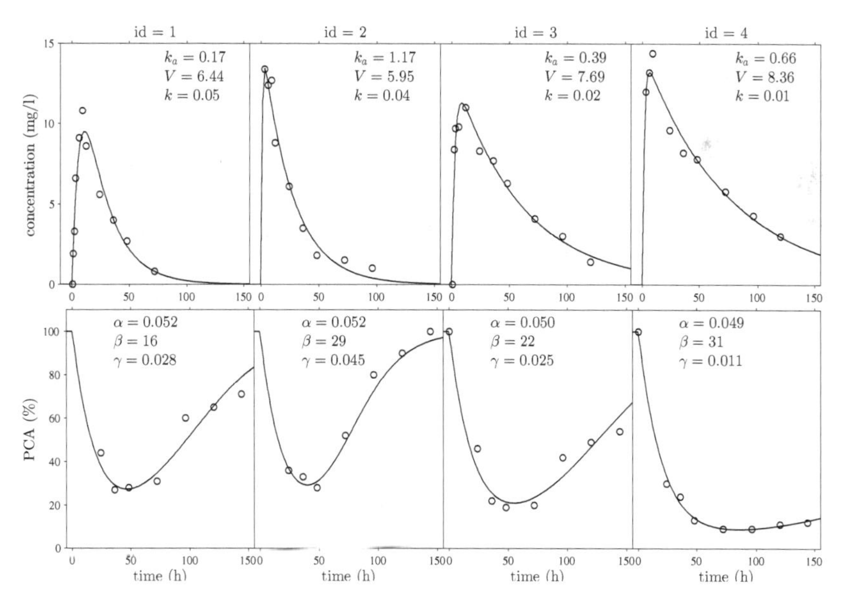

FIGURE 4.27: Top: warfarin PK data and predicted concentration C given by (4.22); bottom: warfarin PD data and predicted PCA P given by (4.23).

In the same way that we jointly modeled these two types of independent continuous data, we can construct joint models using different types of data at the same time, i.e., various combinations of continuous, categorical, count and survival data, if they are independent. We could imagine for instance a joint model for longitudinal data and time-to-event data:

$$\begin{aligned} y_{ij} &= f(t_{ij}, \psi_i^{(1)}) + g(t_{ij}, \psi_i^{(1)})\varepsilon_{ij} \\ \mathbb{P}(T_i > t) &= S(t, \psi_i^{(2)}). \end{aligned}$$

The continuous outcome y_{ij} and the time-to-event T_i are independent if $\psi_i^{(1)}$ and $\psi_i^{(2)}$ are independent.

Remark: In this context, missing data is usually called MCAR (missing completely at random; see Little and Rubin, 2002; Molenberghs and Kenward, 2007). If the event is *dropout*,[4] it is sometimes also called CRD (completely random dropout; see Diggle and Kenward, 1994). This means that the continuous outcome does not provide any information about dropout.

4.6.3 Conditionally independent observations

In this case, the various observation types no longer depend only on disjoint (i.e., independent) individual parameters. We therefore write ψ_i for the overall set of (partially or fully shared) individual parameters. Observations are nevertheless supposed independent when conditioning on ψ_i:

$$\begin{aligned} \mathrm{p}(y_i|\psi_i;\theta) &= \mathrm{p}(y_i^{(1)}, y_i^{(2)}, \ldots, y_i^{(L)}|\psi_i;\theta) \\ &= \prod_{\ell=1}^{L} \mathrm{p}(y_i^{(\ell)}|\psi_i). \end{aligned}$$

In such cases, each observation provides information on the individual parameter vector ψ_i. This is the most common case when we are simultaneously modeling different types of longitudinal data of the form:

$$y_{ij}^{(1)} = f_1(t_{ij}^{(1)}, \phi_i) + g_1(t_{ij}^{(1)}, \phi_i, \xi_i^{(1)})\varepsilon_{ij}^{(1)}, \tag{4.24}$$

$$y_{ij}^{(2)} = f_2(t_{ij}^{(2)}, \phi_i) + g_2(t_{ij}^{(2)}, \phi_i, \xi_i^{(2)})\varepsilon_{ij}^{(2)}. \tag{4.25}$$

Here, predictions f_1 and f_2 both depend on the same vector of individual parameters, which induces dependency between observations $y_i^{(1)}$ and

[4] Participants of a clinical trial may withdraw from the study; this is referred to as dropout.

$y_i^{(2)}$. However, these observations are *conditionally independent* if the residual errors $\varepsilon_{ij}^{(1)}$ and $\varepsilon_{ij}^{(2)}$ are independent.

EXAMPLE 4.12 Pertinent PKPD models aim to establish a link between a drug's concentration and effect. An indirect response model assumes that a drug does not instantaneously affect the PD response. Instead, it affects a precursor which then influences the PD measure. For instance, as warfarin levels increase, prothrombin synthesis is inhibited, which in turn has anti-coagulant effects. Following Holford (1986), such phenomena can be approximated with a very simple ODE-based mathematical model for the PD component (we use the same one-compartment model (4.22) for the PK component):

$$\begin{aligned} R(t, \phi^{(2)}) &= k_{in}/k_{out}, \quad t \leq 0 \\ \dot{R}(t, \phi^{(2)}) &= k_{in}\left(1 - \frac{Imax\, C(t)}{IC_{50} + C(t)}\right) - k_{out}\, R(t), \quad t > 0, \end{aligned} \tag{4.26}$$

where $\phi^{(2)} = (Imax, IC_{50}, k_{in}, k_{out})$.

We can also suppose that vectors $\phi_i^{(1)}$ and $\phi_i^{(2)}$ are independent, but the fact that the effect P predicted by the model is a function of the concentration C introduces dependence between the two observation types because both depend on the PK parameters $\phi_i^{(1)}$.

If the residual errors $(\varepsilon_{ij}^{(1)})$ and $(\varepsilon_{ij}^{(2)})$ defined in (4.24) and (4.25) are independent, then the observations are conditionally independent, i.e., when the predicted concentration $C(t)$ is given, the observed concentrations $\boldsymbol{y}^{(1)}$ do not bring any further information on the distribution of the PD observations $\boldsymbol{y}^{(2)}$.

We will see in Section 8.2 how to use the structural model defined in (4.22) and (4.26) to simultaneously fit the PK and PD for warfarin. We will see that it gives quite similar results to the previous ones in term of fit, using now a PD model that has a biological interpretation. It will therefore be a genuine PKPD joint model.

As before, we can extend this framework to other types of data, considering, for example, categorical observations $(y_{ij}^{(2)})$ for which the probabilities $\mathbb{P}\left(y_{ij}^{(2)} = k\right)$ depend on the prediction of the longitudinal data $f(t_{ij}^{(2)}; \psi_i)$ and consequently ψ_i. We can also consider survival data for which the risk function depends on f:

$$\begin{aligned} y_{ij} &= f(t_{ij}, \psi_i) + g(t_{ij}, \psi_i)\varepsilon_{ij} \\ \mathbb{P}(T_i > t) &= S(t, f(t, \psi_i)). \end{aligned}$$

If, for instance, (y_{ij}) is the measured viral load of an HIV-infected patient, we can assume that the probability of events such as death, seroconversion and dropout depends on the "true" viral load $f(t, \psi_i)$.

Remark: Here, missing data are called MNAR (missing not at random; see Little and Rubin, 2002). If the event is *dropout*, it is sometimes called ID (informative dropout; see Diggle and Kenward, 1994). This means that the probability of dropout depends on some of the individual parameters, but the observation itself of the continuous outcome, which is considered a random variable, does not provide any additional information. In our example, this means that the probability that a patient leaves the study is a function of his true state (i.e., his true but unknown viral load) and not of the random measured viral load values.

4.6.4 Conditionally dependent observations

In this case, there is a dependency structure between different types of observation that no longer allows us to decompose the joint model into a product of models with only one type of observation in each.

This kind of dependency occurs for example when several types of longitudinal data are obtained at the same times with correlated measurement errors. The joint conditional distribution $p_{y_i|\psi_i}$ of the observations is Gaussian if the residual errors are. The dependency structure between observations can then be characterized by the variance-covariance matrix for the errors.

If observations have a hierarchical structure, we can consider a natural decomposition of the joint distribution into a product of conditional distributions:

$$\begin{aligned}\mathrm{p}(y_i|\psi_i;\theta) &= \mathrm{p}(y_i^{(1)}, y_i^{(2)}, \ldots, y_i^{(L)}|\psi_i;\theta) \\ &= \mathrm{p}(y_i^{(1)}|\psi_i;\theta)\mathrm{p}(y_i^{(2)}|y_i^{(1)}, \psi_i;\theta)\ldots\mathrm{p}(y_i^{(L)}|y_i^{(1)}, \ldots, y_i^{(L-1)}, \psi_i;\theta).\end{aligned}$$

Here, the distribution of $y_i^{(2)}$ depends on the observation $y_i^{(1)}$, the distribution of $y_i^{(3)}$ depends on $y_i^{(1)}$ and $y_i^{(2)}$, etc.

For example, we could consider a joint model for longitudinal data and time-to-event data, assuming that the hazard function (or equivalently the survival function) depends on the observed data itself:

$$\begin{aligned}y_{ij} &= f(t_{ij}, \psi_i) + g(t_{ij}, \psi_i)\varepsilon_{ij} \\ \mathbb{P}(T_i > t) &= S(t, (y_{ij}, t_{ij} < t)).\end{aligned}$$

Remark: Here, missing data is called MAR (missing at random; see Little and Rubin 2002). If the event is *dropout*, it is sometimes called RD (random dropout; see Diggle and Kenward, 1994). In our example, where $(y_{ij}, t_{ij} < t)$ is the sequence of measured viral loads before time

t, MAR (or RD) means that the probability that a patient leaves the study depends on his previously-measured viral concentrations.

4.6.5 MLXTRAN for joint models

Model 1: Joint model for continuous PKPD data.

$$\phi_i = (V_i, Cl_i, S0_i, Emax_i, EC50_i)$$
$$\psi_i = (\phi_i, a_1, a_2)$$

$$C(t, \phi_i) = \frac{D}{V_i} e^{-(Cl_i/V_i)(t-t_D)}$$
$$R(\phi_i) = S0_i + \frac{Emax_i\, C(t, \phi_i)}{EC50_i + C(t, \phi_i)}$$
$$y_{ij}^{(1)} | \psi_i \sim \mathcal{N}\left(C(t_{ij}, \phi_i), a_1^2\right)$$
$$y_{ij}^{(2)}) | \psi_i \sim \mathcal{N}\left(E(t_{ij}, \phi_i), a_2^2\right)$$

```
joint1_model.txt

[LONGITUDINAL]
INPUT:
parameter={V,Cl,S0,Emax,EC50,a1,a2}

EQUATION:
C = amtDose/V*exp(-(Cl/V)*(t-tDose))
R = S0 + Emax*C/(EC50+C)

DEFINITION:
y1 = {type=continuous,
      distribution=normal,
      prediction=C, sd=a1}
y2 = {type=continuous,
      distribution=normal,
      prediction=R, sd=a2}
```

Model 2: Joint model for continuous, time-to-event and categorical data.

$$\psi_i = (k_{a,i}, V_i, k_{e,i}, \lambda_i, \alpha_i, \beta_i, \gamma_i, \delta_i, a)$$

$$\dot{Ad}(t, \psi_i) = -k_{a,i}\, Ad(t, \psi_i)$$
$$\dot{Ac}(t, \psi_i) = k_{a,i}\, Ad(t, \psi_i) - k_{e,i}\, Ac(t, \psi_i)$$
$$C(t, \psi_i) = Ac(t, \psi_i)/V_i$$
$$h(t, \psi_i) = \lambda_i e^{\delta_i C(t, \phi_i)}$$

$$\log(y_{ij}^{(1)}) | \psi_i \sim \mathcal{N}\left(\log(C(t, \psi_i)), a^2\right)$$
$$y_i^{(2)} | \psi_i \sim \text{RTTE}(\text{hazard} = h(\ , \psi_i))$$
$$\text{logit}(\mathbb{P}(y_{ij}^{(3)} \leq 1 | \psi_i)) = \alpha_i + \gamma_i C(t, \psi_i)$$
$$\text{logit}(\mathbb{P}(y_{ij}^{(3)} \leq 2 | \psi_i)) = \alpha_i + \beta_i + \gamma_i C(t, \psi_i)$$

```
joint2_model.txt

[LONGITUDINAL]
INPUT:
parameter={ka,V,ke,lambda,alpha,
           beta,gamma,delta,a}

EQUATION:
ddt_Ad=-ka*Ad
ddt_Ac=ka*Ad - ke*Ac
C = Ac/V
h = lambda*exp(delta*C)
lp1 = alpha+gamma*C
lp2 = lp1 + beta

DEFINITION:
y1 = {type=continuous,
      distribution=lognormal,
      prediction=C, sd=a}
y2 = {type=event, hazard=h}
y3 = {type=categorical,
      category={1,2,3},
      logit(P(y3<=1))=lp1,
      logit(P(y3<=2))=lp2}
```

5

Modeling the Individual Parameters

5.1 Introduction

In Chapter 4 we saw a number of models for observations in which the vector of individual parameters ψ_i is given. As we want to work with a population approach, we now suppose that ψ_i comes from some probability distribution p_{ψ_i}.

In this chapter, we are interested in the description, representation and implementation of individual parameter distributions $(p_{\psi_i}, 1 \le i \le N)$. Generally speaking, we assume that individuals are independent. This means that in the following analysis, it suffices to take a closer look at the distribution p_{ψ_i} of a unique individual i.

If p_{ψ_i} is a parametric distribution that depends on a vector θ of *population parameters* and a set of *individual covariates* $c_i = (c_{i,1}, c_{i,2}, \ldots, c_{i,L})$, this dependency can be stated explicitly as

$$\psi_i \sim p_{\psi_i}(\,\cdot\,; c_i, \theta). \tag{5.1}$$

The distribution p_{ψ_i} plays a fundamental role since it describes the *inter-individual variability* of the individual parameter ψ_i. It achieves two things:

1. The definition of a *predicted value* $\tilde{\psi}_i$ of ψ_i for a given vector of covariates c_i and population parameter θ, i.e., a "typical" value of the individual parameter ψ_i for individuals who share the same covariate values in a given population.

2. A description of how the individual parameter ψ_i fluctuates around its predicted value $\tilde{\psi}_i$. In other words, a description of the distribution of the individual parameters for individuals who share the same covariate values c_i.

This means that modeling the individual parameters reduces to describing these two properties of the distribution p_{ψ_i}. We can consider all sorts of discrete and continuous distributions and linear and nonlinear covariate models when defining $\tilde{\psi}_i$. Nevertheless, we must remember that in the modeling context, parameters ψ_i are not actually going to be observed. This means that we will prioritize types of models with structures that let them be both identifiable and interpretable. Distributions related to the normal distribution are presented in Section 5.2, and continuous and categorical covariate models in Section 5.3.

Rather than defining ψ_i using a probability distribution as in (5.1), we can also use equations:

$$\psi_i = M(\beta, c_i, \eta_i),$$

where β is a vector of *fixed effects* and η_i a vector of *random effects*, i.e., a vector of zero-mean random variables: $\mathbb{E}(\eta_i) = 0$. The predicted value $\tilde{\psi}_i$ can then be seen as the value of ψ_i with the random effects set to zero:

$$\tilde{\psi}_i = M(\beta, c_i, \eta_i \equiv 0).$$

We will show that both representations (definitions and equations) can be used with the models presented in Sections 5.2 and 5.3. The pros and cons of the two approaches are discussed in Section 5.6.

Several extensions of this basic model are possible. We can suppose for instance that the individual parameters of a given individual can fluctuate over time. In this case, the model needs to be able to describe the *intra-individual variability* of the individual parameters. We can also suppose that individuals are not independent. The model then requires us to provide the inter-individual dependencies of the individual parameters. Some models incorporating different types of variability are presented in Section 5.5.

A multivariate representation of the distribution of ψ_i is given in Section 5.4 for when the random effects vector η_i is Gaussian. In this case, under fairly general hypotheses we can explicitly calculate the likelihood function

$$\mathcal{L}_{\psi}(\theta) \stackrel{\text{def}}{=} \prod_{i=1}^{N} \mathrm{p}(\psi_i; c_i, \theta).$$

Here, the distribution of the vector of random effects is completely defined by its variance-covariance matrix Ω. Thus, the vector of population parameters θ contains the vector β of fixed effects and the variance-covariance matrix Ω.

5.2 Gaussian models

5.2.1 The normal distribution

Gaussian models have several advantages, including the capacity of describing with ease both the predicted value of a random variable and its fluctuations around this value. Indeed, if we consider a Gaussian random variable ψ with mean μ and standard deviation ω, we can work with two entirely equivalent mathematical representations:

$$\psi \sim \mathcal{N}(\mu, \omega^2) \tag{5.2a}$$

$$\psi = \mu + \eta, \quad \text{where } \eta \sim \mathcal{N}(0, \omega^2). \tag{5.2b}$$

The form (5.2a) provides an explicit description of the distribution of ψ from which we can deduce the probability distribution function (pdf) and other characteristics such as the median, mode and quantiles. Figure 5.1 shows the pdf of a normal distribution with mean μ and standard deviation ω. Each vertical band contains 10% of the distribution.

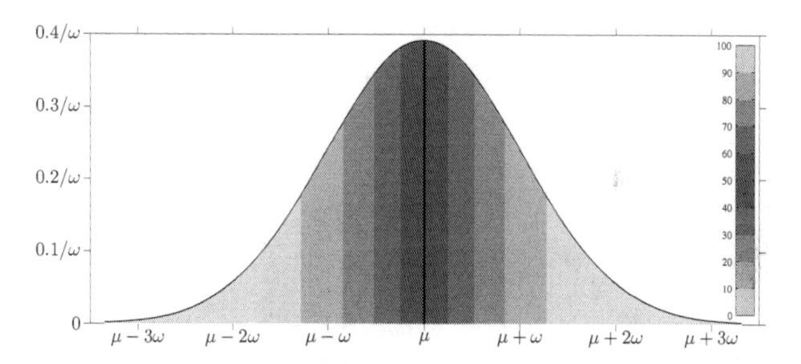

FIGURE 5.1: The $\mathcal{N}(\mu, \omega^2)$ distribution.

This type of graphical representation is powerful and helps us to better visualize the types of values the random variable can take and the values that are more likely than others. Examples of normal distributions with various parameters are shown in Figure 5.2.

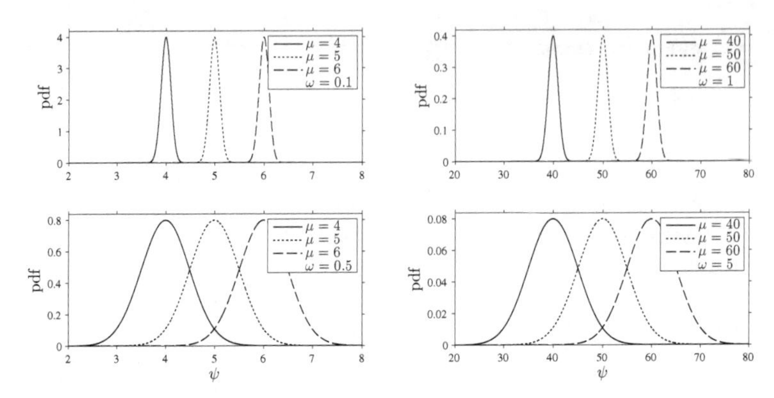

FIGURE 5.2: Different normal distributions.

Representation (5.2b) lets us separate the random and nonrandom components of ψ. If we define as the predicted value the value obtained in the absence of randomness ($\eta = 0$), we get $\tilde{\psi} = \mu$. In the special case of normal distributions, this predicted value is the mean, median and mode of ψ. We can therefore rewrite equations (5.2a) and (5.2b) using $\tilde{\psi}$:

$$\psi \sim \mathcal{N}(\tilde{\psi}, \omega^2)$$
$$\psi = \tilde{\psi} + \eta, \quad \text{where } \eta \sim \mathcal{N}(0, \omega^2).$$

5.2.2 Extensions of the normal distribution

Clearly, not all distributions are Gaussian. To begin with, the normal distribution has support $\mathbb{R}$, unlike many parameters that take values in precise intervals. For instance, some variables take only positive values (e.g., volumes and transfer rate constants) and others are restricted to bounded intervals (e.g., bioavailability).

Furthermore, the Gaussian distribution is symmetric, which is not a property shared by all distributions. One way to extend the use of Gaussian distributions is to consider that some transformation of the parameters in which we are interested is Gaussian, i.e., assume the existence of a monotonic function h such that $h(\psi)$ is normally distributed. Then, there exists some μ and ω such that $h(\psi) \sim \mathcal{N}(\mu, \omega^2)$.

For a given transformation h, we can parametrize the predicted value of ψ using $\tilde{\psi}$. Indeed, the predicted value of $h(\psi)$ is $\mu = h(\tilde{\psi})$, and

$$h(\psi) \sim \mathcal{N}(h(\tilde{\psi}), \omega^2) \tag{5.3a}$$
$$h(\psi) = h(\tilde{\psi}) + \eta, \quad \text{where } \eta \sim \mathcal{N}(0, \omega^2). \tag{5.3b}$$

It is possible to derive the pdf of ψ from (5.3):

$$p_\psi(\psi) = h'(\psi)\, p_{h(\psi)}(h(\psi)) \tag{5.4a}$$

$$= \frac{h'(\psi)}{\sqrt{2\pi\omega^2}} \exp\left\{-\frac{1}{2\,\omega^2}\left(h(\psi) - h(\tilde{\psi})\right)^2\right\}. \tag{5.4b}$$

Let us now see some examples of transformed normal pdfs.

Log-normal distribution: This is widely used for describing distributions of physiological parameters. Note that this choice is usually justified by the fact that it ensures nonnegative values, and rarely because it is shown to properly describe the population distribution of the parameter of interest.

Let ψ be a log-normally distributed random variable with parameters (μ, ω):

$$\log(\psi) \sim \mathcal{N}(\mu, \omega^2).$$

This distribution can be also parametrized with (m, ω), where $m = \tilde{\psi} = e^\mu$. Then, $\log(\psi) \sim \mathcal{N}(\log(m), \omega^2)$ and

$$\mathrm{p}(\psi) = \frac{1}{\psi\sqrt{2\pi\omega^2}}\, e^{-\frac{1}{2\,\omega^2}(\log(\psi)-\log(m))^2}.$$

Figure 5.3 shows some log-normal pdfs obtained with different parameter sets (m, ω).

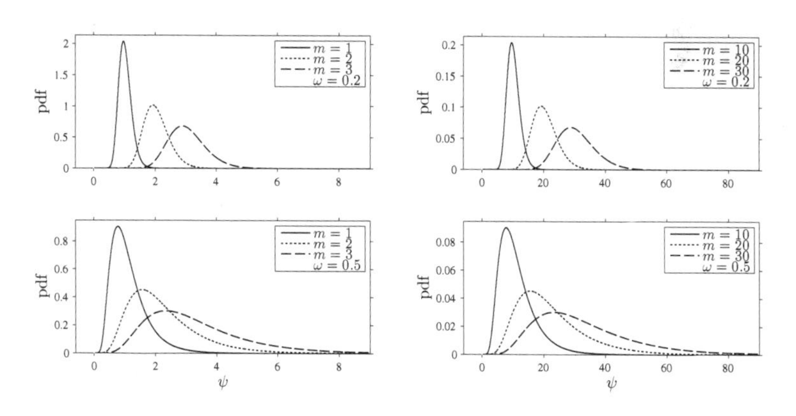

FIGURE 5.3: Log-normal distributions.

We see that for a given standard deviation ω, the pdfs obtained for different m are simply rescaled. On the other hand, for a given m the asymmetry of the distribution increases when the standard deviation ω increases.

Note that the log-normal distribution takes its values in $(0, +\infty)$. It is straightforward to define a rescaled distribution in $(a, +\infty)$ by shifting it:

$$\log(\psi - a) \sim \mathcal{N}(\log(m - a), \omega^2).$$

Power-normal (or Box-Cox) distribution: This is the distribution of a random variable ψ for which the Box-Cox transform of ψ,

$$h(\psi) = \frac{\psi^\lambda - 1}{\lambda}$$

(with $\lambda > 0$) follows a normal distribution $\mathcal{N}(\mu, \omega^2)$ truncated so that $h(\psi) > 0$. It therefore takes its values in $(0, +\infty)$. This distribution converges to a log-normal one when $\lambda \to 0$ and a truncated normal one when $\lambda \to 1$. The main interest of a power-normal distribution is its ability to represent a distribution "between" the log-normal and normal distributions. Here, $m = \tilde{\psi} = (\lambda\mu + 1)^{1/\lambda}$. Figure 5.4 shows several power-normal pdfs obtained with different parameter sets (λ, m, ω).

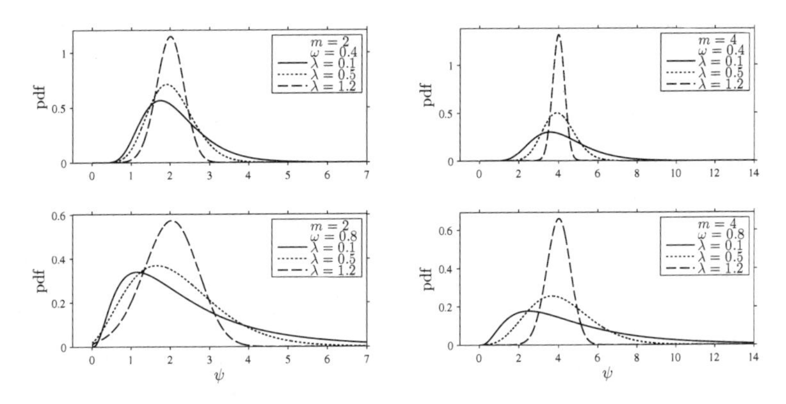

FIGURE 5.4: Power-normal distributions.

Logit-normal and probit-normal distributions: A random variable ψ with a logit-normal distribution takes its values in $(0, 1)$. The logit of ψ is normally distributed, i.e.,

$$\text{logit}(\psi) = \log\left(\frac{\psi}{1 - \psi}\right) \sim \mathcal{N}(\mu, \omega^2),$$

where $m = \tilde{\psi} = 1/(1 + e^{-\mu})$, i.e., $\mu = \text{logit}(m)$.

A random variable ψ with a probit-normal distribution also takes its values in $(0,1)$. The probit[1] of ψ is normally distributed:

$$\text{probit}(\psi) = \Phi^{-1}(\psi) \ \sim \ \mathcal{N}(\mu, \omega^2).$$

Here, $m = \tilde{\psi} = \Phi(\mu)$ and $\mu = \text{probit}(m)$. We can see in Figure 5.5 that the pdfs of the logit and probit distributions with the same m and well-chosen ω are very similar. Thus, these two distributions can be used interchangeably for modeling the distributions of parameters that take values in $(0,1)$.

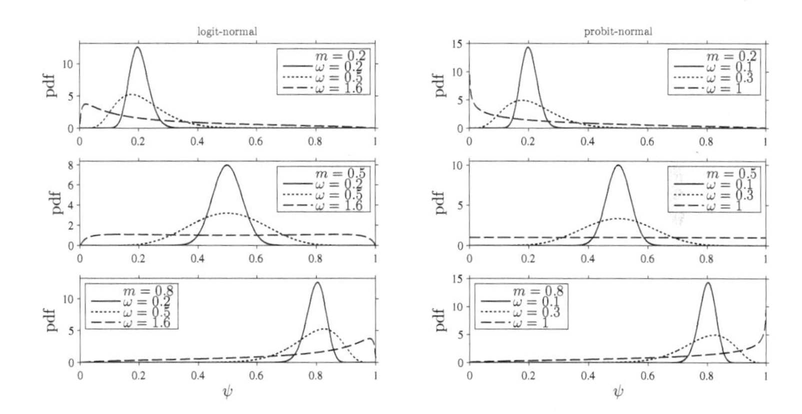

FIGURE 5.5: Logit-normal and probit-normal distributions.

Logit and probit transformations can be generalized to any interval (a, b) by setting

$$\psi_{(a,b)} = a + (b-a)\psi_{(0,1)},$$

where $\psi_{(0,1)}$ is a random variable that takes values in $(0,1)$ with a logit-normal (or probit-normal) distribution. Furthermore, it is easy to show that the probit-normal distribution with $m = 0.5$ and $\omega = 1$ is the uniform distribution on $[0,1]$. Thus, any uniform distribution on an interval can easily be derived from the probit-normal distribution.

Extension to transformed Student's t-distributions: Such extensions (log-t, power-t, etc.) can be obtained simply by replacing the normal distribution for the random effects with a Student's t-distribution. Such extensions can be useful for modeling heavy-tailed distributions. Several Student's t-distributions with different degrees of freedom (d.f.) are shown in Figure 4.10 in Section 4.2.4.3. Student's t-distribution converges to the normal distribution as its d.f. increases, whereas heavy tails are obtained for small d.f.

[1]The probit function is the inverse cumulative distribution function (quantile function) Φ^{-1} associated with the standard normal distribution $\mathcal{N}(0,1)$.

5.2.3 Mlxtran for Gaussian models

We consider in this example four PK parameters F_i, ka_i, V_i and Cl_i, with four different distributions.

$$\theta = (F_{\text{pop}}, ka_{\text{pop}}, V_{\text{pop}}, Cl_{\text{pop}}, \lambda, \omega_F^2, \omega_{ka}^2, \omega_V^2, \omega_{Cl}^2)$$

$$\text{logit}(F_i) \sim \mathcal{N}(\text{logit}(F_{\text{pop}}), \omega_F^2)$$
$$\log(ka_i) \sim \mathcal{N}(\log(ka_{\text{pop}}), \omega_{ka}^2)$$
$$V_i \sim \mathcal{N}(V_{\text{pop}}, \omega_V^2)$$
$$\frac{Cl_i^\lambda - 1}{\lambda} \sim \mathcal{N}(\frac{Cl_{\text{pop}}^\lambda - 1}{\lambda}, \omega_{Cl}^2)$$

Gaussian_model.txt

```
[INDIVIDUAL]
input={F_pop, ka_pop, V_pop, Cl_pop,
       lambda, omega_F, omega_ka,
       omega_V, omega_Cl}

DEFINITION:
F ={distribution=logitnormal,
    reference=F_pop,sd=omega_F}
ka={distribution=lognormal,
    reference=ka_pop,sd=omega_ka}
V={distribution=normal,
   reference=V_pop,sd=omega_V}
Cl={distribution=powernormal,
    power=lambda_Cl,
    reference=Cl_pop,sd=omega_Cl}
```

5.3 Models with covariates

5.3.1 Introduction

For the moment, we are still considering that there is only one scalar parameter ψ_i for each subject i. A covariate model then consists of defining the prediction $\tilde{\psi}_i$ as a function of the subject's covariates c_i and the fixed effects β:

$$\tilde{\psi}_i = m(\beta, c_i). \tag{5.5}$$

We take a statistical approach here. The goal is not necessarily to construct a *causal* model that supposes a cause-effect relationship between covariates and the parameter, but one where the covariates partially describe the parameter's variability.

Consider, for example, a very simple model that posits a linear relationship between the height h_i of subject i and the predicted weight $\tilde{w}_i$:

$$\tilde{w}_i \;=\; m(\beta, h_i) \;=\; \beta_0 + \beta_1 h_i.$$

The parameters $\beta = (\beta_0, \beta_1)$ are population parameters which may vary from one population to the next but are considered fixed within the same homogeneous population. In this model, the height is a covariate that:

1. helps to predict the weight. For an individual of height h_i, we predict the weight $\beta_0+\beta_1 h_i$. We use this model without necessarily supposing that there is a cause-effect relationship between height and weight. We merely assume that having information about height gives us some information about weight.

2. helps to describe variability in the weight. Suppose that we make the arbitrary choice of a "reference individual" in the population who has height $h_{\rm pop}$ and weight $w_{\rm pop}$. Then, the model lets us show the link between the reference height and weight:

$$w_{\rm pop} = \beta_0 + \beta_1 h_{\rm pop}.$$

   Now we can more clearly see the variability in weight around the reference weight as a function of the variation in height around the reference height:

$$\tilde{w}_i - w_{\rm pop} = \beta_1 (h_i - h_{\rm pop}).$$

   If the weight is in kg and the height in cm, for an individual who is 1cm taller than the reference height we predict a weight of β_1 kg above the reference weight.

In more general examples, there is a vector of reference covariates $c_{\rm pop}$. A reference individual is one who would personally have these covariate values. Consequently, $\psi_{\rm pop} = m(\beta, c_{\rm pop})$ is the predicted value of the individual parameter for this virtual individual. The covariate model therefore describes how $\tilde{\psi}_i$ falls around $\psi_{\rm pop}$ as c_i varies around $c_{\rm pop}$:

$$\tilde{\psi}_i - \psi_{\rm pop} = m(\beta, c_i) - m(\beta, c_{\rm pop}). \tag{5.6}$$

For clarity, in the following we distinguish between linear and nonlinear continuous covariate models, and categorical variable models.

5.3.2 Linear models for continuous covariates

In its most simple form, a linear model is one where the individual parameter is modeled as a linear combination of the covariates, i.e.,

$$\tilde{\psi}_i = \beta_0 + \sum_{\ell=1}^{L} \beta_\ell \, c_{i\ell} \, . \tag{5.7}$$

The coefficient β_0 which appears in (5.7) is usually called the *intercept.* Its interpretation is limited by the fact that it is the predicted value of the parameter when all of the covariates are zero, which generally does not mean much. With respect to a reference individual, (5.7) can instead be rewritten as in (5.6):

$$\tilde{\psi}_i = \psi_{\text{pop}} + \beta \cdot (c_i - c_{\text{pop}}).$$

The intercept ψ_{pop} is now the predicted value of the parameter when the covariates are set to their reference values, and therefore, by definition, is the parameter's reference value. More generally, we usually suppose that linearity can be with respect to a transformation h of $\tilde{\psi}_i$:

$$h(\tilde{\psi}_i) = h(\psi_{\text{pop}}) + \beta \cdot (c_i - c_{\text{pop}}). \tag{5.8}$$

Here, h is the transform described in (5.3) such that $h(\psi_i)$ can be supposed Gaussian. As well as covariates such as height and age, c_i may include transformed ones, e.g., log-weight or weight/height^2. By combining (5.3) and (5.8), we obtain the following equivalent representations of ψ_i:

$$\begin{aligned} h(\psi_i) &\sim \mathcal{N}(h(\psi_{\text{pop}}) + \beta \cdot (c_i - c_{\text{pop}}), \omega^2), \\ h(\psi_i) &= h(\psi_{\text{pop}}) + \beta \cdot (c_i - c_{\text{pop}}) + \eta_i\,, \quad \eta_i \sim \mathcal{N}(0, \omega^2). \end{aligned} \tag{5.9}$$

This model gives a clear and easily interpreted decomposition of the variability of $h(\psi_i)$ around $h(\psi_{\text{pop}})$, i.e., of ψ_i around ψ_{pop}:

- The component $\beta \cdot (c_i - c_{\text{pop}})$ describes part of this variability by way of covariates c_i that fluctuate around c_{pop}.
- The random component η_i describes the remaining variability, i.e., variability between subjects that have the same covariate values.

By definition, a mixed effects model combines these two components: fixed and random effects. In linear covariate models, these two effects combine additively.

In the present context, the vector of population parameters is $\theta = (\psi_{\text{pop}}, \beta, \omega^2)$. We can then use (5.4a) to give the pdf of ψ_i:

$$\mathrm{p}(\psi_i; c_i, \theta) = \frac{h'(\psi_i)}{\sqrt{2\pi\omega^2}} \exp\left\{-\frac{1}{2\,\omega^2}\left(h(\psi_i) - h(\psi_{\text{pop}}) - \beta \cdot (c_i - c_{\text{pop}})\right)^2\right\},$$

and the likelihood function:

$$\mathcal{L}_{\psi}(\theta) \;\stackrel{\text{def}}{=}\; \prod_{i=1}^{N} \mathrm{p}(\psi_i; c_i, \theta).$$

The maximum likelihood (ML) estimate of θ has a closed form here since the model is linear. Let

$$\zeta = \begin{pmatrix} h(\psi_{\rm pop}) \\ \beta_1 \\ \vdots \\ \beta_L \end{pmatrix}, \quad h(\boldsymbol{\psi}) = \begin{pmatrix} h(\psi_1) \\ h(\psi_2) \\ \vdots \\ h(\psi_N) \end{pmatrix},$$

$$C = \begin{pmatrix} 1 & c_{1,1} - c_{\rm pop,1} & \dots & c_{1,L} - c_{\rm pop,L} \\ 1 & c_{2,1} - c_{\rm pop,1} & \dots & c_{2,L} - c_{\rm pop,L} \\ \vdots & \vdots & \ddots & \vdots \\ 1 & c_{N,1} - c_{\rm pop,1} & \dots & c_{N,L} - c_{\rm pop,L} \end{pmatrix}.$$

Then,

$$\widehat{\zeta} = (C'C)^{-1} C' h(\boldsymbol{\psi}),$$

and

$$\begin{aligned} \widehat{\omega}^2 &= \frac{1}{N} \| h(\boldsymbol{\psi}) - C\widehat{\zeta} \|^2 \\ &= \frac{1}{N} \sum_{i=1}^{N} \left(h(\psi_i) - h(\widehat{\psi}_{\rm pop}) - \sum_{\ell=1}^{L} \widehat{\beta}_\ell (c_{i,\ell} - c_{{\rm pop},\ell}) \right)^2 . \end{aligned}$$

Remarks

1. Let $d_{i,\ell} = c_{i,\ell} - c_{{\rm pop},\ell}$ and $\eta_i^* = \omega^{-1}\eta_i$. Then (5.9) can be written as

$$h(\psi_i) = h(\psi_{\rm pop}) + \beta_1 d_{i,1} + \beta_2 d_{i,2} + \ldots + \beta_L d_{i,L} + \omega \eta_i^*,$$

   where $\eta_i^* \sim \mathcal{N}(0,1)$. Here, $d_{i,1}, d_{i,2}, \ldots, d_{i,L}$ and η_i^* represent effects that contribute to the fluctuations of $h(\psi_i)$ around $h(\psi_{\rm pop})$. Coefficients β_1, β_2, ..., β_L and ω represent the magnitude of these effects. If the ℓth coefficient is zero, this means that the ℓth covariate has no effect. Similarly, $\omega = 0$ signifies that there is no random effect.

2. The $d_{i,\ell}$ and the standardized random effect η_i^* play similar roles. The difference is essentially that the $d_{i,\ell}$ are "known" in the modeling context, unlike η_i^*. If the context is simulation, all of them can be considered as random variables with their own specific distributions. We can therefore consider a random effect to be like a covariate that is not observed.

EXAMPLE 5.1 In this example, the individual parameter ψ_i is the *volume of distribution* V_i which we can assume to be log-normally distributed. The weight w_i (kg) can be used to explain part of the variability in the volume between individuals:

$$\log(V_i) = \log(V_{\rm pop}) + \beta(\log(w_i) - \log(70)) + \eta_i, \tag{5.10}$$

where $\eta_i \sim \mathcal{N}(0, \omega_V^2)$. Here, the covariate used in the statistical model is the log-weight, and the reference weight we decide to choose is 70kg. Of course, it would be absolutely equivalent to define the covariate as $c_i = \log(w_i/70)$. Then, the reference value of this covariate would become $c_{\rm pop} = 0$ for an individual of 70kg, and model (5.10) is instead written as

$$\log(V_i) = \log(V_{\rm pop}) + \beta \log(w_i/70) + \eta_i.$$

This same model can also be expressed in other ways. For instance, taking the exponential gives a model in terms of V_i:

$$V_i = V_{\rm pop} \left(\frac{w_i}{70}\right)^{\beta} e^{\eta_i}.$$

Here, the predicted volume for an individual with weight w_i is

$$\tilde{V}_i = V_{\rm pop} \left(\frac{w_i}{70}\right)^{\beta}.$$

The right-hand panel of Figure 5.6 shows how the predicted volume $\tilde{V}$ increases with weight w for different values of β. Here, $V_{\rm pop}$ has been set at 10. For β not equal to 0 or 1, the model is not linear. However, the predicted log-volume (left-hand panel) does increase linearly with the log-weight:

$$\log(\tilde{V}_i) = \log(V_{\rm pop}) + \beta \log(w_i/70).$$

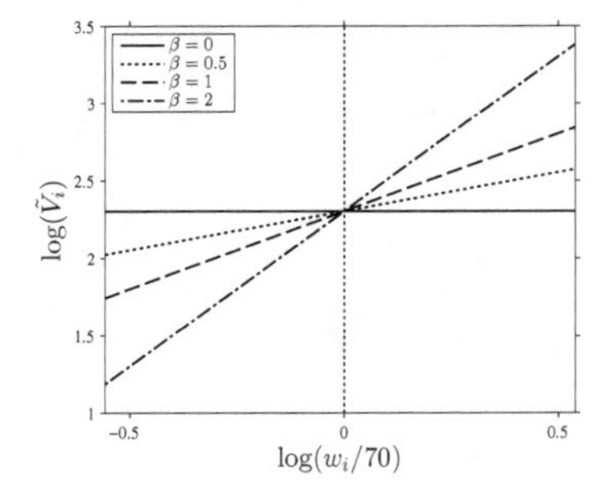

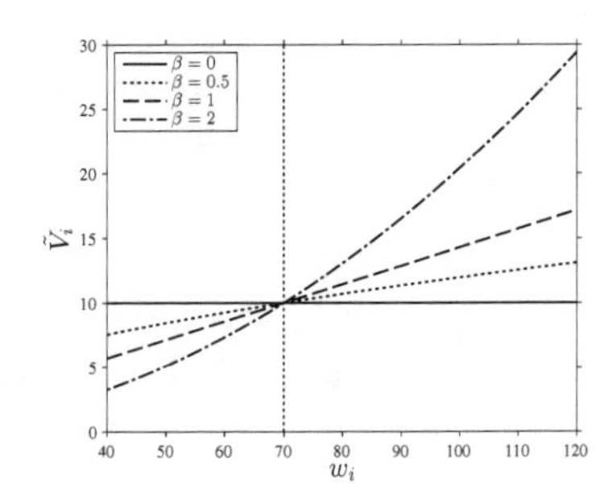

FIGURE 5.6: Examples of covariate models for the volume V assuming that the predicted log-volume is a linear function of the log-weight. Left: $\log(\tilde{V}_i)$ as a function of $\log(w_i)$; right: $\tilde{V}_i$ as a function of w_i.

EXAMPLE 5.2 The model proposed in Example 5.1 is not unique; there exist other possible transformations of the weight that ensure that the predicted volume increases with weight. Setting for example $c_i = w_i - 70$ (as in Figure 5.7, left-hand side) assumes that the predicted log-volume increases linearly with weight:

$$\log(V_i) = \log(V_{\text{pop}}) + \beta(w_i - 70) + \eta_i.$$

Notice that the two proposed covariate models give similar predictions for well chosen values of β

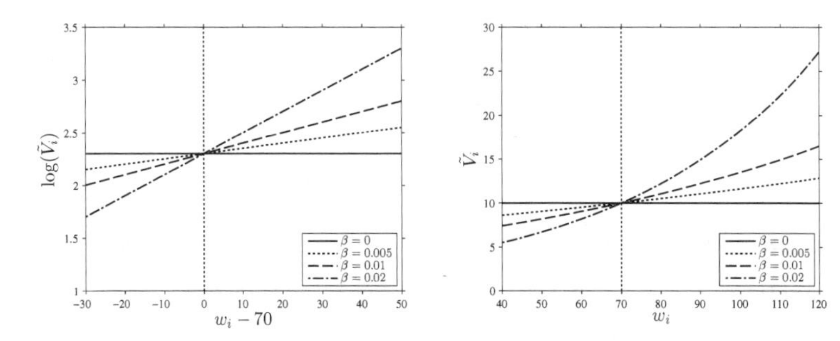

FIGURE 5.7: Examples of covariate models for the volume V assuming that the predicted log-volume is a linear function of the weight. Left: $\log(\tilde{V}_i)$ as a function of $w_i - 70$; right: $\tilde{V}_i$ as a function of w_i.

EXAMPLE 5.3 In this third example, we suppose that the bioavailability F_i has a logit-normal distribution, and age a_i (years) is used as a covariate with a reference age of 40:

$$\begin{aligned}\text{logit}(F_i) &= \text{logit}(\tilde{F}_i) + \eta_{F,i} \\ &= \text{logit}(F_{\text{pop}}) + \beta(a_i - 40) + \eta_{F,i},\end{aligned}$$

where $\eta_{F,i} \sim \mathcal{N}(0, \omega_F^2)$. The predicted logit-bioavailability for an individual of age a_i is then

$$\text{logit}(\tilde{F}_i) = \text{logit}(F_{\text{pop}}) + \beta(a_i - 40).$$

We can derive from this equation an expression for $\tilde{F}_i$:

$$\tilde{F}_i = \frac{F_{\text{pop}}}{F_{\text{pop}} + (1 - F_{\text{pop}})e^{-\beta(a_i - 40)}}.$$

We see in this example how it is much easier to define a model for the transformed parameter $\text{logit}(F_i)$ than for F_i itself. Furthermore, as the logit transform is strictly increasing, both values vary in the same direction with respect to changes in a_i. Figure 5.8 shows how $\tilde{F}_i$ and $\text{logit}(\tilde{F}_i)$ vary with age for several values of β.

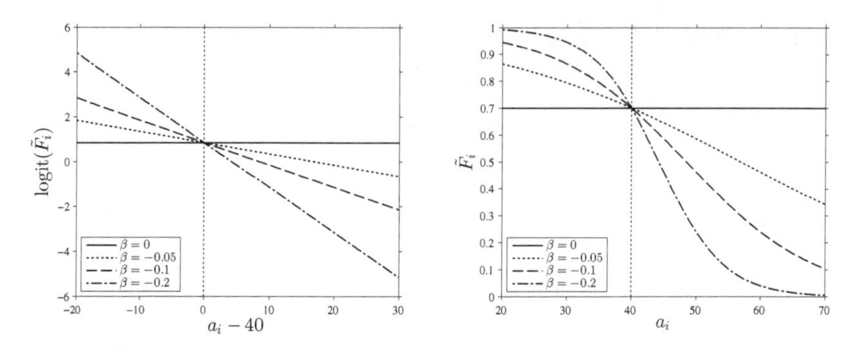

FIGURE 5.8: Examples of covariate models for the bioavailability F assuming that the predicted logit-bioavailability is a linear function of age. Left: logit($\tilde{F}_i$) as a function of $a_i - 40$; right: $\tilde{F}_i$ as a function of a_i.

5.3.3 Nonlinear models for continuous covariates

Nonlinear models allow for much more general relationships between the covariate vector c_i and prediction $\tilde{\psi}_i$. For equation (5.5) we now only assume that there exists some function m and reference value ψ_{pop} such that

$$\begin{aligned}\tilde{\psi}_i &= m(\beta, c_i)\\ \psi_{\text{pop}} &= m(\beta, c_{\text{pop}}).\end{aligned}$$

We can either make the hypothesis that we are still in the Gaussian case, or not.

- If we hypothesize that we are still working with Gaussian models, extending the linear model in (5.9) is straightforward: we suppose that there exists a monotonic transformation h such that

$$\begin{aligned}h(\psi_i) &= h(\tilde{\psi}_i) + \eta_i\\ &= \mu(\beta, c_i) + \eta_i,\end{aligned}$$

  where $\mu(\beta, c_i) = h(m(\beta, c_i))$ is the prediction of $h(\psi_i)$ (while $m(\beta, c_i)$ is the prediction of ψ_i). We can then derive the pdf of ψ_i using (5.4a) as previously:

$$\mathrm{p}(\psi_i; c_i, \theta) = \frac{h'(\psi_i)}{\sqrt{2\pi\omega^2}} \exp\left\{-\frac{1}{2\,\omega^2}(h(\psi_i) - \mu(\beta, c_i))^2\right\}, \tag{5.11}$$

  where $\theta = (\beta, \omega^2)$. The only difference with the Gaussian linear model is that now there is no explicit form available for the ML estimator of θ. Instead, it is defined as the solution of an optimization problem:

$$\hat{\beta} = \arg\min_{\beta} \left\{ \sum_{i=1}^{N} \left(h(\psi_i) - \mu(\beta, c_i)\right)^2 \right\}$$

$$\hat{\omega}^2 = \frac{1}{N} \sum_{i=1}^{N} \left(h(\psi_i) - \mu(\hat{\beta}, c_i)\right)^2 .$$

EXAMPLE 5.4 Consider the following model for ψ_i:

$$\psi_i = \frac{\beta_1 \, e^{\eta_i}}{1 + \beta_2 \, c_i},$$

where $\eta_i \sim \mathcal{N}(0, \omega^2)$. We are therefore assuming that ψ_i is log-normally distributed:

$$\log(\psi_i) \sim \mathcal{N}\left(\log\left(\frac{\beta_1}{1 + \beta_2 \, c_i}\right), \omega^2\right).$$

Here, h is the log function, $\tilde{\psi}_i = \beta_1/(1 + \beta_2 \, c_i)$ and $\psi_{\text{pop}} = \beta_1/(1 + \beta_2 \, c_{\text{pop}})$. The optimization problem to solve for the ML estimator is

$$(\hat{\beta}_1, \hat{\beta}_2) = \arg\min_{\beta_1, \beta_2} \sum_{i=1}^{N} \left(\log(\psi_i) - \log\left(\frac{\beta_1}{1 + \beta_2 \, c_i}\right)\right)^2$$

$$\widehat{\omega}^2 = \frac{1}{N} \sum_{i=1}^{N} \left(\log(\psi_i) - \log\left(\frac{\hat{\beta}_1}{1 + \widehat{\beta}_2 \, c_i}\right)\right)^2 .$$

- For more general distributions of ψ_i, we can simply define ψ_i as a function of fixed and random effects:

$$\psi_i = M(\beta, c_i, \eta_i). \tag{5.12}$$

The prediction $\tilde{\psi}_i$ is obtained when setting $\eta_i = 0$:

$$\tilde{\psi}_i = M(\beta, c_i, \eta_i \equiv 0),$$

and the population value of ψ when $c_i = c_{\text{pop}}$:

$$\psi_{\text{pop}} = M(\beta, c_i \equiv c_{\text{pop}}, \eta_i \equiv 0).$$

If the random effects are supposed Gaussian, there always exists an underlying Gaussian model for the distribution of ψ_i. Let H be the following function obtained by rearranging (5.12) as a function of η_i:

$$\eta_i = H(\beta, c_i, \psi_i).$$

We can then derive the pdf of ψ_i from that of η_i,

$$\mathrm{p}(\psi_i; c_i, \theta) = \frac{\partial}{\partial \psi} H(\beta, c_i, \psi_i) \frac{1}{\sqrt{2\pi\omega^2}} \exp\left\{ -\frac{H^2(\beta, c_i, \psi_i)}{2\,\omega^2} \right\}, \quad (5.13)$$

where $\theta = (\beta, \omega^2)$ is the vector of population parameters of the model. The pdf p_{ψ_i} and the likelihood function $\mathcal{L}_\psi$ have closed forms if and only if the inverse function H can be computed in closed form, which is not always the case.

EXAMPLE 5.5 Suppose that we model ψ_i with

$$\psi_i = \frac{\beta_1\, e^{\eta_i}}{1 + \beta_2\, c_i\, e^{\eta_i}},$$

where $\eta_i \sim \mathcal{N}(0, \omega^2)$. As previously, $\tilde{\psi}_i$ is obtained when η_i is set to 0: $\tilde{\psi}_i = \beta_1/(1 + \beta_2\, c_i)$ and $\psi_{\text{pop}} = \beta_1/(1 + \beta_2\, c_{\text{pop}})$. In this example, it is possible to rearrange the formula for η_i:

$$\eta_i \quad = \log\left(\frac{\psi_i}{\beta_1 - \beta_2\, c_i\, \psi_i} \right).$$

It is therefore possible to explicitly give the distribution of ψ_i and the likelihood $\mathcal{L}_\psi$ using (5.13) with $H(\beta, c_i, \psi_i) = \log\left(\psi_i/(\beta_1 - \beta_2\, c_i\, \psi_i)\right)$.

EXAMPLE 5.6 Let us now propose a model with a small modification with respect to the previous one:

$$\psi_i = \frac{\beta_1 + \eta_i}{1 + \beta_2\, c_i\, e^{\eta_i}}.$$

The predictions $\tilde{\psi}_i$ and ψ_{pop} are both defined as previously, but it is no longer possible to explicitly invert the formula in order to express η_i as a function of ψ_i. Therefore, we cannot explicitly write the likelihood $\mathcal{L}_\psi$ here.

Remarks: Even though the great flexibility of such models appears attractive at first glance, we must remain attentive to what we want to use them for and the tasks we want to perform. In a modeling context, remember that the individual parameters are not observed. The choice of using a complex model for such parameters can pose several problems for model identification and parameter estimation, mainly when the algorithms are based on model linearization. In such cases, users may appreciate the great flexibility when writing the model, but they should be aware of the reduced control they have over the quality of the estimates.

The linear model proposed in (5.8) has certain limits due to the fact that it cannot represent all possible and imaginable models, but it remains sufficiently flexible (due to being able to choose a parameter transform h and covariate transforms) and robust to be successfully used in most situations. MLXTRAN allows us to write any linear or nonlinear covariate model. The model can then be easily used for simulation (using the Simulx function for R and MATLAB, for instance). On the other hand, only linear covariate models can be used for estimation with MONOLIX up to version 4.

5.3.4 Models for categorical covariates

Categorical variables take a finite number of values from a set that is not necessarily numerical or even ordered, e.g., gender, country or ethnicity. The approach taken for continuous covariates extends easily to categorical ones. For simplicity's sake, let us consider a unique covariate c_i that takes its values in $\{a_1, a_2, \ldots, a_K\}$, and a unique parameter ψ_i. Here, a reference covariate value $c_{\rm pop}$ is a reference category, i.e., a specific element a_{k^*} of $\{a_1, a_2, \ldots, a_K\}$. The prediction for ψ_i is thus given by the following model:

$$h(\tilde{\psi_i}) = h(\psi_{\rm pop}) + \beta_1 \mathbb{1}_{c_i=a_1} + \beta_2 \mathbb{1}_{c_i=a_2} + \ldots + \beta_K \mathbb{1}_{c_i=a_K}, \qquad (5.14)$$

with $\beta_{k^*} = 0$ and where $\mathbb{1}$ is the indicator function ($\mathbb{1}_A = 1$ if A is true, 0 otherwise). Thus, (5.14) is equivalent to

$$h(\tilde{\psi_i}) = \begin{cases} h(\psi_{\rm pop}) & \text{if } c_i = a_{k^*} \\ h(\psi_{\rm pop}) + \beta_k & \text{if } c_i = a_k \neq a_{k^*}. \end{cases}$$

We see that if the covariate has K categories, $K-1$ coefficients (β_k) are required for defining the covariate model.

EXAMPLE 5.7 Assume that the individual clearance (of a drug) depends on gender. Here, the gender g_i of individual i is either female or male. We arbitrarily choose female as reference gender. Assuming a log-normal distribution for clearance, the model can be written as follows:

$$\log(Cl_i) = \log(Cl_{\rm pop}) + \beta \mathbb{1}_{g_i=\rm male} + \eta_i,$$

and the predicted clearance as

$$\tilde{Cl}_i = \begin{cases} Cl_{\text{pop}} & \text{if } g_i = \text{female} \\ Cl_{\text{pop}}\, e^{\beta} & \text{if } g_i = \text{male.} \end{cases}$$

EXAMPLE 5.8 Suppose that we want to model the variation in weight between individuals of three countries: India, USA and China. Assuming a normal distribution for weight and India as the reference country, we have

$$w_i = w_{\text{pop}} + \beta_1 \mathbb{1}_{c_i=\text{USA}} + \beta_2 \mathbb{1}_{c_i=\text{China}} + \eta_i .$$

The predicted weight is therefore

$$\tilde{w}_i = \begin{cases} w_{\text{pop}} & \text{if } c_i = \text{India} \\ w_{\text{pop}} + \beta_1 & \text{if } c_i = \text{USA} \\ w_{\text{pop}} + \beta_2 & \text{if } c_i = \text{China.} \end{cases}$$

5.3.5 MLXTRAN for covariate models

Model 1: linear model of covariates.
We consider in this first example a linear model with two covariates:

- weight w_i, a continuous covariate
- gender g_i, a categorical covariate: $g_i \in \{\text{F}, \text{M}\}$.

We consider the following mathematical representation of the model for $\psi_i = (ka_i, V_i, Cl_i)$:

$$\begin{aligned} \log(ka_i) &\sim \mathcal{N}(\log(ka_{\text{pop}}),\, \omega_{ka}^2) \\ \log(V_i) &\sim \mathcal{N}(\log(V_{\text{pop}}) + \beta_{V,w} \log(w_i/70),\, \omega_V^2) \\ \log(Cl_i) &\sim \mathcal{N}(\log(Cl_{\text{pop}}) + \beta_{Cl,w} \log(w_i/70) + \beta_{Cl,g} \mathbb{1}_{g_i=M},\, \omega_{Cl}^2). \end{aligned}$$

Here,

$$\begin{aligned} \theta &= (ka_{\text{pop}}, V_{\text{pop}}, Cl_{\text{pop}}, \omega_{ka}, \omega_V, \omega_{Cl}, \beta_{V,w}, \beta_{Cl,w}, \beta_{Cl,g}) \\ c_i &= (w_i, g_i) \end{aligned}$$

This model can then be implemented with MLXTRAN in the section `[INDIVIDUAL]`.

```
                                    covariate1_model.txt
[INDIVIDUAL]
input={ka_pop, V_pop, Cl_pop, omega_ka, omega_V, omega_Cl,
       beta_V, beta1_Cl, beta2_Cl, weight, gender}

EQUATION:
lw70=log(weight/70)

DEFINITION:
ka = {distribution=lognormal, reference=ka_pop, sd=omega_ka}
V  = {distribution=lognormal, reference=V_pop, sd=omega_V,
      covariate=lw70, coefficient=beta_V}
Cl = {distribution=lognormal, reference=Cl_pop, sd=omega_Cl,
      covariate={lw70,gender}, coefficient={beta1_Cl, beta2_Cl}}
```

Model 2: Nonlinear model for continuous covariates:

$$\theta = (\beta_1, \beta_2, \omega^2)$$

$$\tilde{\psi} = \frac{\beta_1 c_{1,i}}{1 + \beta_2\, c_{2,i}}$$

$$\psi_i \sim \mathcal{N}\left(\tilde{\psi}, \omega^2\right).$$

```
              covariate2_model.txt
[INDIVIDUAL]
input={beta1, beta2, omega, c1, c2}

EQUATION:
predpsi = beta1*c1/(1+beta2*c2)

DEFINITION:
psi = {distribution = normal,
       prediction   = predpsi,
       sd           = omega}
```

5.4 Extensions to multivariate distributions

5.4.1 Gaussian models

We would now like to extend the model defined for a unique individual scalar parameter ψ_i to the case where ψ_i is a vector $(\psi_{i,1}, \psi_{i,2}, \ldots, \psi_{i,d})$ of individual parameters. To begin with, we are going to merely generalize the basic model to each component of ψ_i. To do this, we suppose that there exists a vector of covariates $c_i = (c_{i,1}, \ldots, c_{i,L})$ and:

1. d monotonic transforms $h_1, h_2, \ldots, h_d$
2. d vectors of fixed coefficients $\beta_1, \beta_2, \ldots, \beta_d$
3. d functions $\mu_1, \mu_2, \ldots, \mu_d$
4. d random effects $\eta_{i,1}, \eta_{i,2}, \ldots, \eta_{i,d}$,

such that for each $m = 1, 2, \ldots, d$,

$$\begin{aligned} h_m(\psi_{i,m}) &= h_m(\tilde{\psi}_{i,m}) + \eta_{i,m} \\ &= \mu_m(\beta_m, c_i) + \eta_{i,m}. \end{aligned}$$

In other words, we assume that $h_m(\psi_{i,m})$ is normally distributed and $\mu_m(\beta_m, c_i)$ is the predicted value of $h_m(\psi_{i,m})$. For instance, a linear covariate model supposes that for each $m = 1, 2, \ldots, d$, we have

$$\begin{aligned} h_m(\tilde{\psi}_{i,m}) =& h_m(\psi_{\text{pop},m}) + \beta_{m,1}(c_{i,1} - c_{\text{pop},1}) + \ldots \\ &+ \beta_{m,2}(c_{i,2} - c_{\text{pop},2}) + \beta_{m,L}(c_{i,L} - c_{\text{pop,L}}). \end{aligned} \tag{5.15}$$

Dependency can be introduced between parameters by supposing that the random effects $(\eta_{i,m})$ are not independent. In the special case where the random effects are Gaussian, this means considering them to be linearly correlated: let $\eta_i = (\eta_{i,1}, \eta_{i,2}, \ldots, \eta_{i,d})^t$ and suppose there exists a $d \times d$ variance-covariance matrix Ω such that

$$\begin{aligned} \mathbb{E}\left(\eta_i\right) &= (0, 0, \ldots, 0)^t \\ \mathbb{E}\left(\eta_i \eta_i^t\right) &= \Omega. \end{aligned}$$

Here,

$$\Omega = \begin{pmatrix} \omega_1^2 & \omega_{1,2} & \ldots & \omega_{1,d} \\ \omega_{1,2} & \omega_2^2 & \ldots & \omega_{2,d} \\ \vdots & \vdots & \ddots & \vdots \\ \omega_{1,d} & \omega_{2,d} & \ldots & \omega_d^2 \end{pmatrix},$$

where ω_m^2 is the variance of $\eta_{i,m}$ and $\omega_{m,m'}$ the covariance between $\eta_{i,m}$ and $\eta_{i,m'}$.

It will be useful in the following to have a diagonal decomposition of Ω. To this end, let us define the correlation matrix $R = (R_{m,m'}, 1 \leq m, m' \leq d)$ of the vector η_i:

$$R_{m,m'} = \begin{cases} 1 & \text{if } m = m' \\ \rho_{m,m'} = \frac{\omega_{m,m'}}{\omega_m \omega_{m'}} & \text{otherwise,} \end{cases}$$

and let $D = (D_{m,m'})$ be a diagonal matrix which contains the standard deviations (ω_m):

$$D_{m,m'} = \begin{cases} \omega_m & \text{if } m = m' \\ 0 & \text{otherwise.} \end{cases}$$

Then, we have the diagonal decomposition: $\Omega = D\,R\,D$.

EXAMPLE 5.9 Consider the growth model $f(t, \psi_i) = a_i + b_i(1 - e^{-k_i t})$ introduced in Section 1.1 and where $\psi_i = (a_i, b_i, k_i)$. We suppose that a_i and b_i are log-normally distributed and k_i fixed in the population:

$$\begin{aligned} \log(a_i) &= \log(a_{\text{pop}}) + \eta_{a,i} \\ \log(b_i) &= \log(b_{\text{pop}}) + \eta_{b,i} \\ k_i &= k_{\text{pop}}. \end{aligned}$$

Furthermore, we make the assumption that $\eta_{a,i}$ and $\eta_{b,i}$ are correlated with correlation:

$$\begin{aligned} \rho_{a,b} &= \text{Corr}\left(\eta_{a,i}, \eta_{b,i}\right) \\ &= \text{Corr}\left(\log(a_i), \log(b_i)\right). \end{aligned}$$

Assuming that $k_i = k_{\text{pop}}$ for any i implies that $\eta_{k,i} = 0$, and thus $\omega_k = 0$. The correlation matrix R and the variance-covariance matrix Ω of $(\eta_{a,i}, \eta_{b,i}, \eta_{k,i})$ are therefore:

$$R = \begin{pmatrix} 1 & \rho_{a,b} & 0 \\ \rho_{a,b} & 1 & 0 \\ 0 & 0 & 1 \end{pmatrix}, \quad \Omega = DRD = \begin{pmatrix} \omega_a^2 & \omega_a \omega_b \, \rho_{a,b} & 0 \\ \omega_a \omega_b \, \rho_{a,b} & \omega_b^2 & 0 \\ 0 & 0 & 0 \end{pmatrix}.$$

Warning: Here, $\rho_{a,b}$ does not denote the linear correlation between initial weight and weight gain, but that between the log-transform of these parameters.

5.4.2 The probability distribution function

We now have all the elements needed for computing the pdf of $\psi_i = (\psi_{i,1}, \psi_{i,2}, \ldots, \psi_{i,d})$ when here $\theta = (\beta_1, \ldots, \beta_d, \Omega)$.

- If Ω is a positive-definite matrix, it can be inverted, and a straightforward extension to the pdf proposed in (5.11) for one scalar variable gives

$$\begin{aligned} \mathrm{p}(\psi_i; c_i, \theta) = &\left(\prod_{m=1}^{d} h'_m(\psi_{i,m}) \right) (2\pi)^{-\frac{d}{2}} |\Omega|^{-\frac{1}{2}} \\ &\times \exp\left\{ -\frac{1}{2} (h(\psi_i) - \mu(\beta, c_i))^t \Omega^{-1} (h(\psi_i) - \mu(\beta, c_i)) \right\}, \end{aligned} \tag{5.16}$$

  where $h(\psi_i)$ is the column vector $(h_1(\psi_{i,1}), h_2(\psi_{i,2}), \ldots, h_d(\psi_{i,d}))^t$ and $\mu(\beta, c_i)$ the column vector $(\mu_1(\beta_1, c_i), \mu_2(\beta_2, c_i), \ldots, \mu_d(\beta_d, c_i))^t$.

- If some of the random effects have zero variance, Ω is not positive-definite. The pdf in (5.16) no longer applies to the complete d-vector

ψ_i but only to the d_1-vector subset $\psi_i^{(1)}$ of ψ_i whose matrix Ω_1 is positive-definite. The distribution of the remaining fixed parameters $\psi_i^{(0)}$ is a Dirac delta distribution. Let I_0 be the indices of the parameters $\psi_i^{(0)}$ and I_1 those of the parameters $\psi_i^{(1)}$, i.e., $\omega_m = 0$ if $m \in I_0$ and $\omega_m > 0$ if $m \in I_1$. Then,

$$\mathrm{p}(\psi_i; c_i, \theta) = \mathrm{p}(\psi_i^{(0)}; c_i, \theta)\ \mathrm{p}(\psi_i^{(1)}; c_i, \theta),$$

where

$$\mathrm{p}(\psi_i^{(0)}; c_i, \theta) = \prod_{m \in I_0} \delta_{\{h(\psi_{i,m}) = \mu_m(\beta_m, c_i)\}} \tag{5.17}$$

$$\mathrm{p}(\psi_i^{(1)}; c_i, \theta) = \left(\prod_{m \in I_1} h'_m(\psi_{i,m}) \right) (2\pi)^{-\frac{d_1}{2}} |\Omega_1|^{-\frac{1}{2}} \tag{5.18}$$

$$\times \exp\left\{ -\frac{1}{2} (h(\psi_i) - \mu(\beta, c_i))^{(1)^t} \Omega_1^{-1} (h(\psi_i) - \mu(\beta, c_i))^{(1)} \right\},$$

with $(h(\psi_i) - \mu(\beta, c_i))^{(1)}$ the same as $(h(\psi_i) - \mu(\beta, c_i))$ but with the I_0 entries removed.

- There exist other situations where Ω is not positive-definite. This is the case, for instance, when two random effects are equal: $\eta_{i,m} = \eta_{i,m'}$ for any i. For them, we can calculate a joint distribution:

$$\mathrm{p}(\psi_{i,m}, \psi_{i,m'}, \eta_{i,m}; \beta_m, \beta_{m'}, \omega_m^2, c_i) = \\ \mathrm{p}(\psi_{i,m} | \eta_{i,m}; \beta_m, c_i)\ \mathrm{p}(\psi_{i,m'} | \eta_{i,m}; \beta_{m'}, c_i)\ \mathrm{p}(\eta_{i,m}; \omega_m^2),$$

where

$$\mathrm{p}(\psi_{i,m} | \eta_{i,m}; \beta_m, c_i) = \delta_{\{h(\psi_{i,m}) = \mu_m(\beta_m, c_i) + \eta_{i,m}\}}$$

$$\mathrm{p}(\psi_{i,m'} | \eta_{i,m}; \beta_{m'}, c_i) = \delta_{\{h(\psi_{i,m'}) = \mu_{m'}(\beta_{m'}, c_i) + \eta_{i,m}\}}$$

$$\mathrm{p}(\eta_{i,m}; \omega_m^2) = \frac{1}{\sqrt{2\,\pi\omega_m^2}} \exp\left\{ -\frac{\eta_{i,m}^2}{2\omega_m^2} \right\}.$$

All kinds of combinations are possible, including parameters with and without variability, algebraic relationships between random effects, etc. In all possible cases it is possible to find an adequate decomposition that lets us build a pdf. This pdf turns out to play a fundamental role for tasks such as population parameter estimation with maximum likelihood when we start with observations $\boldsymbol{y} = (y_i, 1 \leq i \leq N)$ and the individual parameters (ψ_i) are not observed.

We will see in Chapter 9 that these types of degenerate models cannot be used as they are for certain tasks such as estimation. In these cases, it will be necessary to work with modified versions of the joint distribution $\mathrm{p}(\boldsymbol{y}, \boldsymbol{\psi})$ of the observations and parameters.

5.4.3 MLXTRAN for multivariate normal distributions

We consider the following model for $\psi_i = (A_i, B_i, C_i, D_i)$:

$$
\begin{aligned}
A_i &= A_{\text{pop}} + \eta_{A,i}, & \eta_{A,i} &\underset{\text{i.i.d.}}{\sim} \mathcal{N}(0, \omega_A^2) \\
B_i &= B_{\text{pop}} + \eta_{B,i}, & \eta_{B,i} &\underset{\text{i.i.d.}}{\sim} \mathcal{N}(0, \omega_B^2) \\
\log(C_i) &= \log(C_{\text{pop}}) + \eta_{C,i}, & \eta_{C,i} &\underset{\text{i.i.d.}}{\sim} \mathcal{N}(0, \omega_C^2) \\
\text{logit}(D_i) &= \text{logit}(D_{\text{pop}}) + \eta_{D,i}, & \eta_{D,i} &\underset{\text{i.i.d.}}{\sim} \mathcal{N}(0, \omega_D^2).
\end{aligned}
$$

The correlation matrix for $(\eta_{A,i}, \eta_{B,i}, \eta_{C,i}, \eta_{D,i})'$ is a symmetric block one:

$$
R = \begin{pmatrix} 1 & r_1 & r_2 & 0 \\ r_1 & 1 & r_3 & 0 \\ r_2 & r_3 & 1 & 0 \\ 0 & 0 & 0 & 1 \end{pmatrix}.
$$

Implementation with MLXTRAN:

```
correlation_model.txt

[INDIVIDUAL]
input={A_pop,B_pop,C_pop,D_pop,omega_A,omega_B,
       omega_C,omega_D,r1,r2,r3}

DEFINITION:
A = {distribution=normal, reference=A_pop, sd=omega_A}
B = {distribution=normal, reference=B_pop, sd=omega_B}
C = {distribution=lognormal, reference=C_pop, sd=omega_C}
D = {distribution=logitnormal, reference=D_pop, sd=omega_D}

correlationCoefficient = {r(A,B)=r1, r(A,C)=r2, r(B,C)=r3}
```

5.5 Additional levels of variability

5.5.1 Modeling inter-occasion variability

Up to now, the distribution p_{ψ_i} or equivalently the equation

$$\psi_i = M(\beta, c_i, \eta_i), \tag{5.19}$$

describes only the inter-individual variability of the individual parameters (ψ_i). This model therefore assumes that:

- the individual parameter ψ_i for individual i remains constant during the whole study.

- the N individuals in the study are independent, i.e., the parameters $(\psi_i, 1 \leq i \leq N)$ are mutually independent.

We will now see that these hypotheses can be weakened by considering additional levels of variability.

Let us look at the first assumption and consider introducing *intra-individual variability* of individual parameters into the model. A first simple model consists of splitting the study into K time periods or "occasions" and assuming that individual parameters can vary from occasion to occasion but remain constant within occasions. Then, we can try to explain part of the *intra-individual* variability of the individual parameters by piecewise-constant covariates, i.e., "occasion-dependent" or "occasion-varying" (varying from occasion to occasion and constant within an occasion) ones. The remaining part must then be described by random effects.

We will need some additional notation for describing this new statistical model. Let

- ψ_{ik} be the vector of individual parameters of individual i for occasion k, where $1 \leq i \leq N$ and $1 \leq k \leq K$.

- c_{ik} be the vector of covariates of individual i for occasion k. Some of these covariates remain constant (gender, group treatment, ethnicity, etc.) and others can vary (weight, treatment, etc.).

Let $\psi_i = (\psi_{i1}, \psi_{i2}, \ldots, \psi_{iK})$ be the sequence of K individual parameters for individual i. The model for ψ_i is now a joint distribution:

$$\psi_i \sim p_{\psi_i}(\,\cdot\,; c_{i1}, c_{i2}, \ldots, c_{iK}, \theta).$$

We also need to define:

- $\eta_i^{(0)}$, the vector of random effects which describes the random *inter-individual variability* of the individual parameters and

- $\eta_{ik}^{(1)}$, the vector of random effects which describes the random *intra-individual variability* of the individual parameters in occasion k, for each $1 \leq k \leq K$.

Here and in the following, the superscript (0) is used to represent *inter-individual variability*, i.e., variability at the individual ("reference") level, while superscript (1) represents *inter-occasion variability*, i.e., variability at the "occasion" level for each individual. Then, for any individual i and occasion k, model (5.19) becomes

$$\psi_{ik} = M(\beta, c_{ik}, \eta_i^{(0)}, \eta_{ik}^{(1)}). \quad (5.20)$$

As previously, the prediction $\tilde{\psi}_{ik}$ of ψ_{ik} is obtained in the absence of random effects:

$$\begin{aligned} \tilde{\psi}_{ik} &= M(\beta, c_{ik}, \eta_i^{(0)} \equiv 0, \eta_{ik}^{(1)} \equiv 0) \\ &= m(\beta, c_{ik}). \end{aligned}$$

If $\eta_i^{(0)} \neq 0$, then the parameters ψ_{ik} defined in (5.20) are no longer independent because they all depend on the same random effect $\eta_i^{(0)}$. The joint distribution p_{ψ_i} will therefore depend on the model M and in particular on the way in which the model integrates the random effects $\eta_i^{(0)}$ and $\eta_{ik}^{(1)}$. Let us look at this in more detail.

1. Assume first an additive model for the random effects. Here, $\eta_i^{(0)}$ and $\eta_{ik}^{(1)}$ can be grouped into a random effect η_{ik}, where

$$\eta_{ik} = \eta_i^{(0)} + \eta_{ik}^{(1)}. \quad (5.21)$$

Figure 5.9 gives an example for one individual with three time periods, when the random effect is additive.

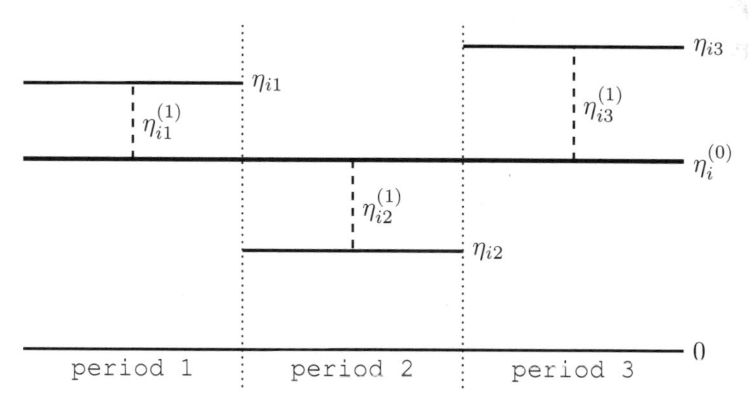

FIGURE 5.9: Possible decomposition of the random effects of a single subject over three time periods.

If we also assume that $\eta_i^{(0)}$ and $\eta_{ik}^{(1)}$ are normally distributed with variance-covariance matrices $\Omega^{(0)}$ and $\Omega^{(1)}$, then η_{ik} is also normally distributed and the covariance between η_{ik} and $\eta_{ik'}$ is

$$\text{Cov}(\eta_{ik}, \eta_{ik'}) = \begin{cases} \Omega^{(0)} + \Omega^{(1)} & \text{if } k = k' \\ \Omega^{(0)} & \text{otherwise.} \end{cases} \tag{5.22}$$

Model (5.20) then reduces to $\psi_{ik} = M(\beta, c_{ik}, \eta_{ik})$, where now the ψ_{ik} are not independent.

2. Assume now a Gaussian model of the form

$$\begin{aligned} h(\psi_{ik}) &= h(\tilde{\psi}_{ik}) + \eta_{ik} & (5.23) \\ &= h(\tilde{\psi}_{ik}) + \eta_i^{(0)} + \eta_{ik}^{(1)}. & (5.24) \end{aligned}$$

Here, the $h(\psi_{i1}), \ldots, h(\psi_{iK})$ are correlated Gaussian vectors whose variance-covariance structure is that of the (η_{ik}) defined in (5.22).

3. Assume furthermore a linear covariate model. For the sake of simplicity, we consider a unique covariate; extension to multiple covariates, including categorical and continuous covariates, is straightforward. An initial covariate model deduced from the basic linear model proposed in (5.9) can be written

$$h(\psi_{ik}) = h(\psi_{\text{pop}}) + \beta(c_{ik} - c_{\text{pop}}) + \eta_i^{(0)} + \eta_{ik}^{(1)}. \tag{5.25}$$

EXAMPLE 5.10 Consider the model for the volume of distribution introduced in Example 5.1, which assumes a linear relationship between the log-weight and log-volume. If the weight does not vary from occasion to occasion, we can consider the following model:

$$\log(V_{ik}) = \log(V_{\text{pop}}) + \beta \log(w_i/70) + \eta_{ik}.$$

Rewriting this as

$$V_{ik} = V_{\text{pop}} \left(\frac{w_i}{70}\right)^{\beta} e^{\eta_i^{(0)}} e^{\eta_{ik}^{(1)}}$$

helps us to deduce that:

- V_{pop} is the reference volume for the whole population
- $V_{\text{pop}}(w_i/70)^{\beta}$ is the predicted volume at any occasion for any individual with weight w_i
- $V_{\text{pop}}(w_i/70)^{\beta} e^{\eta_i^{(0)}}$ is the typical volume of individual i over time
- $V_{\text{pop}}(w_i/70)^{\beta} e^{\eta_i^{(0)}} e^{\eta_{ik}^{(1)}}$ is the volume of individual i in occasion k.

We can then decompose the part of the variability explained by the covariate c into inter-individual and intra-individual components, exactly as we did with the random effects. Let c_{pop} be the reference value of covariate c in the population as previously, and also let c_i be some reference (or typical) value for individual i. Then we can write

$$\begin{aligned} c_{ik} - c_{\text{pop}} &= (c_i - c_{\text{pop}}) + (c_{ik} - c_i) \\ &= d_i^{(0)} + d_{ik}^{(1)}, \end{aligned}$$

where $d_i^{(0)}$ describes the variability of the reference individual value c_i around the reference population value c_{pop}, and $d_{ik}^{(1)}$ the fluctuations of the sequence of individual covariate values (c_{ik}) around c_i. Here is an illustration of this for one individual and three time periods.

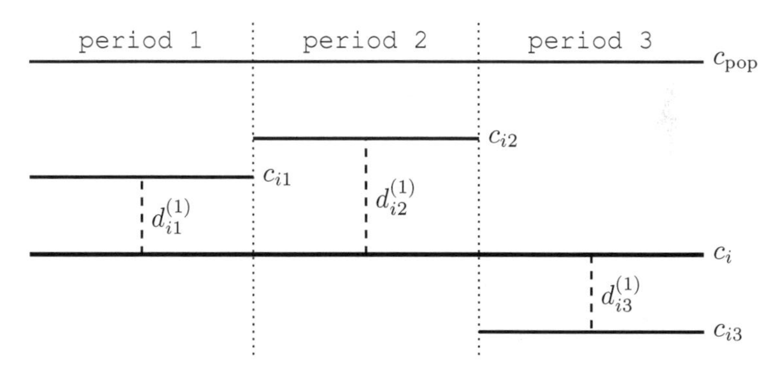

FIGURE 5.10: Decomposition of a time-varying covariate for a single subject over three time periods.

It is instructive now to write model (5.25) with the following decomposition:

$$h(\psi_{ik}) - h(\psi_{\text{pop}}) = \left(\beta(c_i - c_{\text{pop}}) + \eta_i^{(0)}\right) + \left(\beta(c_{ik} - c_i) + \eta_{ik}^{(1)}\right). \quad (5.26)$$

On the right-hand side the first term gives the inter-individual (or intra-individual) variability and the second the inter-occasion variability for the individual. If a covariate c does not vary from occasion to occasion, it is the same as saying that for each k, $c_{ik} = c_i$. It may also be that some random effects do not exhibit inter-occasion variability, i.e., $\eta_{ik}^{(1)} = 0$. Therefore, an individual parameter ψ_i does not exhibit inter-occasion variability if and only if both $c_{ik} - c_i = 0$ and $\eta_{ik}^{(1)} = 0$.

In general the goal is to construct a model based on the perceived variability of each of these two terms:

- The inter-individual variability (IIV) model: choose a model for the covariates that do not change from occasion to occasion, and a variance-covariance structure for the random effects $\eta_i^{(0)}$.

- The inter-occasion variability (IOV) model: choose a model for the covariates that change from occasion to occasion, and a variance-covariance structure for the random effects $\eta_{ik}^{(1)}$.

EXAMPLE 5.11 Consider again our model for the volume of distribution, where now the weight of individual i varies over time:

$$\log(V_{ik}) = \log(V_{\text{pop}}) + \beta \log(w_{ik}/70) + \eta_{ik}.$$

Here, w_{ik} is the typical weight of individual i at occasion k. Let w_i be the typical weight of individual i for the whole study. We can then rewrite the model as

$$\log(V_{ik}) = \log(V_{\text{pop}}) + \left(\beta \log(w_i/70) + \eta_i^{(0)}\right) + \left(\beta \log(w_{ik}/w_i) + \eta_{ik}^{(1)}\right),$$

or

$$V_{ik} = V_{\text{pop}} \left(\frac{w_i}{70}\right)^{\beta} e^{\eta_i^{(0)}} \left(\frac{w_{ik}}{w_i}\right)^{\beta} e^{\eta_{ik}^{(1)}}.$$

Here,

- $V_{\text{pop}}(w_i/70)^{\beta}$ is the predicted volume at any occasion for any individual with typical weight w_i
- $V_{\text{pop}}(w_{ik}/70)^{\beta}$ is the predicted volume at occasion k for any individual with weight w_{ik} at occasion k
- $V_{\text{pop}}(w_i/70)^{\beta} e^{\eta_i^{(0)}}$ is the typical volume of individual i over time.

Model (5.26) assumes that the inter-individual and intra-individual variability of the covariate have the same magnitude of effect on the parameter, i.e., an increase of one unit of c_{ik} with respect to c_i has the same effect as an increase of one unit of c_i with respect to c_{pop}. If we would rather not make this hypothesis, we can weight differently the covariates $(c_i - c_{\text{pop}})$ and $(c_{ik} - c_i)$:

$$h(\psi_{ik}) = h(\psi_{\text{pop}}) + \beta(c_i - c_{\text{pop}}) + \gamma(c_{ik} - c_i) + \eta_i^{(0)} + \eta_{ik}^{(1)}. \quad (5.27)$$

EXAMPLE 5.12 Consider a model that supposes a linear relationship between income and happiness. Denote ψ_{ik} the happiness score (on some scale) for subject i in year k, and c_{ik} his income (in K€) in year k. Model (5.26) supposes that for each subject and year k, a difference in annual income of 1K€ with respect to the reference income in the population generates an increase of β happiness. There is no reason to expect that the intra-individual variability (fluctuation in an individual's salary) has the same effect on happiness. Indeed, an increase in annual salary of 1K€ for some individuals might lead to more happiness than the fact of having a salary of 1K€ more than the reference salary. Model (5.27) lets us take this into account, assuming for example that $\gamma > \beta$.

5.5.2 Extensions to multiple levels of variability

Extension of the proposed approach to nested levels of variability is straightforward. We illustrate this with several examples.

1. Suppose that an occasion can be split into several suboccasions. For instance, imagine that the same study (that lasts several days) is repeated each year. In this case, we might want to take into account year-by-year variability *and* day-by-day variability. To do this, we can introduce an additional level of intra-individual (or inter-occasion) variability into the model:

$$\psi_{ikl} = M(\beta, c_{ikl}, \eta_i^{(0)}, \eta_{ik}^{(1)}, \eta_{ikl}^{(2)}).$$

   Here, c_{ikl} is the value of covariate c for subject i during suboccasion l of occasion k, and $\eta_i^{(0)}$, $\eta_{ik}^{(1)}$ and $\eta_{ikl}^{(2)}$ describe different levels of random variability of the parameter. As in (5.21), we can assume an additive model where the different levels of random effect can be grouped as a single one named η_{ikl}. Now both the explained and the unexplained parts of the variability can be decomposed into inter-individual and two intra-individual components:

$$\begin{aligned}
c_{ikl} - c_{\text{pop}} &= (c_i - c_{\text{pop}}) + (c_{ik} - c_i) + (c_{ikl} - c_{ik}) \\
&= d_i^{(0)} + d_{ik}^{(1)} + d_{ikl}^{(2)} \\
\eta_{ikl} &= \eta_i^{(0)} + \eta_{ik}^{(1)} + \eta_{ikl}^{(2)}.
\end{aligned}$$

2. Consider instead that the individuals are allocated to different centers or studies. Then, possible variability between centers or studies also needs to be taken into account by the statistical model.

   Let $\ell = 1, 2, \ldots, L$ be the set of subgroups or studies. To keep things simple, first consider the case where there is only one occasion. Let $\psi_{\ell i}$ be the vector of individual parameters of individual i from study ℓ. Then, $\psi_{\ell i}$ can be characterized by a model that takes into account the *inter-study* variability:

$$\psi_{\ell i} = M(\beta, c_{\ell i}, \eta_\ell^{(-1)}, \eta_{\ell i}^{(0)}),$$

where $c_{\ell i}$ is the vector of covariates for individual i from study ℓ, and $\eta_{\ell}^{(-1)}$ and $\eta_{\ell i}^{(0)}$ the random effects that describe the random components of the *inter-study* and *inter-individual* variability (within the same study). Note that some components of $c_{\ell i}$ might be specific to study ℓ and have no dependency on any given individual.

3. We can include in the model any combination of *inter-group*, *inter-individual* and *inter-occasion* variability with any combination of interactions. Consider for example a cross-over study with K occasions performed in L centers and assume the following levels of random variability:

   - Center: $\eta_{\ell}^{(-1)}$; $1 \leq \ell \leq L$,
   - Center and individual: $\eta_{\ell i}^{(0)}$; $1 \leq i \leq N$,
   - Center, individual and occasion: $\eta_{\ell ik}^{(1)}$; $1 \leq k \leq K$.

   Now, if we decide to assume an additive model for the random effects, all the random components of the variability can be combined as a unique vector of random effects:

$$\eta_{\ell ik} = \eta_{\ell}^{(-1)} + \eta_{\ell i}^{(0)} + \eta_{\ell ik}^{(1)}.$$

   For example, if we were considering an animal study, we might want to group animals with the same father (equivalent to "center") and then try and characterize variability of some animal feature by a "father" effect, an "animal" effect and an "occasion" effect.

5.5.3 Mlxtran for multiple levels of variability

Model 1: One additional level of variability.
We assume only IIV for (A_{ik}), only IOV for (B_{ik}) and both IIV and IOV for (C_{ik}):

$$A_{ik} = A_{\text{pop}} + \eta_{A,i}^{(0)}, \qquad \eta_{A,i}^{(0)} \underset{\text{i.i.d.}}{\sim} \mathcal{N}(0, \omega_A^2)$$

$$B_{ik} = B_{\text{pop}} + \eta_{B,ik}^{(1)}, \qquad \eta_{B,ik}^{(1)} \underset{\text{i.i.d.}}{\sim} \mathcal{N}(0, \gamma_B^2)$$

$$C_{ik} = C_{\text{pop}} + \eta_{C,i}^{(0)} + \eta_{C,ik}^{(1)}, \qquad \eta_{C,i}^{(0)} \underset{\text{i.i.d.}}{\sim} \mathcal{N}(0, \omega_C^2), \quad \eta_{C,ik}^{(1)} \underset{\text{i.i.d.}}{\sim} \mathcal{N}(0, \gamma_C^2).$$

The levels of variability *individual* (0) and *occasion* (1) are assumed nested.

```
                                         level1_model.txt
[INDIVIDUAL]
input={A_pop, B_pop, C_pop, omega_A, gamma_B, omega_C, gamma_C}
level={id, occ}

DEFINITION:
A ={distribution=normal,mean=A_pop,level={id},sd=omega_A}
B ={distribution=normal,mean=B_pop,level={id*occ},sd=gamma_B}
C ={distribution=normal,mean=C_pop,level={id,id*occ},
    sd={omega_C,gamma_C}}
```

Model 2: Two additional levels of variability.
$A_{\ell ik}$ varies with *center*, $B_{\ell ik}$ with *center* and *individual* and $C_{\ell ik}$ with *center*, *individual* and *occasion*:

$$
\begin{aligned}
A_{\ell ik} &= A_{\text{pop}} + \eta_{A,\ell}^{(-1)}, \qquad \eta_{A,\ell}^{(-1)} \underset{\text{i.i.d.}}{\sim} \mathcal{N}(0,\tau_A^2) \\
B_{\ell ik} &= B_{\text{pop}} + \eta_{B,\ell i}^{(0)}, \qquad \eta_{B,\ell i}^{(0)} \underset{\text{i.i.d.}}{\sim} \mathcal{N}(0,\omega_B^2) \\
C_{\ell ik} &= C_{\text{pop}} + \eta_{C,\ell}^{(-1)} + \eta_{C,\ell i}^{(0)} + \eta_{C,\ell ik}^{(1)}, \quad \text{with} \\
& \qquad \eta_{C,\ell}^{(-1)} \underset{\text{i.i.d.}}{\sim} \mathcal{N}(0,\tau_C^2), \quad \eta_{C,\ell i}^{(0)} \underset{\text{i.i.d.}}{\sim} \mathcal{N}(0,\omega_C^2), \quad \eta_{C,\ell ik}^{(1)} \underset{\text{i.i.d.}}{\sim} \mathcal{N}(0,\gamma_C^2).
\end{aligned}
$$

Here *center*, *individual* and *occasion* are nested.

```
                                         level2_model.txt
[INDIVIDUAL]
input={A_pop,B_pop,C_pop,tau_A,omega_B,tau_C,omega_C,gamma_C}
level={center, id, occ}

DEFINITION:
A ={distribution=normal,mean=A_pop,level={center},sd=tau_A}
B ={distribution=normal,mean=B_pop,level={center*id},sd={omega_B}}
C ={distribution=normal,mean=C_pop,
    level={center,center*id,center*id*occ},sd={tau_C,omega_C,gamma_C}}
```

5.6 Different mathematical representations and implementations of the same model

The statistical component of a model can be decomposed into two submodels: a model that describes the variability of the observations and one that describes the variability of the individual parameters. Each submodel needs to be described, represented and implemented. Different mathematical representations of the same model lead to different implementations. The choice of the mathematical representation – and then the implementation – should be driven by the task we want to execute. Let us illustrate this with a very simple statistical model used for modeling variability in a single individual parameter.

5.6.1 Description of the statistical model

Let us consider the example of wanting to describe the distribution of the volume in a population using weight as a covariate. The first step consists of describing with extreme precision the statistical model we want to use:

1. Individuals in the population are mutually independent.
2. The volume is log-normally distributed.
3. The log-volume predicted by the model is a linear function of the log-weight.
4. The reference weight in the population is 70kg.
5. The variance of the log-volume is constant.

5.6.2 Representation of the statistical model

Since this model involves probability distributions, we will use a probabilistic model to represent it. Let V_i and w_i be the volume and weight of individual i. Statement 1 implies that only the distribution $\mathrm{p}(V_i; w_i)$ for individual i needs to be represented. A probability distribution can be mathematically represented by a series of definitions and equations. This mathematical representation is not unique. We can use, for instance, any of these three representations:

$$V_i = V_{\text{pop}} \left(\frac{w_i}{70}\right)^{\beta} e^{\eta_i} \quad \text{where} \quad \eta_i \sim \mathcal{N}(0, \omega^2) \tag{5.28a}$$

$$\log(V_i) \sim \mathcal{N}(\log(\tilde{V}_i), \omega^2) \quad \text{where} \quad \tilde{V}_i = V_{\text{pop}} \left(\frac{w_i}{70}\right)^{\beta} \tag{5.28b}$$

$$\log(V_i) \sim \mathcal{N}(\log(V_{\text{pop}}) + \beta c_i\,,\, \omega^2) \quad \text{where} \quad c_i = \log\left(\frac{w_i}{70}\right). \tag{5.28c}$$

Here, ω is the standard deviation of the log-volume, V_{pop} a reference value for the volume in the population for a reference individual of 70kg, and $V_{\text{pop}}(w_i/70)^{\beta}$ the predicted volume for an individual with weight w_i.

These three representations combine equations and definitions. The equations allow us to define the variables via algebraic equations, while the definitions characterize the random variables using probability distributions.

5.6.3 Which representation for which task?

Representations (5.28a), (5.28b) and (5.28c) provide three different mathematical representations of the same probabilistic model. This means that when written in text, anyone with some basic knowledge in statistics and mathematics will be able to derive the same information from any of them.

However, if we want to use the model to perform tasks using specific software, the information passed to the software needs to be of a form that the software can understand with respect to each given task. It is not always true that any representation paired with any implementation can be used to perform any task. Let us illustrate this on our example for three basic tasks: simulation, likelihood computation and covariate model assessment.

Simulation. If we assume that the software we use is able to simulate normal random variables with any given mean and standard deviation, then any representation of the model can be used for simulation:

- Using (5.28a), η_i is first simulated as a random normal variable with mean 0 and variance ω^2. Then the volume V_i is calculated as a function of η_i.
- Using (5.28b) or (5.28c), $\log(V_i)$ can be directly simulated as a random normal variable with mean $\log(V_{\rm pop}) + \beta \log(w_i/70)$, or equivalently $\log(V_{\rm pop}(w_i/70)^{\beta})$, and standard deviation ω^2. Then $V_i = \exp(\log(V_i))$.

In summary, what is required for simulation is the capacity to express the variable to be simulated as a function of some random variable that can be directly simulated by the software. In conclusion, any of the three representations can be used for simulation.

Likelihood computation. Deriving the likelihood of $\theta = (V_{\rm pop}, \beta, \omega^2)$ requires computation of the pdf of V_i or some function of it. Here, it is straightforward to derive the likelihood from the pdf of V_i, which is log-normally distributed.

$$
\begin{aligned}
L_1(\theta; V_1, \ldots, V_N) & \\
&= \mathrm{p}(V_1, V_2, \ldots, V_N; \theta) \\
&= \prod_{i=1}^{N} \mathrm{p}(V_i; \theta) \\
&= \prod_{i=1}^{N} \frac{1}{\sqrt{2\pi\omega^2} V_i} \exp\left\{ -\frac{1}{2\omega^2} \left(\log(V_i) - \log\left(V_{\rm pop} \left(\frac{w_i}{70} \right)^{\beta} \right) \right)^2 \right\}.
\end{aligned}
$$

It is also straightforward to derive the likelihood from the pdf of $\log(V_i)$, which is normally distributed:

$$\begin{aligned} L_2(\theta; \log(V_1), \ldots, \log(V_N)) \\ &= \mathrm{p}(\log(V_1), \ldots, \log(V_N); \theta) \\ &= \prod_{i=1}^{N} \frac{1}{\sqrt{2\pi\omega^2}} \exp\left\{ -\frac{1}{2\omega^2} \left(\log(V_i) - \log\left(V_{\mathrm{pop}} \left(\frac{w_i}{70} \right)^{\beta} \right) \right)^2 \right\}. \end{aligned}$$

These likelihoods L_1 and L_2 are equal up to a constant $\prod_i V_i$. No matter what the definition on which the likelihood is based, it is nonetheless necessary to provide some information about the pdf of V_i for computing the likelihood. In this very basic example, the minimal set of information on the model that needs to be passed to the software via code to be able to compute the likelihood is

- The log-volume is normally distributed.
- The mean of $\log(V_i)$ is $\log\left(V_{\mathrm{pop}}\,(w_i/70)^{\beta}\right)$.
- The standard deviation of $\log(V_i)$ is ω.

Then, the likelihood can be easily computed if the software is able to compute a normal pdf for a given mean and standard deviation.

In our example, only the model representations given in (5.28b) and (5.28c) can be used for computing the likelihood in closed form. Indeed, both explicitly describe the probability distribution of $\log(V_i)$ and provide all the required information. In contrast, the representation given in (5.28a) does not provide any explicit information about the distribution of V_i. Deriving the pdf of V_i from (5.28a) would therefore require an interpreter to "understand" the formula and a tool that could perform symbolic computation.

Covariate model assessment. Our model hypothesizes a linear relationship between the log-weight and log-volume. To assess if this is valid, we might consider using some visual diagnostic checks on the plot of the (predicted or simulated) log-volume against log-weight to see whether this linear relationship seems plausible. Specific statistical procedures can also be used for testing the linearity hypothesis.

Thus, both displaying an appropriate goodness of fit plot and using an appropriate statistical test require knowledge of the explicit relationship between the covariate and the parameter, i.e., the software needs to "know" this relationship. Neither of the representations of the model based on equations (5.28a) and (5.28b) explicitly spell out this relationship to the software. Of course, we can rewrite (5.28b) as

$$\begin{aligned} \mu_i &= \log(V_{\text{pop}}) + \beta \log(w_i/70) \\ \log(V_i) &\sim \mathcal{N}(\mu_i, \omega), \end{aligned}$$

and clearly "see" that the predicted log-volume is a linear function of the log-weight. The issue is that without a powerful interpreter, this information is not available to the software, so it cannot automatically run these tasks. Therefore, we must explicitly "tell" the software that the model is linear and provide lists of covariates and coefficients, as can be done with a MLXTRAN script derived from (5.28c).

5.6.4 Implementation of the statistical model

Implementation of models (5.28a, 5.28b, 5.28c) with MLXTRAN means the direct usage of these definitions and equations with a language very close to the mathematical one. The model in (5.28a) can be implemented in the following way:

```
DEFINITION:
eta = {distribution=normal, mean=0, sd=omega}

EQUATION:
V = Vpop*((w/70)^beta)*exp(eta)
```

The model in (5.28b) can be implemented as:

```
EQUATION:
Vpred = Vpop*(w/70)^beta

DEFINITION:
V = {distribution=lognormal, prediction=Vpred, sd=omega}
```

The model in (5.28c) can be implemented as:

```
EQUATION:
c = log(w/70)

DEFINITION:
V = {distribution=lognormal, reference=Vpop,
     covariate=c, coefficient=beta, sd=omega}
```

6

Extensions

We have so far reviewed the most frequently used models for describing both the individual parameters (ψ_i) and the observations (y_i), but several extensions can be considered.

For instance, if we assume that a population consists of several homogeneous subpopulations, mixture models can be very useful for describing different types of mixtures such as mixtures of distributions, mixtures of structural models and mixtures of residual models (see Section 6.1).

A stochastic component can also be added to a model by assuming certain underlying stochastic dynamics, characterized by either a hidden Markov model (see Section 6.2) or a system of stochastic differential equations (see Section 6.3).

6.1 Mixture models

6.1.1 Introduction

Mixed effects models are frequently used for modeling longitudinal data when data is obtained from different individuals from the same population. These models allow us to take into account between-subject variability. One complicating factor arises when data is obtained from a population with some underlying heterogeneity. If we assume that the population consists of several homogeneous subpopulations, a straightforward extension of mixed effects models is a finite mixture of mixed effects models.

As an example, the use of a mixture of mixed effects models is particularly relevant when the response of patients to a drug therapy is heterogeneous. In any clinical efficacy trial, patients who respond well, partially or not at all can be considered different subpopulations with quite different profiles.

The introduction of a categorical covariate (e.g., sex, genotype, treatment, status, etc.) into such a model already supposes that the whole population can be decomposed into subpopulations. The covariate then serves as a *label* for assigning each individual to a subpopulation. In practice, the covariate can either be known or not.

Mixture models usually refer to models for which the categorical covariate is unknown, but whichever the case, the joint model that brings together all the parts (observations, individual parameters, covariates, labels, design, etc.) is the same. The difference appears when having to perform certain tasks and in the methods needed to implement them. For instance, the task of simulation makes no distinction between the two situations because all variables are simulated, whereas model building is different depending on whether the labels are known or unknown: we have supervised learning if the labels are known and unsupervised otherwise.

There exist several types of mixture models useful in the context of mixed effects models, including mixtures of distributions, mixtures of residual error models and mixtures of structural models. Indeed, heterogeneity in the response variable cannot be always adequately explained only by inter-patient variability of certain parameters. It may therefore be necessary to introduce diversity into the structural models themselves:

- *Between-subject model mixtures* assume that there exist subpopulations of individuals. Different structural models describe the response of each subpopulation, and each subject belongs to one of these subpopulations. One can imagine for example different structural models for responders, nonresponders and partial responders to a given treatment.

- *Within-subject model mixtures* assume that there exist subpopulations (of cells, viruses, etc.) within each patient. In this case, different structural models can be used to describe the response of different subpopulations, but the proportion of each subpopulation depends on the patient.

6.1.2 Mixtures of mixed effects models

For the sake of simplicity, we will consider a basic model that involves individual parameters $\boldsymbol{\psi} = (\psi_i, 1 \leq i \leq N)$ and observations $\boldsymbol{y} = (y_i, 1 \leq i \leq N)$, where $y_i = (y_{ij}, 1 \leq j \leq n_i)$. Then, the easiest way to model a finite mixture model is to introduce a label sequence $\boldsymbol{z} = (z_i; 1 \leq i \leq N)$ that takes its values in $\{1, 2, \ldots, M\}$ such that $z_i = m$ if subject i belongs to subpopulation m.

In some situations, the label set $\boldsymbol{z}$ is known and can be used as a categorical covariate in the model. If $\boldsymbol{z}$ is known and if we consider it the realization of a random vector, the model is the conditional distribution

$$\mathrm{p}(\boldsymbol{y}, \boldsymbol{\psi}|\boldsymbol{z};\theta) = \mathrm{p}(\boldsymbol{y}|\boldsymbol{\psi}, \boldsymbol{z})\mathrm{p}(\boldsymbol{\psi}|\boldsymbol{z};\theta).$$

If $\boldsymbol{z}$ is unknown, it can modeled as a random vector, and the model is the joint distribution

$$\mathrm{p}(\boldsymbol{y}, \boldsymbol{\psi}, \boldsymbol{z};\theta) = \mathrm{p}(\boldsymbol{y}, \boldsymbol{\psi}|\boldsymbol{z};\theta)\mathrm{p}(\boldsymbol{z};\theta).$$

We therefore consider that $\boldsymbol{z} = (z_i)$ is a set of independent random variables taking its values in $\{1, 2, \ldots, M\}$ where for $i = 1, 2, \ldots, N$, $\mathbb{P}(z_i = m)$ is the probability that individual i belongs to group m. Simple models can assume that the (z_i) are identically distributed, i.e., $\mathbb{P}(z_i = m)$ does not depend on i for $m = 1, \ldots, M$. However, more complex models can be considered, assuming for instance that an individual's probabilities depend on individual covariates.

EXAMPLE 6.1 The Hepatitis C virus (HCV) can be divided into six distinct genotypes. Genotype 1 is the most difficult to treat, whereas individuals with genotypes 2 and 3 are almost three times more likely to respond to therapy involving a combination of alpha interferon and ribavirin.

Suppose we want to divide patients infected with HCV into three outcome groups: patients who respond, partially respond or do not respond. It is plausible to assume that an individual's probabilities for ending up in each of these groups depend on his genotype, which therefore can be used as an individual covariate to help explain $\mathbb{P}(z_i = m)$.

In its most general form, a mixture of mixed effects models assumes that there exist M joint distributions $\mathrm{p}_1, \ldots, \mathrm{p}_M$ and M vectors of parameters $\theta_1, \ldots, \theta_M$ such that for any individual i, the joint distribution of y_i and ψ_i is

$$\mathrm{p}(y_i, \psi_i;\theta) = \sum_{m=1}^{M} \mathbb{P}(z_i = m)\, \mathrm{p}_m(y_i, \psi_i;\theta_m),$$

where p_m is the joint distribution of (y_i, ψ_i) in group m and $\theta = (\theta_1, \ldots, \theta_M)$. The distribution of observations y_i is therefore itself a mixture of M distributions:

$$\begin{aligned}
\mathrm{p}(y_i;\theta) &= \int \mathrm{p}(y_i, \psi_i;\theta)\, d\psi_i \\
&= \sum_{m=1}^{M} \mathbb{P}(z_i = m) \int \mathrm{p}_m(y_i, \psi_i, \theta_m)\, d\psi_i \\
&= \sum_{m=1}^{M} \mathbb{P}(z_i = m)\, \mathrm{p}_m(y_i;\theta_m).
\end{aligned}$$

The mixture can be in terms of the distribution of the individual parameters p_{ψ_i} and/or the conditional distribution of the observations $p_{y_i|\psi_i}$. Let us now see some examples of mixtures models.

1. A latency structure can be introduced at the individual parameter level:

$$\begin{aligned} \mathrm{p}(y_i, \psi_i; \theta) &= \mathrm{p}(y_i|\psi_i)\mathrm{p}(\psi_i; \theta) \\ &= \mathrm{p}(y_i|\psi_i) \left(\sum_{m=1}^{M} \mathbb{P}(z_i = m)\, \mathrm{p}_m(\psi_i; \theta_m) \right), \end{aligned}$$

   where $\mathrm{p}_m(\psi_i; \theta_m)$ is the distribution of the individual parameters in group m. For example, a mixture of linear Gaussian models for the individual parameters assumes that there exist M population parameters $\psi_{\mathrm{pop},1}, \ldots, \psi_{\mathrm{pop},M}$, M vectors of coefficients $\beta_1, \ldots, \beta_M$, M variance-covariance matrices $\Omega_1, \ldots, \Omega_M$ and M transforms $h_1, \ldots, h_M$ such that

$$h_m(\psi_i) \mid z_i = m \quad \sim \quad \mathcal{N}(h_m(\psi_{\mathrm{pop},m}) + \beta_m \cdot c_i \,,\, \Omega_m). \qquad (6.1)$$

   This is the most general representation possible because it allows the transformation, population parameters, covariate model and variance-covariance structure of the random effects all to vary from one group to the next. A more simpler representation would have one or several of these fixed across groups. If we assume, for instance, that only the reference value of the parameter changes, then (6.1) becomes

$$h(\psi_i) \mid z_i = m \quad \sim \quad \mathcal{N}(h(\psi_{\mathrm{pop},m}) + \beta \cdot c_i \,,\, \Omega).$$

2. A latency structure can be introduced at the level of the conditional distribution of the observations (y_{ij}):

$$\begin{aligned} \mathrm{p}(y_i, \psi_i; \theta) &= \mathrm{p}(y_i|\psi_i)\mathrm{p}(\psi_i; \theta) \\ &= \left(\sum_{m=1}^{M} \mathbb{P}(z_i = m)\, \mathrm{p}_m(y_i|\psi_i) \right) \mathrm{p}(\psi_i; \theta), \end{aligned}$$

   where $\mathrm{p}_m(y_i|\psi_i)$ is the conditional distribution of the observations in group m. For example, the model for continuous data

$$y_{ij} = f\,(t_{ij}; \psi_i, z_i) + g\,(t_{ij}; \psi_i, z_i)\, \varepsilon_{ij}$$

   with $\varepsilon_{ij} \sim \mathcal{N}(0, 1)$, can be equivalently represented as

$$y_{ij}| \, z_i = m \quad \sim \quad \mathcal{N}(f_m(t_{ij}; \psi_i),\; g_m(t_{ij}; \psi_i)^2)$$

for each $m = 1, \ldots, M$. A mixture of conditional distributions is therefore reduced to a mixture of structural models and/or residual errors. To give a precise example, a mixture of constant error models would assume that

$$y_{ij} = f\left(t_{ij}; \psi_i\right) + \left(\sum_{m=1}^{M} \mathbb{1}_{z_i=m} a_m\right) \varepsilon_{ij},$$

where a_m is the standard deviation of the residual errors in group m. Another possible alternative is between-subject model mixtures (BSMM), which assume that the structural model is a mixture of M different structural models:

$$f\left(t_{ij}; \psi_i, z_i\right) = \sum_{m=1}^{M} \mathbb{1}_{z_i=m} f_m\left(t_{ij}; \psi_i\right).$$

Remark: It may be too simplistic to assume that each individual is represented by only one well-defined model from the mixture. For instance, in a pharmacological setting there may be subpopulations of cells or viruses *within each patient* that react differently to a drug treatment. In this case, it makes sense to consider that the mixture of models happens *within* each individual. Such within-subject model mixtures (WSMM) require additional vectors of individual parameters $\pi_i = (\pi_{1,i}, \ldots, \pi_{M,i})$ representing the proportions of the M models within each individual i:

$$f\left(t_{ij}; \psi_i, z_i\right) = \sum_{m=1}^{M} \pi_{m,i} f_m\left(t_{ij}; \psi_i\right).$$

The proportions $(\pi_{m,i})$ are now individual parameters in the model and the problem is transformed into a standard mixed effects model. These proportions are assumed to be positive and to sum to 1 for each patient. We can then define $\pi_{m,i}$ in order to satisfy these constraints. One possible way to do this is

$$\pi_{m,i} = \frac{\gamma_{m,i}}{\sum_{\ell=1}^{M} \gamma_{\ell,i}},$$

where $\log(\gamma_{m,i}) \sim \mathcal{N}(\log(\gamma_{m,\text{pop}}), \omega_m^2)$.

6.1.3 Example 1: A mixture of normal distributions

We consider here a simple pharmacokinetic (PK) model for a single oral administration:

$$f(t; ka_i, V_i, Cl_i) = \frac{D\, ka_i}{V ka_i - Cl_i)} \left(e^{-(Cl_i/V_i)\, t} - e^{-ka_i\, t}\right),$$

where the absorption rate constant ka_i and clearance Cl_i of patient i have log-normal distributions:

$$\log(ka_i) \sim \mathcal{N}(\log(1), 0.3^2)$$
$$\log(Cl_i) \sim \mathcal{N}(\log(4), 0.3^2),$$

and the distribution of the volume V_i is a mixture of two log-normal distributions:

$$\log(V_i) \sim 0.35\ \mathcal{N}(\log(70), 0.3^2) + 0.65\ \mathcal{N}(\log(42), 0.3^2).$$

Figure 6.1 shows the distributions p_1 and p_2 of the volume in the two groups and the mixture of these two distributions.

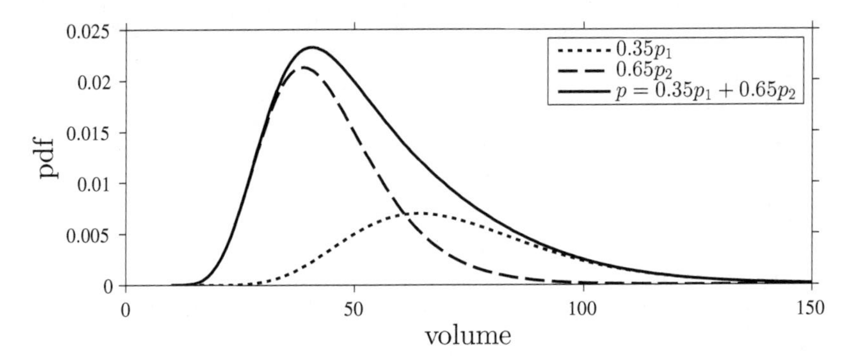

FIGURE 6.1: Two weighted log-normal distributions $0.35p_1$ and $0.65p_2$ and the mixture of p_1 and p_2: $p = 0.35p_1 + 0.65p_2$.

Here, the structural model f is a function of time and $f(t;\psi_i)$ the predicted concentration of the drug in individual i at time t, with $\psi_i = (ka_i, V_i, Cl_i)$. The probability distribution of $f(\,\cdot\,;\psi_i)$ then represents the inter-individual variability of predicted concentration of the drug across the population. Figure 6.2 shows prediction intervals for the concentration $f(\,\cdot\,;\psi_i)$ for one individual i randomly chosen in the population. This plot allows us to visualize the impact of the inter-individual variability of the individual PK parameters on exposure to the drug.

In this example, the distribution of $f(\,\cdot\,;\psi_i)$ is itself a mixture of two distributions since the distribution of ψ_i is a mixture of distributions due to V_i. It is then interesting to visualize the distribution of the predicted concentration in each subpopulation. Indeed, any individual i will have either a log-volume from $\mathcal{N}(\log(70), 0.3^2)$ (with probability 0.35) or a log-volume from $\mathcal{N}(\log(42), 0.3^2)$ (with probability 0.65), so in order to see what really happens to a single individual i, we need to split the data into two plots: 35% of the individuals will have concentration curves distributed as on the left of Figure 6.3 and 65% as on the right.

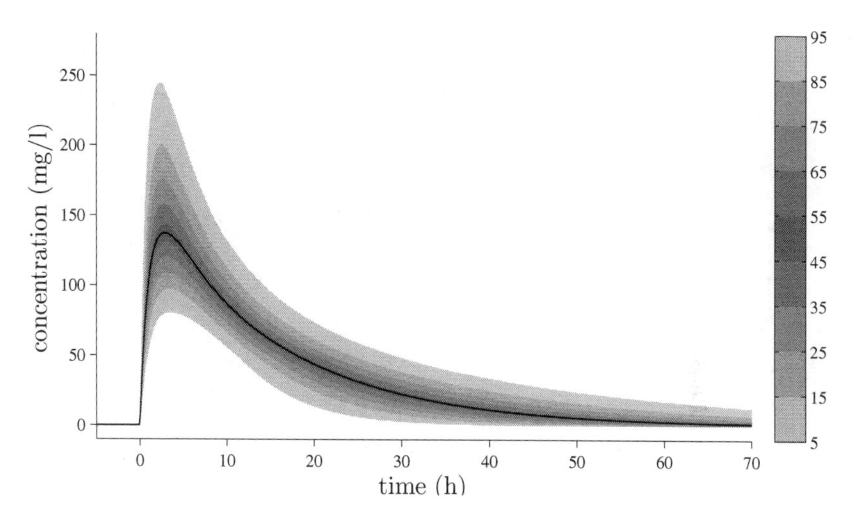

FIGURE 6.2: Probability distribution for the predicted concentration curve $f(\,\cdot\,;\psi_i)$.

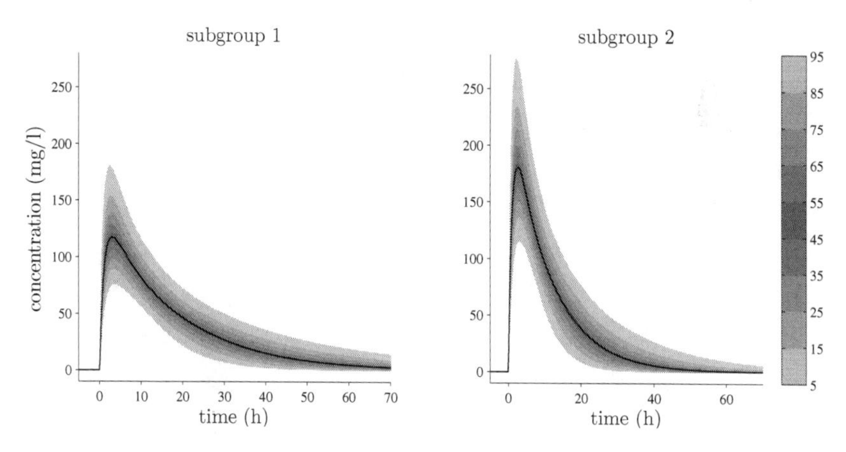

FIGURE 6.3: Probability distribution of the predicted concentration curves $f(\,\cdot\,;\psi_i)$ in the two subpopulations.

6.1.4 Example 2: A mixture of structural models

We will work here with the example given in Mbogning et al. (2012) where we are interested in a study of treated human immunodeficiency virus (HIV) infected patients; the output data are the evolution in their viral loads. Figure 6.4 gives examples of patients with one of three "typical" viral load progressions:

- *Non-responders* (1) show no decline in viral load.
- *Responders* (2) exhibit a sustained viral load decline.
- *Partial responders* (3 and 4) exhibit an initial drop in viral load, then a rebound to higher levels.

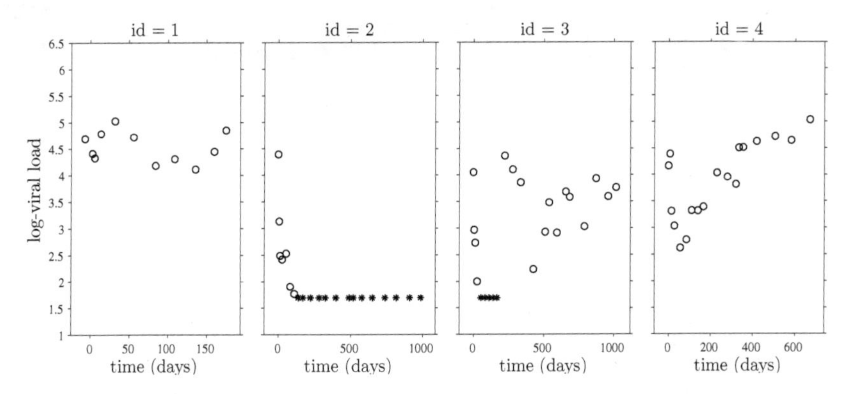

FIGURE 6.4: Viral load progression for four HIV-infected patients. (1) non-responder; (2) responder; (3) and (4) partial responders. The $*$ symbol indicates below level of quantification data.

Remarks:

- Since viral loads generally evolve exponentially over time, they are most commonly expressed on a logarithmic scale.
- There is a detection limit at 50 HIV RNA copies/ml, corresponding to a log-viral load of 1.7, i.e., data are left-censored. These points are shown with a $*$.

Within a few months of HIV infection, patients typically enter a steady state of chronic infection and have a stabilized concentration of HIV-1 in blood plasma. This concentration is modeled as a baseline A_0. When antiretroviral treatment starts, the viral load of patients who respond shows an initial rapid exponential decay usually followed by a slower second phase of exponential decay. This two-phase decay in viral load can be approximated by the bi-exponential model $A_1 e^{-\lambda_1 t} + A_2 e^{-\lambda_2 t}$ (Samson et al., 2006).

After the decrease in viral load some subjects show a rebound, which may be due to several factors (nonadherence to the therapy, emergence of drug-resistant virus strains, etc.). We can extend the bi-exponential model to these patients by adding a third phase, characterized by a logistic growth process $A_3/(1 + e^{-\lambda_3(t-\tau)})$, where τ is its inflection point.

We can then consider three simple models, corresponding to each of the three types of viral load progression:

$$\begin{aligned}
f_1(t_{ij}, \psi_i) &= A_{0,i} \\
f_2(t_{ij}, \psi_i) &= A_{1,i} e^{-\lambda_{1,i} t_{ij}} + A_{2,i} e^{-\lambda_{2,i} t_{ij}} \\
f_3(t_{ij}, \psi_i) &= A_{1,i} e^{-\lambda_{1,i} t_{ij}} + A_{2,i} e^{-\lambda_{2,i} t_{ij}} + \frac{A_{3,i}}{1 + e^{-\lambda_{3,i}(t_{ij} - \tau_i)}}.
\end{aligned}$$

The log-transformed viral load can then be modeled using a BSMM:

$$\log(y_{ij}) = \sum_{m=1}^{3} \mathbb{I}_{z_i = m} \log(f_m(t_{ij}, \psi_i)) + a\varepsilon_{ij},$$

where y_{ij} is the viral load for patient i at time t_{ij} and $\psi_i = (A_{0,i}, A_{1,i}, A_{2,i}, A_{3,i}, \lambda_{1,i}, \lambda_{2,i}, \lambda_{3,i}, \tau_i)$ the vector of individual parameters.

Figure 6.5 displays the predicted viral loads for the four patients using model f_1 for patient 1, f_2 for patient 2 and f_3 for patients 3 and 4, with the following parameters[1]

id	A_0	A_1	A_2	A_3	λ_1	λ_2	λ_3	τ
1	92	–	–	–	–	–	–	–
2	–	66	5	–	0.14	2×10^{-5}	–	–
3	–	53	6	28	0.15	1.5×10^{-5}	0.15	200
4	–	77	10	100	0.1	1.5×10^{-5}	0.013	270

Not all observed viral load progressions fall so easily into one of the three classes, as seen in the patients shown in Figure 6.6.

[1]These values and the predicted class for each patient were obtained using MONOLIX.

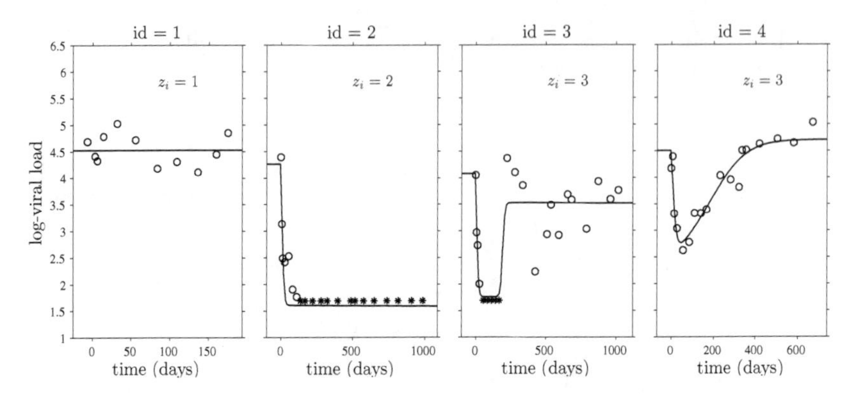

FIGURE 6.5: Observed and predicted viral load progression for four HIV-infected patients.

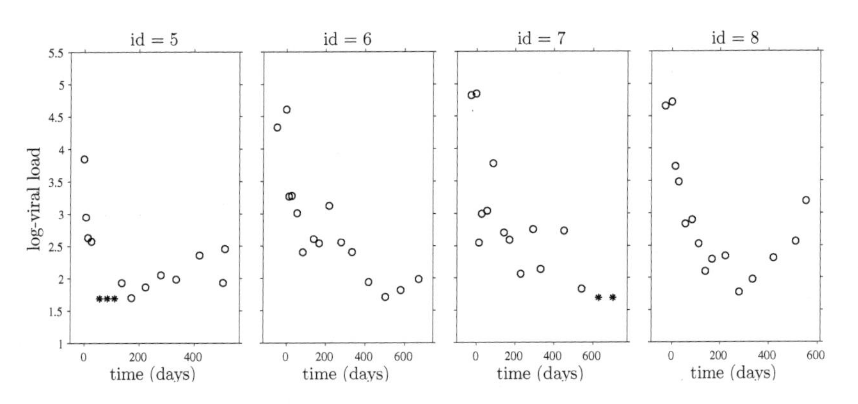

FIGURE 6.6: Viral load data for four patients with ambiguous progressions.

In these cases, it does not seem quite so reasonable to model the data under the BSMM assumption that each patient must belong uniquely to one class. Instead, it is perhaps more natural to suppose that each patient is partially responding, partially nonresponding and partially rebounding to the given drug treatment. The goal becomes to find the relative strength of each process in each patient, and WSMMs are ideal tools for this:

$$\log\left(y_{ij}\right) = \sum_{m=1}^{3} \pi_{m,i} \log\left(f_m\left(t_{ij}, \psi_i\right)\right) + a\varepsilon_{ij}.$$

Without going into further detail, Figure 6.7 displays the observed and predicted viral loads computed with MONOLIX for these four individuals when each individual has a mixture of the three viral load progressions.

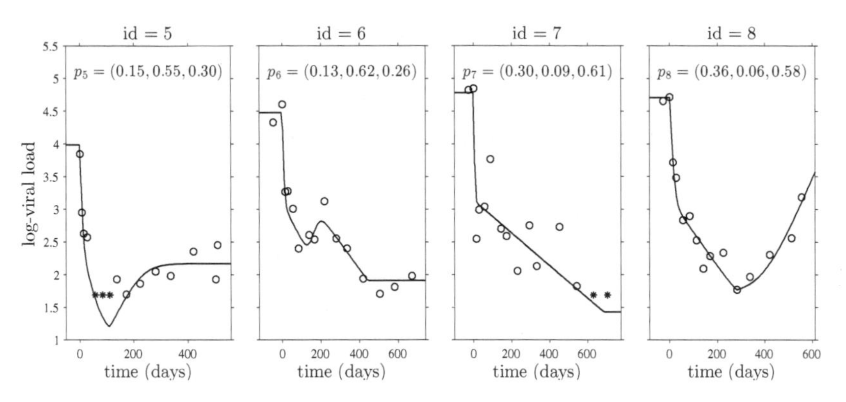

FIGURE 6.7: Observed and predicted viral load progression for four patients using within-subject model mixtures.

6.2 Hidden Markov models

6.2.1 Introduction

Markov chains are a useful tool for analyzing categorical longitudinal data. However, sometimes the Markov process cannot be directly observed and only some output, dependent on the (hidden) state, is seen. More precisely, we assume that the distribution of this observable output depends on the underlying hidden state. Such models are called hidden Markov models (HMMs; see Cappé et al., 2005; Rabiner, 1989). HMMs can be applied to many domains and have turned out to be particularly useful in several biological contexts. For example, they are helpful when characterizing diseases for which the existence of several discrete stages of illness is a realistic assumption, e.g., epilepsy (Albert, 1991) and migraines (Anisimov et al., 2007).

In this section, we will consider a parametric framework with Markov chains in a discrete and finite state space $\mathbf{K} = \{1, \ldots, K\}$.

6.2.2 Mixed hidden Markov models

HMMs were developed to describe how a given system moves from one state to another over time in situations where the successive visited states are unknown and a set of observations is the only available information to describe the system's dynamics. HMMs can be seen as a variant of mixture models that allow for possible memory in the sequence of hidden states. An HMM is thus defined as a pair of processes $(z_j, y_j, j = 1, 2, \ldots)$, where the latent sequence (z_j) is a Markov chain and the distribution of observation y_j at time t_j depends on state z_j (see Figure 6.8).

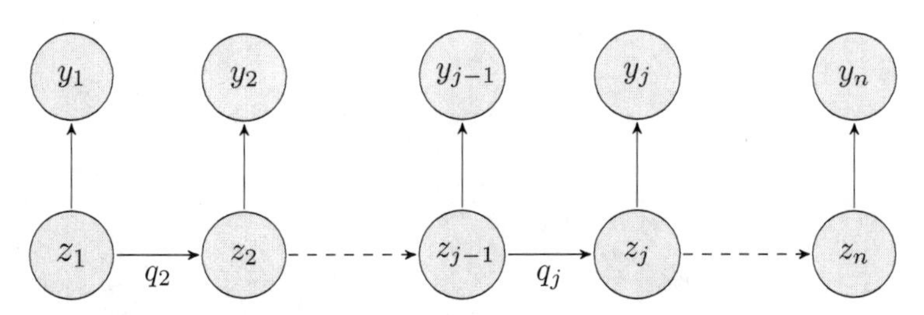

FIGURE 6.8: Dynamics of a hidden Markov model.

In the population approach, HMMs for several individuals can be simultaneously defined by considering *mixed* HMMs (Altman, 2007; Delattre and Lavielle, 2012; Maruotti, 2011; Reuter et al., 2004). Let $y_i = (y_{i,1}, \ldots, y_{i,n_i})$ and $z_i = (z_{i,1}, \ldots, z_{i,n_i})$ denote, respectively, the sequences of observations and hidden states for individual i.

We suppose that the joint distribution of (z_i, y_i) is a parametric one that depends on a vector of parameters ψ_i and can be decomposed as

$$\mathrm{p}(z_i, y_i|\psi_i) = \mathrm{p}(z_i|\psi_i)\,\mathrm{p}(y_i|z_i, \psi_i).$$

For each individual i, z_i is a Markov chain whose probability distribution is defined by

- the distribution $\pi_i = (\pi_i^k,\ k = 1, 2, \ldots, K)$ of the first state $z_{i,1}$:

$$\pi_i^k = \mathbb{P}(z_{i,1} = k|\psi_i)\,.$$

- the sequence of *transition matrices* $(Q_{ij},\ j = 2, 3, \ldots)$, where for each j, $Q_{ij} = (q_{ij}^{\ell,k}\ ;\ 1 \leq \ell, k \leq K)$ is a matrix of size $K \times K$ such that $q_{ij}^{\ell,k} = \mathbb{P}(z_{ij} = k|z_{i,j-1} = \ell, \psi_i)$.

The conditional distribution $p_{y_i|z_i,\psi_i}$ depends on the model chosen for the observations; for each state, observation y_{ij} has a certain distribution. Let us now see some examples.

6.2.3 Probability distribution function for the observations

Assuming that the N individuals are independent, the joint pdf is given by

$$\mathrm{p}(y_1, \ldots, y_N | \psi_1, \ldots, \psi_N) = \prod_{i=1}^{N} \mathrm{p}(y_i | \psi_i).$$

Then, computing the conditional distribution of the observations $p_{y_i|\psi_i}$ for any individual i requires integration of the joint conditional distribution $p_{z_i,y_i|\psi_i}$ over all states:

$$\begin{aligned}
\mathrm{p}(y_i|\psi_i) &= \sum_{z_i \in \mathbf{S}} \mathrm{p}(z_i, y_i|\psi_i) \\
&= \sum_{z_i \in \mathbf{S}} \mathrm{p}(z_i|\psi_i)\,\mathrm{p}(y_i|z_i, \psi_i) \\
&= \sum_{z_i \in \mathbf{S}} \left\{ \pi_i^{z_{i,1}} \mathrm{p}(y_{i,1}|z_{i,1}, \psi_i) \prod_{j=2}^{n} \left(q_{ij}^{z_{i,j-1}, z_{ij}}\, \mathrm{p}(y_{ij}|z_{ij}, \psi_i) \right) \right\}.
\end{aligned}$$

Though this looks complicated, it turns out that a forward recursion of the Baum-Welch algorithm provides a quick way to numerically compute it (Cappé et al., 2005; Rabiner, 1989).

6.2.4 Examples

In a continuous data model, one possibility is that the residual error model is a hidden Markov model that can randomly switch between K possible residual error models.

EXAMPLE 6.2 In this example, we consider a 2-state Markov chain. A constant error model is assumed in each state:

$$\begin{aligned}
y_{ij} &= \sin(\alpha\, t_{ij}) + a_{1,i}\varepsilon_{ij} \quad \text{if } z_{ij} = 1 \\
y_{ij} &= \sin(\alpha\, t_{ij}) + a_{2,i}\varepsilon_{ij} \quad \text{if } z_{ij} = 2.
\end{aligned}$$

Figure 6.9 shows simulated data from this model for two individuals. Only the observations are shown in the top two plots. Clearly it is not trivial to visually identify the two states. In the lower panel, the structural model is displayed and observations drawn from state 1 (resp. state 2) are displayed with dots (resp. crosses). Now the model is easier to understand; in particular we can see how the residual variability changes with time for these two individuals. Unfortunately however, this is not a realistic situation with hidden Markov models because only the values are observed, not the symbols.

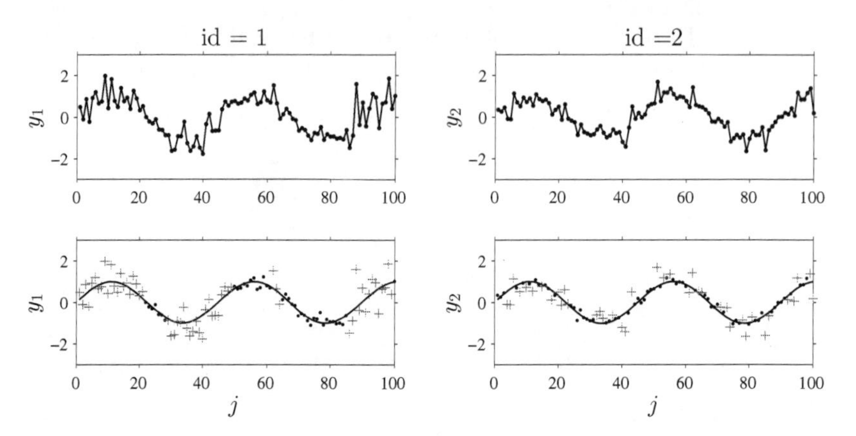

FIGURE 6.9: 2-state Markov chains for two individuals. Different constant error models are used in each state. Top: only the observations are displayed; bottom: the structural model is displayed with a solid line and the 2 states are represented differently (state 1 with dots and state 2 with crosses). Individual 1: $a_{1,1} = 0.1$, $a_{2,1} = 0.6$, $q_1^{12} = 0.1$, $q_1^{21} = 0.1$; individual 2: $a_{1,2} = 0.1$, $a_{2,2} = 0.6$, $q_2^{12} = 0.4$, $q_2^{21} = 0.6$.

In Poisson models for count data, the Poisson parameter might randomly switch between K intensities. This type of model has been used to describe the evolution of seizures in epileptic patients.

EXAMPLE 6.3 Instead of assuming a unique Poisson distribution for the observed numbers of seizures, this model assumes that patients go through alternating periods of low and high epileptic susceptibility. Therefore, we consider what is called a 2-state Poisson mixed-HMM:

$$
\begin{aligned}
y_{ij} &\sim \text{Poisson}(\lambda_{1,i}) \quad \text{if } z_{ij} = 1 \\
y_{ij} &\sim \text{Poisson}(\lambda_{2,i}) \quad \text{if } z_{ij} = 2.
\end{aligned}
$$

Again, only the upper plots of Figure 6.10 are seen in reality because the states are unknown. Note that we can see for the first individual that simply defining a fixed cutoff value between the two states would not work because there is significant overlap in the two distributions.

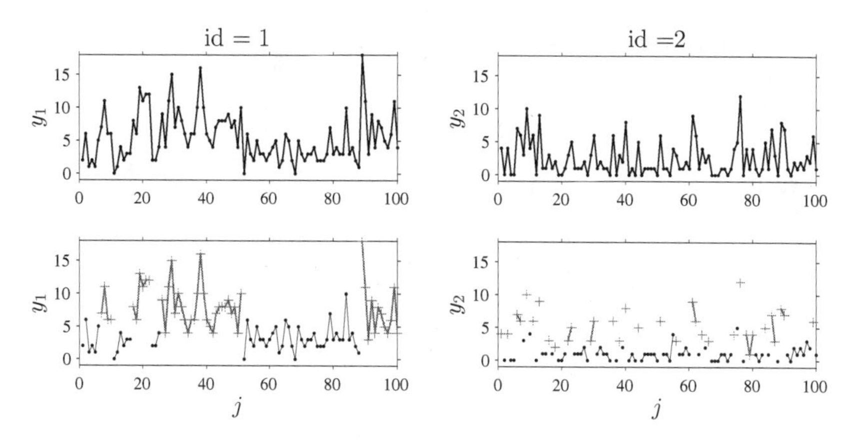

FIGURE 6.10: 2-state Poisson mixed-HMM for two individuals. Different Poisson distributions are used in each state. Top: only the observations are displayed; bottom: the two states are represented differently (state 1 with dots and state 2 with crosses). Only consecutive observations in the same state are connected. Individual 1: $\lambda_{1,1} = 2$, $\lambda_{2,1} = 8$, $q_1^{12} = 0.1$, $q_1^{21} = 0.1$; Individual 2: $\lambda_{1,2} = 1$, $\lambda_{2,2} = 5$, $q_2^{12} = 0.4$, $q_2^{21} = 0.6$.

6.3 Stochastic differential equation-based models

6.3.1 Introduction

Diffusion models are known to be a useful tool for modeling stochastic dynamics phenomena and are widely used in various fields including finance, physics, biology, physiology and control. In the population approach, a mixed effects diffusion model aims to describe each individual series of observations using a system of stochastic differential equations (SDE) while also taking into account variability between individuals (Delattre and Lavielle, 2013; Ditlevsen and Gaetano, 2005; Donnet and Samson, 2008; Klim et al., 2009).

For the sake of simplicity, we will first consider a diffusion model for a single individual involving a quite general dynamical system with linear transfers, and illustrate it with several PK examples. We will then show that the extension to mixed diffusion models is fairly straightforward.

Note that the conditional distribution $p_{y|\psi}$ of the observations usually does not have a closed-form expression. When the underlying system is a Gaussian linear dynamical one, the conditional pdf $\mathrm{p}(y_i|\psi_i)$ of the observations can be computed using the *Kalman filter* (Grewal and Andrews, 2011). When the system is not linear, the *extended Kalman filter* (EKF) provides an approximation of the conditional pdf.

6.3.2 Diffusion models

We assume that one diffusion trajectory is observed with noise at discrete time points $t_1 < \ldots < t_j < \ldots < t_n$. Let us note $(X(t), t \geq 0) \in \mathbb{R}^p$ the underlying dynamical process and $y_j \in \mathbb{R}$ a noisy function of $X(t_j)$, $j = 1, \ldots, n$. The general form of the diffusion model is given by

$$\begin{cases} dX(t) &= b(X(t), \psi)dt + \gamma(X(t), \psi)dW(t) \\ y_j &= c(X(t_j), \psi) + \varepsilon_j \\ \varepsilon_j &\underset{i.i.d.}{\sim} \mathcal{N}(0, a^2(\psi)), \quad j = 1, \ldots, n, \end{cases} \tag{6.2}$$

with initial condition $X(0) = x \in \mathbb{R}^p$. Here, $(W(t), t > 0)$ is a standard Wiener process in $\mathbb{R}^p$ and $\varepsilon_j \in \mathbb{R}$ represents the measurement error occurring at the jth observation, independent of $W(t)$. The measurement function $c: \mathbb{R}^p \times \mathbb{R}^d \to \mathbb{R}$, drift function $b: \mathbb{R}^p \times \mathbb{R}^d \to \mathbb{R}^p$ and diffusion function $\gamma: \mathbb{R}^p \times \mathbb{R}^d \to \mathcal{M}_p(\mathbb{R})$, where $\mathcal{M}_p(\mathbb{R})$ is the set of $p \times p$ matrices with real elements, are known functions that depend on an unknown parameter $\psi \in \mathbb{R}^d$.

We can in fact consider an SDE-based model as a ODE-based one with a stochastic component.

EXAMPLE 6.4 The ODE

$$dA_c(t) = -kA_c(t)dt \tag{6.3}$$

can be used to describe the kinetics of a drug administered by rapid injection (iv bolus) into plasma. Here, $A_c(t)$ represents the drug amount in plasma at time t after injection, and k the elimination rate constant. Figure 6.11 (left) displays the typical evolution of the amount found in the central compartment when $k = 4$.

Imagine now that we want to describe the evolution of the drug amount over time by means of SDEs rather than ODEs in order to better describe the *intra-individual variability* of the observed process. We can assume, for example, that system (6.3) is randomly perturbed by an additive Wiener process:

$$dA_c(t) = -kA_c(t)dt + \gamma dW(t).$$

Figure 6.11 (right) displays three kinetics for the amount in the central compartment simulated from this model with $k = 4$ and $\gamma = 2$.

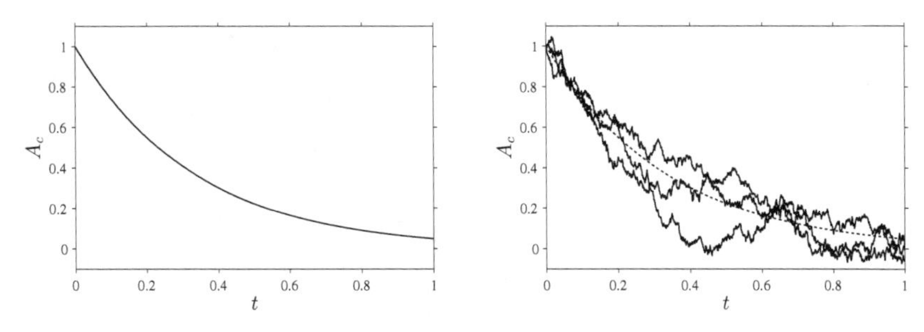

FIGURE 6.11: Drug amount kinetics. Left: ODE model; right: SDE model for three individuals.

These kinetics are clearly stochastic. Nevertheless, they are not realistic because:

- they give an overly erratic description of the evolution of the drug concentration within compartments of the human body.
- they do not comply with certain constraints on biological dynamics (concentration should be positive and decreasing over time).

A more relevant model might consider that some parameters randomly fluctuate over time, rather than the observed variable itself. We could model for example the elimination rate "constant" k as a stochastic process $k(t)$ that randomly varies around a typical value k^*.

More generally, we can describe fluctuations within a linear dynamical system by considering transfer rates as diffusion processes rather than the observed processes themselves.

6.3.3 Diffusion models for dynamical systems with linear transfers

Dynamical systems are of importance in many fields. For example, they can be used to model viral dynamics, population flows, interactions between cells and drug pharmacokinetics. Dynamical systems involving linear transfers between different entities are usually modeled by means of a system of ODEs with the following general form

$$dA(t) = K\, A(t)dt, \tag{6.4}$$

where $A(t)$ is a vector whose lth component represents the condition of the lth entity at time t and $K = (K^{l\,l'}, 1 \leq l, l' \leq p)$ is a deterministic matrix defined as

$$\begin{cases} K^{l\,l'} = k^{l\,l'} & \text{if} \quad l \neq l' \\ K^{l\,l} = -k^{l\,0} - \sum_{l'} k^{l\,l'} & \text{otherwise,} \end{cases} \tag{6.5}$$

where $k^{l\,l'}$ represents the transfer rate from entity l to entity l' and k^{l0} the elimination rate from entity l. An example of such a dynamical system with three components is shown in Figure 6.12.

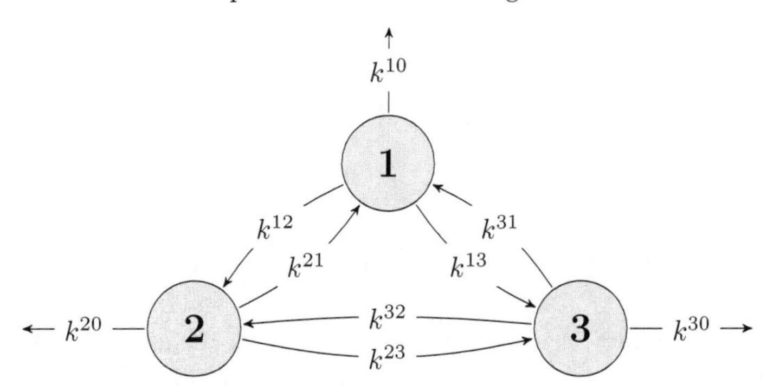

FIGURE 6.12: Dynamical system with three components (circles) and linear transfers between them (arrows).

In this particular example, the matrix K would be

$$K = \begin{pmatrix} -k^{10} - k^{12} - k^{13} & k^{21} & k^{31} \\ k^{12} & -k^{20} - k^{21} - k^{23} & k^{32} \\ k^{13} & k^{23} & -k^{30} - k^{31} - k^{32} \end{pmatrix}.$$

The model defined by equations (6.4) and (6.5) is a deterministic one which assumes that transfers take place at the same rate at all times. This is often a restrictive assumption since in reality, dynamical systems tend to exhibit some random behavior. It is therefore reasonable to consider that transfers are not constant but randomly fluctuate over time. This new assumption leads to the following dynamical system:

$$dA(t) = K(t)A(t)dt,$$

where K has the same structure as in (6.5) but now some components $k^{l\,l'}$ are stochastic processes which take nonnegative values and randomly fluctuate around a typical value $k^{l\,l'^*}$. Let us illustrate the construction of these types of diffusion models using some specific examples from pharmacokinetics.

EXAMPLE 6.5 We consider in this example iv bolus administration with stochastic linear elimination. We will first extend the ODE-based model defined in (6.3) by assuming that k is a diffusion process which takes nonnegative values and fluctuates around a typical value k^*. In this example, nonnegativity of $k(t)$ is ensured by defining the logarithm of the transfer rate as an Ornstein-Uhlenbeck diffusion process:

$$d\log k(t) = -\alpha\left(\log k(t) - \log k^*\right)dt + \gamma dW(t),$$

where W is a standard one-dimensional Wiener process. This results in the following diffusion system:

$$dX(t) = b(X(t))dt + \gamma(X(t))dW(t),$$

where

$$X(t) = \begin{pmatrix} A_c(t) \\ \log k(t) \end{pmatrix}, \quad b(x) = \begin{pmatrix} -x_1 \exp(x_2) \\ -\alpha(x_2 - \log k^*) \end{pmatrix}, \quad \gamma(x) = \begin{pmatrix} 0 & 0 \\ 0 & \gamma \end{pmatrix}.$$

Note that in this specific example, the Jacobian matrix of the drift function b has a simple form:

$$B(x) = \begin{pmatrix} -\exp(x_2) & -x_1 \exp(x_2) \\ 0 & -\alpha \end{pmatrix}.$$

Figure 6.13 shows four simulated processes $k(t)$ and the associated amount processes $A_c(t)$.

We measure the concentration at times $(t_j, 1 \leq j \leq n)$:

$$y_j = \frac{A_c(t_j)}{V} + a\,\varepsilon_j.$$

The parameter vector of the model is therefore $\psi = (V, k^*, \alpha, \gamma, a)$. We see in this example that the simulated kinetics are much more realistic than those obtained with the previous model because:

- the elimination rate process $k(t)$ is a stochastic process that takes non-negative values.
- even though the amount process is stochastic, it is smooth and decreases monotonically with time.

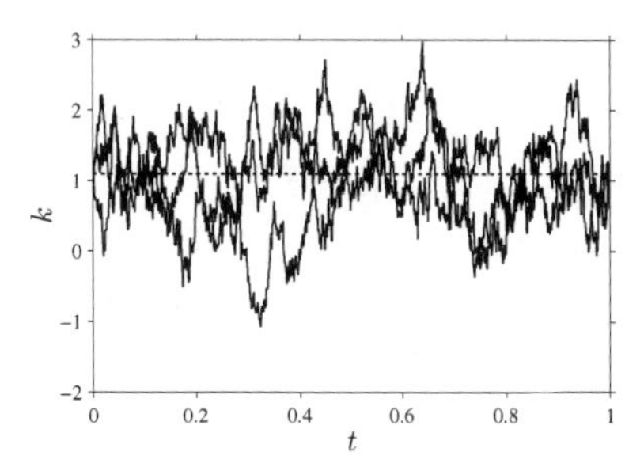

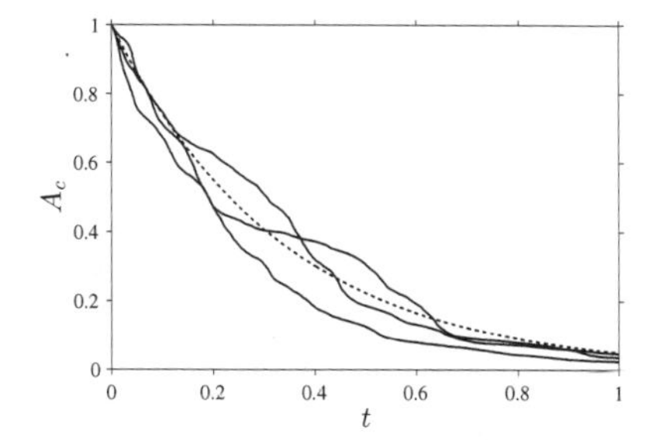

FIGURE 6.13: Four simulated processes $k(t)$ and the associated amount processes $A_c(t)$.

EXAMPLE 6.6 Consider now a one compartment model for oral administration:

$$\frac{d}{dt}\begin{pmatrix} A_d(t) \\ A_c(t) \end{pmatrix} = \begin{pmatrix} -k_a & 0 \\ k_a & -k_e \end{pmatrix}\begin{pmatrix} A_d(t) \\ A_c(t) \end{pmatrix}, \tag{6.6}$$

where $A_d(t)$ and $A_c(t)$ represent, respectively, the drug amount at time t in the depot and central compartments. Assume now that the elimination constant is driven by a stochastic process, solution of the stochastic differential equation:

$$dk_e(t) = -\alpha(k_e - k_e{}^*)dt + \gamma\sqrt{k_e(t)}dW(t),$$

where W is a standard one-dimensional Wiener process. Then (6.6) becomes

$$dX(t) = b(X(t))dt + \gamma(X(t))dW(t).$$

Here,

$$X(t) = \begin{pmatrix} A_d(t) \\ A_c(t) \\ k_e(t) \end{pmatrix}, \quad b(x) = \begin{pmatrix} -k_a x_1 \\ k_a x_1 - x_3 x_2 \\ -\alpha(x_3 - k_e{}^*) \end{pmatrix}, \quad \gamma(x) = \begin{pmatrix} 0 & 0 & 0 \\ 0 & 0 & 0 \\ 0 & 0 & \gamma\sqrt{x_3} \end{pmatrix},$$

and the parameter vector for the model is $\psi = (V, k_a, k^*, \alpha, \gamma, a)$.

In both examples, the diffusion model can be easily extended to the population approach by defining the system's parameters ψ as an individual random vector.

6.3.4 Mixed effects diffusion models

Let us now consider model (6.2) with observations coming from several subjects. An adequate adaptation of model (6.2) in this context consists of considering as many dynamical systems as there are individuals, and defining the parameters of the individual's dynamical systems as independent random variables in such a way as to correctly reflect variability between different trajectories.

To standardize notation, we consider N subjects randomly chosen from a population and note n_i the number of observations for individual i, so that $t_{i,1} < \ldots < t_{i,n_i}$ are subject i's observation time points. $(X_i(t),\, t \geq 0) \in \mathbb{R}^p$ and $y_{ij} \in \mathbb{R}$ will denote, respectively, individual i's diffusion and observation $X_i(t_{ij})$. The y_{ij}, $i = 1, \ldots, N$, $j = 1, \ldots, n_i$, are governed by a mixed effects model based on a p-dimensional real-valued system of SDEs of the general form:

$$\begin{cases} dX_i(t) = b(X_i(t), \psi_i)dt + \gamma(X_i(t), \psi_i)dW_i(t) \\ y_{ij} = c(X_i(t_{ij}), \psi_i) + \varepsilon_{ij} \\ \varepsilon_{ij} \underset{i.i.d.}{\sim} \mathcal{N}(0, a^2(\psi_i)) \;,\; j = 1, \ldots, n_i, \;\; i = 1, \ldots, N, \end{cases}$$

and initial conditions $X_i(0) = x_{0,i} \in \mathbb{R}^p$ for $i = 1, \ldots, N$. The ψ_i are unobserved independent p-dimensional random subject-specific parameters drawn from a distribution p_ψ which depends on a set of population parameters θ. The $(W_1(t), t > 0), \ldots, (W_N(t), t > 0)$ are standard independent Wiener processes and the ε_{ij} are independent Gaussian random variables representing residual errors in such a way that the ψ_i, W_i and ε_{ij} are mutually independent. The measurement function c, drift function b and diffusion function γ are known functions common to the N subjects that depend on the unknown parameters ψ_i.

For example, a straightforward extension of the dynamical system with linear transfers defined in (6.4) and (6.5) consists of considering individual transfer rates $k_i^{l\,l'}$ and individual volatilities γ_i for individual i at time t_{ij}. Assuming that the N individuals are independent, the joint pdf is given by

$$\mathrm{p}(y_1, \ldots, y_N | \psi_1, \ldots, \psi_N) = \prod_{i=1}^{N} \mathrm{p}(y_i | \psi_i).$$

Computing the conditional distribution p of the observations for any individual i requires calculation of the conditional distribution of each observation given the past:

$$\mathrm{p}(y_i | \psi_i) \quad = \quad \mathrm{p}(y_{i1} | \psi_i) \prod_{j=2}^{n_i} p(y_{ij} | y_{i,1}, \ldots, y_{i,j-1}, \psi_i).$$

Except in some very specific classes of mixed effects diffusion models, the transition density $\mathrm{p}(y_{ij} | y_{i,1}, \ldots, y_{i,j-1}, \psi_i)$ does not have a closed-form expression since it involves the transition densities of the underlying diffusion processes X_i. When the underlying system is a Gaussian linear dynamical one, this density is Gaussian with mean and variance that can be computed using the Kalman filter. When the system is not linear, an initial solution comes from approximating this density by a Gaussian one and using the extended Kalman filter for quickly computing its mean and variance (Delattre and Lavielle, 2013). In comparison to this, particle filters do not require making approximations of the transition density, but are quite demanding in terms of simulation requirements and computation time (see Zechner et al., 2014 for an application in quantitative biology).

Part III

Using Models

In Part II of the book we learned how to define models. Now we want to look at the practical aspects of modeling using such models. In other words, aspects of how a modeler can decide which models for observations and individual parameters give good approximations of how the data changes with time and varies between individuals. In this part of the book, we are therefore going to present several useful statistical methods for modeling, and examples of implementing and using them in practice.

The tasks of identifying, evaluating and choosing models are presented in Chapter 7 along with statistical methods useful for these tasks. Being at ease with these tasks and methods is critical for modelers, especially when it comes to knowing the method to use for a given task, as well as its features. For example, it is important to know the properties of a chosen estimator, understand when Bayesian methods are applicable, know the limits of methods based on model linearization as opposed to exact methods, know how to analyze diagnostic plots constructed by software tools, etc.

We are not pretending to be providing a "how-to toolbox" for model construction; we merely present a set of tools for modelers to help construct models. Hence, the examples provided in Chapter 8 illustrate approaches and methods presented in the book but do not pretend to describe the actual data modeling process; this itself relies on the talent of expert modelers in each domain.

All examples and illustrations presented here were undertaken using MONOLIX, the modeling software in which all methods presented are implemented. The data and MONOLIX scripts used to analyze them are readily available from the supporting web site `http://www.math.u-psud.fr/~lavielle/book`

Some proposed methods – maximum likelihood estimation in nonlinear mixed effects models for instance – are complicated to implement in practice. Algorithms for how to do so are presented in Chapter 9, in particular the SAEM (Stochastic Approximation Expectation Maximization) algorithm, known to be particularly adept at parameter estimation in mixed models. This chapter is aimed at those who are considering implementing such algorithms or simply want to understand how – and why – they work. We will not go into theoretical properties (i.e., convergence of SAEM and Metropolis-Hastings) here.

7

Tasks and Methods

7.1 Introduction

Data modeling is by definition the main task confronted by modelers. The main goal of this chapter is to introduce several statistical methods available to modelers, for both parameter estimation in and evaluation of mixed effects models.

In the modeling context we usually assume that we have data that includes observations $\boldsymbol{y}$, measurement times $\underline{\boldsymbol{t}}$ and possibly additional regression variables $\boldsymbol{x}$. There may also be individual covariates $\boldsymbol{c}$ and in pharmacological applications a dose regimen $\boldsymbol{u}$. However, for clarity in the notation that follows, we will omit the design variables $\underline{\boldsymbol{t}}$, $\boldsymbol{x}$ and $\boldsymbol{u}$, and the covariates $\boldsymbol{c}$.

Here, we find ourselves in the classical framework of incomplete data models. Indeed, only $\boldsymbol{y} = (y_{ij})$ is observed in the joint model $\mathrm{p}(\boldsymbol{y}, \boldsymbol{\psi}; \theta)$. Modeling means estimation of population and individual parameters, model diagnostics and model selection.

Throughout this section we are going to use the pharmacokinetics (PK) of warfarin (Holford, 1986) to illustrate various tasks that can be undertaken when modeling, and statistical methods to perform them. Observed longitudinal data (y_{ij}, $1 \leq i \leq N, 1 \leq j \leq n_i$) are the PK data introduced in the Example 4.11 and shown in Figure 4.26. We will consider a one-compartment PK model for oral administration, assuming first-order absorption and linear elimination processes (see Appendix C for a short introduction to PK modeling):

$$C(t, \phi) = \frac{D\, ka}{V\, ka - Cl}\left(e^{-(Cl/V)\,t} - e^{-ka\,t}\right). \tag{7.1}$$

Here, the PK parameters are $\phi = (ka, V, Cl)$. We then assume a normal distribution for the observed concentration, with a constant error model:

$$y_{ij} | \psi_i \sim \mathcal{N}(C(t_{ij}, \phi_i), a^2), \tag{7.2}$$

where $\psi_i = (\phi_i, a)$. The PK parameters (ka_i, V_i, Cl_i) are log-normally distributed. Furthermore, a linear relationship between log-weight and log-volume is assumed. The reference weight in the population is set as $w_{\rm pop} = 70$kg. We therefore have

$$\begin{aligned} \log(ka_i) &\sim \mathcal{N}(\log(ka_{\rm pop}), \omega_{ka}^2) \\ \log(V_i) &\sim \mathcal{N}(\log(V_{\rm pop}) + \beta_V \log(w_i/70), \omega_V^2) \\ \log(Cl_i) &\sim \mathcal{N}(\log(Cl_{\rm pop}), \omega_{Cl}^2). \end{aligned} \tag{7.3}$$

We will use this model, which we call $\mathcal{M}_0$, to illustrate the estimation methods presented in Section 7.2 and model evaluation methods in Section 7.3. We will see in Section 7.3.4 how to improve this model, thus providing an introduction to the model building process. How to load the data and implement models using MONOLIX is detailed in Appendix D.

Even though this chapter is dedicated to modeling, other tasks such as visualization and simulation deserve a mention. Indeed, first of all, before deciding to model data, it is essential to look at it, graphically. This is especially the case for longitudinal data when we want to see how an outcome varies with time or as a function of another variable. We may also want to visualize how individual covariates are distributed, detect if there are relationships between variables, compare data from different groups, etc. It may also be useful to be able to visualize the model itself by looking at how the structural model changes when we vary one or several parameters. This is important for truly understanding the structural model, i.e., what is behind the given mathematical equations, in particular when dealing with things such as complex dynamical systems defined by differential equations. Although essential, these data and model visualization tasks do not require any specific methods worth presenting here. Therefore, we will not consider them here, but tools for data and model exploration such as DATXPLORE and MLXPLORE are presented briefly in Appendix D.

Simulation is another important task, useful for example for simulating clinical trials. The process of clinical trial simulation (CTS) is known to be very helpful for improving the efficiency of the drug development process by allowing optimization of trial designs. It also makes possible the use of virtual patients to analyze drug effectiveness and safety (Holford et al., 2010). The simulation techniques we use for the models that interest us here do not involve any specific difficulties and are strongly linked to the hierarchical structure of the probabilistic models we use, as described in Chapter 3. They are used by Simulx – both an R and MATLAB function – that uses MLXTRAN for implementing models. Examples of the use of Simulx are provided in Appendix D.

7.2 Estimation

7.2.1 Maximum likelihood estimation of population parameters

Maximum likelihood estimation of the vector of population parameters θ consists of maximizing with respect to θ the *observed likelihood function* defined by

$$\mathcal{L}_{\boldsymbol{y}}(\theta) \stackrel{\text{def}}{=} \mathrm{p}(\boldsymbol{y};\theta) = \int \mathrm{p}(\boldsymbol{y},\boldsymbol{\psi};\theta)\,d\boldsymbol{\psi}. \tag{7.4}$$

Suppose that there exists a parameter vector θ^* such that observations have been generated by the model parametrized by θ^*, i.e., $\boldsymbol{y} \sim p_y(\cdot\,;\,\theta^*)$. Then, under very general conditions, maximum likelihood (ML) estimation possesses several attractive limit properties as the number of individuals N increases (Lehmann and Casella, 1998):

- consistency: the sequence of ML estimates converges in probability to the true parameter value θ^*.
- asymptotic normality: as the sample size increases, the distribution of the ML estimate tends to the normal distribution with mean θ^* and covariance matrix equal to the inverse of the Fisher information matrix (see Section 7.2.2).
- efficiency: it achieves the Cramer-Rao lower bound when N tends to infinity. This means that no consistent estimator has lower asymptotic mean squared error than the ML estimator.

The models of interest to us and for which we want to calculate the ML estimate are ones that combine a model for the observations (see Chapter 4) with a model for the individual parameters (see Chapter 5). One of the main goals in the population approach is to estimate the distribution of the individual parameters $\mathrm{p}(\psi_i;\theta)$. In particular, if the parameter vector ψ_i is normal, $\psi_i \sim \mathcal{N}(\psi_{\mathrm{pop}},\Omega)$, we would like to estimate the population parameter vector ψ_{pop} (which simultaneously represents the mean, median and mode of the distribution of ψ_i) and the variance-covariance matrix Ω.

Remark: If the distribution of ψ_i is the transformation of a normal one (e.g., log-normal, logit-normal), i.e., if there exists a function h such $h(\psi_i) \sim \mathcal{N}(h(\psi_{\mathrm{pop}}),\Omega)$, then it is important to note that:

- the ML estimate $\hat{\psi}_{\mathrm{pop}}$ of the reference parameter ψ_{pop} is usually neither the mean nor the mode of the estimated population distribution. It is in fact the median (see Appendix B, Proposition 1).

- the ML estimate of $h(\psi_{\rm pop})$ is $h(\hat{\psi}_{\rm pop})$. Thus, the estimated distribution of $h(\psi_i)$ is the normal distribution with mean $h(\hat{\psi}_{\rm pop})$.

After formally defining the ML estimate $\widehat{\theta}$ as the value that maximizes the integral defined in (7.4), we need to be able to calculate it. This task requires an algorithm to help us to maximize $\int \mathrm{p}(\boldsymbol{y}, \boldsymbol{\psi}; \theta)\, d\boldsymbol{\psi}$ with respect to θ. The stochastic approximation expectation-maximization (SAEM) algorithm as implemented in MONOLIX has appealing practical and theoretical properties. It has been shown to be extremely efficient for a wide variety of complex models: categorical data, count data, time-to-event data, mixture models, hidden Markov models, stochastic differential equation-based models and censored data. Furthermore, convergence of SAEM has been rigorously proved (Allassonnière et al., 2010; Delyon et al., 1999; Kuhn and Lavielle, 2005).

The SAEM algorithm and its implementation are described in Section 9.2. It is not necessary to completely master all parts of the algorithm in order to use it. However, in practical situations, it is important to keep in mind some of its key properties.

- SAEM is an iterative algorithm:
  - Initial estimates must be provided by the user. Even though SAEM is relatively insensitive to initial parameter values, it is always preferable to provide as good as possible initial values to minimize the number of iterations required and also increase the probability of converging to the global maximum of the likelihood.
  - SAEM as implemented in MONOLIX has two phases. The goal of the first is to get to a neighborhood of the solution in only a few iterations. A *simulated annealing* version of SAEM accelerates this process when the initial value is far from the actual solution. The second phase consists of convergence to the located maximum with behavior that becomes increasingly deterministic, like a gradient algorithm.

- SAEM is a stochastic algorithm:
  - We cannot claim that SAEM *always* converges (i.e., with probability 1) to the global maximum of the likelihood. We can only say that it converges under quite general hypotheses to a maximum – global or perhaps local – of the likelihood. A large number of simulation studies have shown that SAEM converges with high probability to a "good" solution – it is hoped the global maximum – after a small number of iterations.

– The trajectory of the outputs of SAEM depends on the sequence of random numbers used by the algorithm. This sequence is entirely determined by the "seed." In this way, two runs of SAEM using the same seed will produce exactly the same results. If different seeds are used, the trajectories will be different but convergence occurs to the same solution under quite general hypotheses.

Let us now use SAEM to calculate the ML estimate in our example. The vector of population parameters is

$$\theta = (ka_{\rm pop}, V_{\rm pop}, Cl_{\rm pop}, \beta_V, \omega_{ka}, \omega_V, \omega_{Cl}, a).$$

Running SAEM requires several choices to be made (initial estimates, number of iterations, number of Markov chains, simulated annealing, etc. See Section 9.2 for more details). Here, when we run SAEM using as initial value $\theta_0 = (1, 7, 0.2, 0, 1, 1, 1, 1)$ and the default settings proposed in MONOLIX, it converges easily and quickly to the ML estimate. Figure 7.1 displays the sequences of estimates (θ_k) computed after each SAEM iteration.

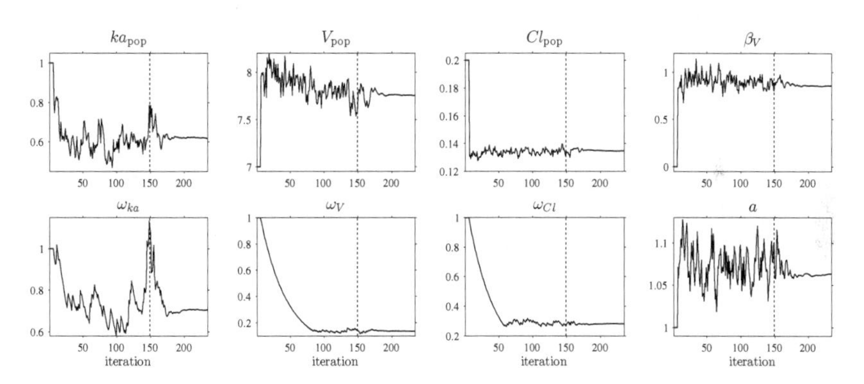

FIGURE 7.1: Convergence of SAEM. The vertical dotted line indicates where the algorithm switches from the first phase to the second.

The estimated values of the components of θ are:

```
ka_pop       0.615
V_pop        7.75
beta_V       0.859
Cl_pop       0.135
omega_ka     0.704
omega_V      0.136
omega_Cl     0.283
a            1.06
```

Remark: In this example, SAEM converges to the same solution even when provided with poor initial values for $ka_{\rm pop}$, $V_{\rm pop}$, $Cl_{\rm pop}$ such as

(1, 1, 1) or even (100, 100, 100). However, this appealing practical property of the algorithm should not stop modelers from trying to choose good initial values!

In general, we see that parameter estimation can actually be seen as estimating the reference values of the parameters and the standard deviations of the random effects. In addition to these summary values, Section 5.2 showed that it is useful to graphically represent each entire distribution for visualization's sake. Indeed, the interpretation of certain parameters is not always simple. Of course, we know what a normal distribution represents and in particular its mean, median and mode, which are in fact identical. However, these three measures of central tendency can be different for asymmetric distributions such as the log-normal one. Furthermore, interpreting dispersion terms such as ω_{ka}, ω_V and ω_{Cl} is not at all obvious when the parameter distributions are not normal. Figure 7.2 shows the probability distribution function (pdf) of the three PK parameters here. We see in particular that the distribution of ka_i clearly appears to be asymmetric. Our three measures of central tendency are quite different here, the mode, median and mean taking, respectively, the values 0.372, 0.615 and 0.788.

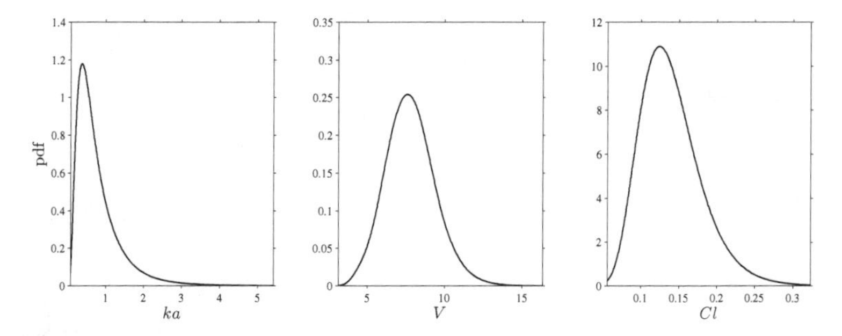

FIGURE 7.2: Estimated population distributions of the individual parameters of the model.

Remark: The coefficient of variation (CV) is the ratio of the standard deviation to the mean. For a parameter whose distribution is log-normal with parameters (μ, ω), we can show that $CV = \sqrt{e^{\omega^2} - 1}$. If ω^2 is fairly small, we can approximate the CV by ω. In our example, the CVs for ka, V and Cl are, respectively, 80%, 14% and 29%. We see that the approximation of CV by ω is quite good for V and Cl but not so much so for ka. Do not forget however that this approximation is only valid in the case of log-normal distributions. It does not carry over to any other distributions such as logit-normal or probit-normal ones. Only by looking at plots of their pdfs or by calculating some quantiles of interest can we begin to get an idea of dispersion in their parameters.

7.2.2 Estimation of the Fisher information matrix

The variance of the maximum likelihood estimate (MLE) $\hat{\theta}$, and thus confidence intervals, can be derived from the observed Fisher information matrix (FIM), itself derived from the observed likelihood (i.e., the pdf of observations $\boldsymbol{y}$):

$$I_{\boldsymbol{y}}(\hat{\theta}) \stackrel{\text{def}}{=} -\frac{\partial^2}{\partial \theta^2} \log(\mathcal{L}_{\boldsymbol{y}}(\hat{\theta})).$$

As can be seen in Appendix B.2, the variance-covariance matrix of $\hat{\theta}$ can then be estimated by the inverse of the observed FIM. Standard errors (s.e.) for each component of $\hat{\theta}$ are the standard deviations, i.e., the square root of the diagonal elements of the variance-covariance matrix.

A stochastic approximation algorithm using a Markov chain Monte Carlo (MCMC) algorithm is implemented in MONOLIX for estimating the FIM (see Section 9.4 for more details). This method is extremely general and can be used for many data and model types (continuous, categorical, time-to-event, mixtures, etc.). In the case of continuous data, it is also possible to use a method based on model linearization. This method is generally much faster than stochastic approximation and also gives good estimates of the FIM.

In the case of our example, results for the two methods are quite similar, so only those obtained with model linearization will be presented here. MONOLIX displays for each estimated parameter its estimated relative standard error (r.s.e.), i.e., the estimated standard error divided by the value of the estimated parameter.

```
warfarinPK_M0

              parameter      s.e. (lin)    r.s.e.(%)   p-value
ka_pop          0.615          0.14           23
V_pop           7.750          0.25            3
beta_V          0.859          0.16           18        3.1e-008
Cl_pop          0.135          0.0073          5
omega_ka        0.704          0.18           25
omega_V         0.136          0.028          21
omega_Cl        0.283          0.041          14
a               1.060          0.056           5
```

We can use the estimated standard error $\widehat{\text{s.e.}}(\hat{\beta}_V)$ to perform a Wald test of whether $\beta_V = 0$. In fact, under this hypothesis, the distribution of the Wald statistic $\hat{\beta}_V/\widehat{\text{s.e.}}(\hat{\beta}_V)$ can be approximated by a normal distribution with mean 0 and variance 1. The p-value of the Wald test displayed in the table is the value of $\mathbb{P}\Big(|\mathcal{N}(0,1)| > |\hat{\beta}_V|/\widehat{\text{s.e.}}(\hat{\beta}_V)\Big)$.

The FIM can also be used for detecting overparametrization of the structural model. This is because if the model is poorly identifiable, certain estimators will be relatively correlated and the FIM will be poorly conditioned and difficult to invert. Suppose, for example, that we want to fit a 3-compartment PK model (see Appendix C) to the same warfarin data. The distribution process is now characterized by five parameters (three volumes and two inter-compartmental clearances). The output is shown in the table.

```
          parameter     s.e. (lin)    r.s.e.(%)
ka_pop       0.603          0.14            24
Cl_pop       0.134         0.011             8
V1_pop         7.6           1.9            25
Q2_pop        13.4      7.6e+005     5.65e+006
V2_pop      0.0115           3.6     3.09e+004
Q3_pop         152      1.8e+007     1.18e+007
V3_pop       0.036           3.4     9.36e+003

______________________________________________
correlation matrix of the estimates(linearization)

Eigenvalues (min, max, max/min): 0.0039  2.2  5.5e+002
```

The parameters ka and Cl which characterize the absorption and eliminations processes and the volume $V1$ of the central compartment are still correctly estimated in this example but the large standard errors for the remaining parameters mean that the data does not allow us to estimate them well. We can also see that the correlation matrix of the estimates of the fixed effects is poorly conditioned due to strong dependencies between the parameters. We thus have an available empirical criterion for detecting a lack of identifiability in a model.

It is easy to build a confidence interval with level $1 - \alpha$ for the parameter ψ_{pop} starting from the s.e. obtained for that parameter:

$$CI_{1-\alpha}(\psi_{\text{pop}}) = [\hat{\psi}_{\text{pop}} + q_{\alpha/2}\widehat{\text{s.e.}}(\hat{\psi}_{\text{pop}}) \ , \ \hat{\psi}_{\text{pop}} + q_{1-\alpha/2}\widehat{\text{s.e.}}(\hat{\psi}_{\text{pop}})],$$

where q_α is the quantile of order α for a standard normal distribution.

When transformed normal distributions are used, it may sometimes be better to construct confidence intervals for parameters of the Gaussian model, then deduce those of the original parameter. Consider for example an individual parameter ψ_i such that $h(\psi_i) \sim \mathcal{N}(h(\psi_{\text{pop}}), \omega^2)$ where h is a monotonic transformation, and let $\mu_{\text{pop}} = h(\psi_{\text{pop}})$. We will see in Section 9.2 that it is this parametrization that is used in MONOLIX for estimating the model's parameters and their s.e. We can therefore construct a new confidence interval of level $1 - \alpha$ for μ_{pop}:

$$CI_{1-\alpha}(\mu_{\text{pop}}) = [\mu_{\text{pop},\alpha/2} \ , \ \mu_{\text{pop},1-\alpha/2}],$$

where $\mu_{\text{pop},\alpha/2} = \hat{\mu}_{\text{pop}} + q_{\alpha/2}\widehat{\text{s.e.}}(\hat{\mu}_{\text{pop}})$ and $\mu_{\text{pop},1-\alpha/2} = \hat{\mu}_{\text{pop}} +$

$q_{1-\alpha/2}\widehat{\text{s.e.}}(\hat{\mu}_{\text{pop}})$. We can then deduce a confidence interval for ψ_{pop}:

$$\widetilde{CI}_{1-\alpha}(\psi_{\text{pop}}) = [h^{-1}(\mu_{\text{pop},\alpha/2})\ ,\ h^{-1}(\mu_{\text{pop},1-\alpha/2})].$$

This helps us obtain asymmetric intervals and also to satisfy constraints such as when $\psi_{\text{pop}} > 0$ and we use a log-transform, or when $0 < \psi_{\text{pop}} < 1$ and we use a logit-transform.

In our running example, the s.e. for $\log(ka_{\text{pop}})$, $\log(V_{\text{pop}})$ and $\log(Cl_{\text{pop}})$ are, respectively, 0.2184, 0.0320 and 0.0538. The two tables show for each parameter the 90% confidence intervals obtained. These intervals are quite similar for V_{pop} and Cl_{pop} but a little different for ka_{pop}.

	$CI_{90\%}(\psi_{\text{pop}})$	
ka_{pop}	0.3942	0.8362
V_{pop}	7.3467	8.1629
Cl_{pop}	0.1229	0.1467

	$\widetilde{CI}_{90\%}(\psi_{\text{pop}})$	
ka_{pop}	0.4296	0.8811
V_{pop}	7.3573	8.1738
Cl_{pop}	0.1234	0.1473

Other parametrizations can be derived from the original one of ka, V, β_V, Cl. Suppose for instance that we want to estimate the half-life $t_{1/2} = \log(2)V/Cl$ instead of the clearance Cl. Using the estimated values for V_{pop} and Cl_{pop}, we find that the estimated population half-life is $\widehat{t_{1/2}}_{\text{pop}} = 39.88\,h$. Parameters ka and β_V are not affected by this transformation as there exists in effect a bijection between (V, Cl) and $(V, t_{1/2})$.

The variance-covariance matrix of the estimates of the new vector of fixed effects $(V_{\text{pop}}, t_{1/2\text{pop}})$ is $\tilde{\Gamma} = J^t \Gamma J$ (see Appendix B.2), where J is the Jacobian matrix for this transformation, i.e.,

$$J = \begin{pmatrix} 1 & \log(2)/Cl_{\text{pop}} \\ 0 & -\log(2)V_{\text{pop}}/Cl_{\text{pop}}^2 \end{pmatrix} = \begin{pmatrix} 1 & 5.1421 \\ 0 & -295.82 \end{pmatrix},$$

and Γ the variance of the estimates of $(V_{\text{pop}}, Cl_{\text{pop}})$ in the original parametrization:

$$\Gamma = 10^{-4}\begin{pmatrix} 615.34 & -1.2876 \\ -1.2876 & 0.5260 \end{pmatrix}.$$

We therefore obtain

$$\tilde{\Gamma} = \begin{pmatrix} 0.0615 & 0.3545 \\ 0.3545 & 6.6220 \end{pmatrix}.$$

The variance and therefore the s.e. remain unchanged for V_{pop}, while the s.e. of $\hat{t_{1/2}}_{\text{pop}}$ is $2.57\,h$.

As a final note, we remark that the Fisher information is also widely used in optimal experimental design (Fedorov and Leonov, 2013). Minimizing the variance of the estimator corresponds to maximizing the information. Consequently, estimators and designs can be evaluated by looking at certain summary statistics of the variance-covariance matrix such as the determinant and trace.

7.2.3 Bootstrapping

The bootstrap is a technique useful for estimating the distribution of statistics such as the empirical mean and variance without using asymptotic theory and with very few assumptions on the data distribution (Efron and Tibshirani, 1994). Suppose, for example, that we are looking to estimate the distribution of the empirical mean $\bar{x}$ of a sequence of independent and identically distributed (i.i.d.) random variables $\boldsymbol{x} = (x_1, x_2, \ldots, x_n)$ with mean μ. $\bar{x}$ is thus a random variable whose distribution and, in particular, variance depends on the distribution of the x_i. Bootstrapping consists of resampling the data with replacement to obtain $\boldsymbol{x}^{(1)} = (x_1^{(1)}, x_2^{(1)}, \ldots, x_n^{(1)})$ and computing the empirical mean $\bar{x}^{(1)}$ of $\boldsymbol{x}^{(1)}$. The same process is repeated M times and the M empirical means $\bar{x}^{(1)}$, $\bar{x}^{(2)}$, ..., $\bar{x}^{(M)}$ are then used to create an empirical estimate of the distribution of $\bar{x}$.

In the mixed effects model context, bootstrap methods have been proposed for estimating the standard errors of the population parameter estimates (Das and Krishen, 1999; Thai et al., 2014). Here we describe only the two most relevant methods: the *case bootstrap* and *parametric bootstrap.*

The case bootstrap consists of resampling with replacement from the entire dataset associated with each individual (covariates, design and observations); the original data is used to create M bootstrap resamples $\boldsymbol{y}^{(1)}$, ..., $\boldsymbol{y}^{(M)}$. We then estimate the model's parameters with these, following the same method used for the original data, leading to M vectors of estimated parameters $\hat{\theta}^{(1)}, \hat{\theta}^{(2)}, \ldots, \hat{\theta}^{(M)}$: for $m = 1, 2, \ldots M$,

$$\hat{\theta}^{(m)} = \arg\max_{\theta} \mathrm{p}(\boldsymbol{y}^{(m)}; \theta).$$

The empirical distribution of the $\hat{\theta}^{(m)}$ can then be used to estimate the distribution of $\hat{\theta}$.

The parametric bootstrap on the other hand consists of using the original design $(\boldsymbol{u}, \underline{\boldsymbol{t}})$ and covariates $\boldsymbol{c}$ of the N subjects for the M bootstrap samples. For each of these samples, the estimated model for the individual parameters is used for drawing N vectors of individual parameters, and the estimated model for the observations for drawing N

vectors of observations; i.e., for $m = 1, 2, \ldots, M$ and $i = 1, 2, \ldots, N$,

$$\psi_i^{(m)} \sim \mathrm{p}(\,\cdot\,;\; c_i, \hat{\theta})$$
$$y_i^{(m)} \sim \mathrm{p}(\,\cdot\,|\psi_i^{(m)};\; u_i, t_i).$$

As for the case bootstrap, population parameters are estimated using each bootstrap sample.

One of the most common reasons given to justify the use of the bootstrap is that it makes few hypotheses on the statistical model. This justification is debatable in the mixed effects context because it is precisely a parametric model being used to fit the observed data, one which involves strong hypotheses on both the distributions of the individual parameters and the observations. There is therefore no good reason why these assumptions used to compute population parameter estimates should not also be used to estimate the distribution of these estimates.

The parametric bootstrap is by definition based entirely on the use of a parametric model; it is clearly most useful when using parametric models with fixed designs. The parametric bootstrap helps answer the legitimate question of every modeler: "If I use this model, with what precision can I hope to estimate the model's parameters using the given data, and given the design used to generate them?"

From a statistical point of view, the question is to know whether asymptotic theory – which allows us in particular to approximate the distribution of estimators by a normal distribution with variance equal to the inverse of the FIM – is usable with finite sample sizes. It should be kept in mind that although bootstrapping is asymptotically consistent, it does not provide general finite-sample guarantees. Even though only the asymptotic properties of these estimators are theoretically known, their nonasymptotic properties can be investigated by simulation in the mixed effects model context (Thai et al., 2014).

Table 7.1 gives a comparison of the s.e. obtained using the FIM with those obtained using the bootstrap for the warfarin data. Here, $M = 1000$ bootstrap samples were used for each method.

We see that the case bootstrap gives quite different results from the other methods for certain parameters such as parameter a from the residual error model. This can partly be explained by the fact that the design is unbalanced (the number of observations per individual varies from 6 to 17). Consequently, the bootstrap samples involve different numbers of observations and are difficult to compare.

We can also see that the FIM gives estimates of the s.e. close to those obtained using parametric bootstrap and is therefore entirely suitable for investigating uncertainty in estimators associated with a given design.

TABLE 7.1: Standard errors of parameter estimates obtained using three different methods.

	ka	V	β_V	Cl	ω_{ka}	ω_V	ω_{Cl}	a
se_{FIM}	0.13	0.25	0.16	0.0072	0.17	0.028	0.040	0.056
se_{case}	0.24	0.31	0.17	0.0077	0.23	0.032	0.041	0.166
se_{param}	0.14	0.26	0.16	0.0084	0.19	0.034	0.039	0.060

se_{FIM}: Fisher info. matrix; se_{case}: case bootstrap; se_{param}: parametric bootstrap.

This can be seen more clearly in Figure 7.3 which shows the empirical distributions of the estimators $(\hat{\theta}^{(m)})$ obtained by parametric bootstrap. Here, the estimators have been centered using the "true" value $\widehat{\theta}$ used for the simulations and standardized by the s.e. estimated using the FIM. We see that for most parameters, this empirical distribution is quite close to the asymptotic one, i.e., the standard normal distribution.

Note that these useful statistical properties of the FIM have also been noted when working with PK (Thai et al., 2014), categorical data (Savic et al., 2011) and count data (Savic and Lavielle, 2009) models.

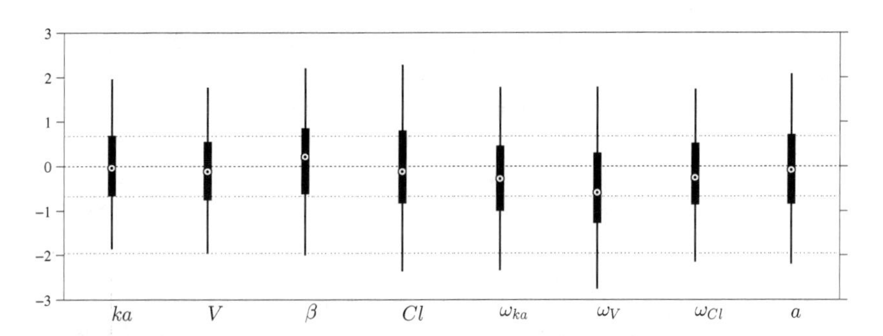

FIGURE 7.3: Empirical distribution of the standardized estimates $(\hat{\theta}^{(m)} - \widehat{\theta})/\widehat{\text{s.e.}}(\widehat{\theta})$. Dots are the medians of the distributions; extremities of the thick segments are the order 25% and 75% quantiles; extremities of the thinner lines are the order 2.5% and 97.5% quantiles. Dotted lines are the 2.5%, 25%, 50%, 75% and 97.5% quantiles of the standard normal distribution.

7.2.4 Bayesian estimation of population parameters

The *Bayesian approach* considers θ as a random vector with a *prior distribution* p_θ (Congdon, 2006; Gelman et al., 2003; Robert, 2007). We can then define the posterior distribution of θ:

$$\begin{aligned} \mathrm{p}(\theta|\boldsymbol{y}) &= \frac{\mathrm{p}(\theta)\mathrm{p}(\boldsymbol{y}|\theta)}{\mathrm{p}(\boldsymbol{y})} \\ &= \frac{\mathrm{p}(\theta)\int \mathrm{p}(\boldsymbol{y},\boldsymbol{\psi}|\theta)\,d\boldsymbol{\psi}}{\mathrm{p}(\boldsymbol{y})}. \end{aligned}$$

We can estimate this conditional distribution and derive statistics (posterior mean, standard deviation, quantiles, etc.) and the so-called *maximum a posteriori* (MAP) estimate of θ:

$$\begin{aligned} \hat{\theta}^{\mathrm{MAP}} &= \arg\max_{\theta} \mathrm{p}(\theta|\boldsymbol{y}) \\ &= \arg\max_{\theta} \left\{\mathcal{LL}_{\boldsymbol{y}}(\theta) + \log(\mathrm{p}(\theta))\right\}. \end{aligned}$$

The MAP estimate maximizes a penalized version of the observed likelihood. In other words, MAP estimation is the same as penalized maximum likelihood estimation. Suppose for instance that θ is a scalar parameter and the prior is a normal distribution with mean θ_0 and variance γ^2. Then, the MAP estimate is the solution of the following minimization problem:

$$\hat{\theta}^{\mathrm{MAP}} = \arg\min_{\theta} \left\{-2\mathcal{LL}_{\boldsymbol{y}}(\theta) + \frac{1}{\gamma^2}(\theta - \theta_0)^2\right\}.$$

This is a trade-off between the MLE which minimizes the deviance, $-2\mathcal{LL}_{\boldsymbol{y}}(\theta)$, and θ_0 which minimizes $(\theta - \theta_0)^2$. The weight given to the prior directly depends on the variance of the prior distribution: the smaller γ^2 is, the closer to θ_0 the MAP is. In the limiting case, $\gamma^2 = 0$; this means that θ is fixed at θ_0 and no longer needs to be estimated.

Both the Bayesian and frequentist approaches have their supporters and detractors. But rather than being dogmatic and following the same rule-book every time, we need to be pragmatic and ask the right methodological questions when confronted with a new problem. We have to remember that Bayesian methods have been extremely successful in recent times, in particular for numerical calculations. For instance, (Bayesian) MCMC methods allow us to estimate almost any conditional distribution from any hierarchical model, whereas frequentist approaches such as maximum likelihood estimation can be much more difficult to implement.

All things considered, the problem comes down to knowing whether the data contains sufficient information to answer a given question, and whether some other information may be available to help answer it. This is the essence of the art of modeling: find the right compromise between the confidence we have in the data and our prior knowledge of the problem. Each problem is different and requires a specific approach. For instance, if all the patients in a clinical trial have essentially the same weight, it is pointless to estimate a relationship between weight and the model's PK parameters using the trial data. A modeler would be better served trying to use prior information based on physiological knowledge rather than just some statistical criterion.

Generally speaking, if prior information is available it should be used, on the condition of course that it is relevant. Systematically using priors for parameters is not always meaningful. Can we reasonable suppose that we have access to such information? For continuous data for example, what does putting a prior on the residual error model's parameters mean in reality? A reasoned statistical approach consists of including prior information only for certain parameters (those for which we have real prior information) and having confidence in the data for the others.

MONOLIX allows this hybrid approach which reconciles the Bayesian and frequentist approaches. A given parameter can be

- a fixed constant if we have absolute confidence in its value or the data does not allow it to be estimated, essentially due to lack of identifiability.
- estimated by maximum likelihood, either because we have great confidence in the data or no information on the parameter.
- estimated by introducing a prior and calculating the MAP estimate or estimating the posterior distribution.

We put aside dealing with the fixed components of θ in the following. Here are some possible scenarios:

1. *Combined maximum likelihood and maximum a posteriori estimation*: split θ into (θ_E, θ_M) where θ_E are the components of θ to be estimated with MLE and θ_M those with a prior distribution whose posterior distribution is to be maximized. Then, the following $(\hat{\theta}_E, \hat{\theta}_M)$ maximizes the penalized likelihood of (θ_E, θ_M):

$$\begin{aligned}(\hat{\theta}_E, \hat{\theta}_M) &= \arg\max_{\theta_E, \theta_M} \log(\mathrm{p}(\boldsymbol{y}, \theta_M; \theta_E)) \\ &= \arg\max_{\theta_E, \theta_M} \left\{\mathcal{LL}_{\boldsymbol{y}}(\theta_E, \theta_M) + \log(\mathrm{p}(\theta_M))\right\},\end{aligned}$$

   where $\mathcal{LL}_{\boldsymbol{y}}(\theta_E, \theta_M) \stackrel{\text{def}}{=} \log\left(\mathrm{p}(\boldsymbol{y}|\theta_M; \theta_E)\right)$.

2. *Combined maximum likelihood and posterior distribution estimation*:

split θ into (θ_E, θ_R) where θ_E are the components of θ to be estimated with MLE and θ_R those with a prior distribution whose posterior distribution is to be estimated. The following strategy can be used for estimating θ_E and θ_R:

a. Compute the maximum likelihood of θ_E:

$$\begin{aligned}\hat{\theta}_E &= \arg\max_{\theta_E} \log(\mathrm{p}(\boldsymbol{y}; \theta_E)) \\ &= \arg\max_{\theta_E} \int \mathrm{p}(\boldsymbol{y}, \theta_R; \theta_E) d\theta_R.\end{aligned}$$

b. Estimate the conditional distribution $\mathrm{p}(\theta_R | \boldsymbol{y}; \hat{\theta}_E)$.

It is then straightforward to extend this approach to more complex situations where some components of θ are estimated with MLE, others using MAP estimation and others still by estimating their conditional distributions.

Let us return to our running example, in which the parameter ka is the hardest to estimate by maximum likelihood. This is due to a lack of information in the data as seen in Figure 4.26: 19 of the 32 patients have no measured data in the first 24 hours after taking the drug. These subjects therefore give little information on the absorption process for the drug and thus ka_{pop}. Now suppose that we know that the value of ka_{pop} is close to 1. We can then introduce a log-normal prior for ka_{pop}:

$$\log(ka_{\text{pop}}) \sim \mathcal{N}(\log(1), \gamma^2).$$

No other prior is used for the other model parameters; they will therefore be estimated by maximum likelihood.

MONOLIX allows us to compute the MAP estimate of ka_{pop} for various values of γ. As expected, the mode of the posterior distribution converges to the maximum likelihood estimate of ka_{pop} when γ increases.

γ	0	0.02	0.04	0.1	0.3	$+\infty$
$\hat{ka}_{\text{pop}}^{\text{MAP}}$	1	0.991	0.963	0.809	0.623	0.615

Using the same prior distributions, we can now estimate the posterior distributions of ka_{pop}. Figure 7.4 shows that the posterior distribution converges to the prior distribution when the standard deviation γ decreases.

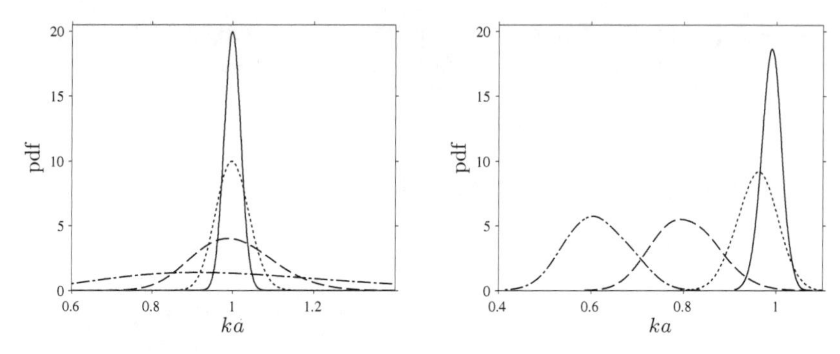

FIGURE 7.4: Prior distributions (left) and posterior distributions (right) of ka_{pop} for different values of γ. Solid line: $\gamma = 0.02$, dotted line: $\gamma = 0.03$, dashed line: $\gamma = 0.2$, dash-dot line: $\gamma = 0.3$.

7.2.5 Estimation of the individual parameters

Once θ has been estimated, the conditional distribution $\mathrm{p}(\psi_i|y_i;\hat{\theta})$ of the vector of individual parameters ψ_i can be estimated for each individual i using the Metropolis-Hastings (MH) algorithm described in Section 9.3. For each i, this algorithm generates a sequence $(\psi_i^{(k)}, 1 \leq k \leq K)$ which converges in distribution to the conditional distribution $\mathrm{p}(\psi_i|y_i;\hat{\theta})$ and can be used for estimating any summary statistic of it (mean, standard deviation, quantiles, etc.).

The MH algorithm therefore allows us to define an initial estimator of the individual parameter ψ_i that approximates the conditional mean $\mathbb{E}(\psi_i|y_i;\hat{\theta})$:

$$\hat{\psi}_i^{\text{mean}} = \frac{1}{K}\sum_{k=1}^{K} \psi_i^{(k)}.$$

We could also define as estimator of ψ_i the mode of the conditional distribution:

$$\hat{\psi}_i^{\text{mode}} = \arg\max_{\psi_i} \mathrm{p}(\psi_i|y_i;\hat{\theta}).$$

The choice of using the conditional mean $\hat{\psi}_i^{\text{mean}}$ or conditional mode $\hat{\psi}_i^{\text{mode}}$ is arbitrary. By default, MONOLIX uses the conditional mode for computing predictions, taking the philosophy that the "most likely" values of the individual parameters are the most suited for computing the "most likely" predictions. Figure 7.5 shows the individual concentrations predicted by the model for three individuals whose individual parameters have been estimated by their conditional modes.

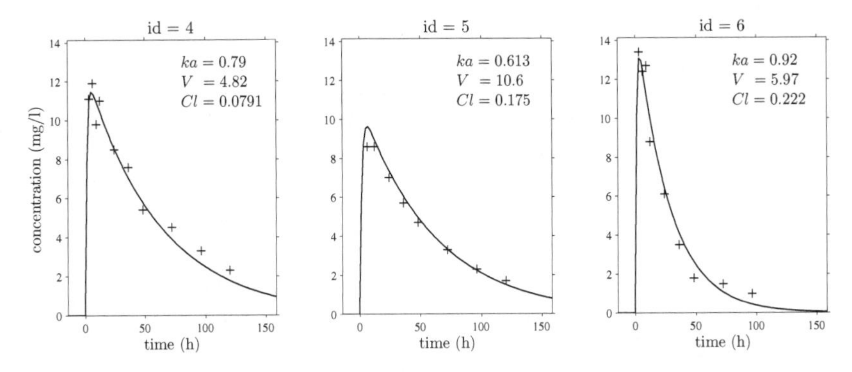

FIGURE 7.5: Observed and predicted concentrations for 3 individuals using the estimated conditional modes of the individual PK parameters.

Remark: In this example, the use of conditional means estimated by MONOLIX gives predictions close to those obtained using conditional modes.

This approach, consisting of estimating the population parameter vector θ using the data (e.g., ML estimator) then using conditional distributions for each individual parameter, can be seen as an *empirical Bayes* approach (Casella, 1985; Gelman et al., 2003). In effect, we suppose that for each observation vector y_i we have a parametric distribution indexed by some parameter ψ_i. In the Bayesian context, we give ψ_i a *prior* distribution p_{ψ_i} which leads us to be able to define a posterior distribution $p_{\psi_i|y_i}$. In the population approach, the prior p_{ψ_i} is a parametric distribution indexed by a vector of *hyper-parameters* θ which we estimate using a maximum likelihood approach on the data. We will see in Section 7.3 that outputs generated from the conditional distributions $\mathrm{p}(\psi_i|y_i;\hat{\theta})$ should be used, rather than conditional means or modes, to construct model diagnostic tools.

7.3 Model evaluation

7.3.1 Introduction

Defining the expression "model evaluation" is a harder task than it may appear at first glance (Comets and Brendel, 2010). Intuitively, it would seem to suggest evaluating the performance of a model based on the observed data, the same data that was used to build the model. This may or may not be reasonable, but what do we mean then by the "performance" of a model?

Do we mean its ability to characterize and explain the phenomena being studied, in which case the goal is to use the model to understand the phenomena? Or do we mean the model's predictive performance when the model is used to predict the phenomena's behavior, either in the future or under new experimental conditions?

What it comes down to is this: do we want to use the model to understand or to predict? This is the key question to ask before even starting to think about what tools to use and tasks to execute.

Here, we will be for the most part focused on the ability of a model to explain the phenomena and data. Therefore, the first goal will be to check whether the data are in agreement with the model, and vice versa. In this process, model diagnostics can be used to eliminate model candidates that do not seem capable of reproducing the observed data (Comets and Brendel, 2010; Karlsson and Savic, 2007). As is the usual case in statistics, it is not because a model has not been rejected that it is necessarily the "true" one. All that we can say is that the experimental data does not allow us to reject it. It is merely one of perhaps many models that cannot be rejected. Indeed, we can usually find several models that get past this first diagnostic step and are therefore not rejected.

What to do, then, when several possible models are retained? Well, we can try to select the "best" one (or best ones if no leader distinguishes itself from the rest). This means developing a model selection process which allows us to compare models. But with what criteria?

In a purely explanatory context, Occam's razor is a useful parsimony principle which states that among competing hypotheses, the one with the fewest assumptions should be selected. In the modeling context, this means that among valid competing models, the most simple one should be selected.

Model diagnostic tools are for the most part graphical, i.e., visual; we "see" when something is not right between a chosen model and the data it is hypothesized to describe. Model selection tools, on the other hand, are analytical: we calculate the value of some criterion that allows us to compare models with each other. However, it is absolutely critical to keep in mind the limits of such tools. They are not decision-making tools. It is not a p-value or some information criterion that will automatically allow a decision as to what model to choose. It is always the modeler who must have the last word! This person uses the model diagnostics and selection tools in order to guide his choice, but in the end, it is he who must make the final decision.

Here, we will not look at model selection techniques based on the various models' predictive performances. One such approach consists of splitting the data into three sets: a *learning set* for fitting the model, a *validation set* for choosing between models and a *test set* to assess the quality of the predictions made by the chosen model (Hastie et al., 2011). Instead, we will only consider *internal evaluation*, where the same data set is used for building the model and validating it.

Throughout this chapter, we will illustrate the techniques we introduce with MONOLIX on the warfarin PK example. This does not mean a complete presentation of all diagnostic plots available in MONOLIX along with all their options, but more of a run through some of them in order to illustrate a typical model diagnostics workflow.

7.3.2 Model diagnostics

7.3.2.1 Model diagnostics and statistical tests

Suppose first that a model has been defined by a modeler and its parameters either chosen or estimated. What we call the "model" is therefore a joint probability distribution along with some parameter values. Let us note $\mathcal{M}_0$ the model we wish to evaluate. We place ourselves in the framework of statistical testing and would like to perform the following hypothesis test (Comets and Brendel, 2010):

$$H_0: \quad \text{``}\mathcal{M} = \mathcal{M}_0\text{''} \qquad \text{vs} \qquad H_1: \quad \text{``}\mathcal{M} \neq \mathcal{M}_0\text{''}.$$

"Passing" the test does not mean that we accept H_0 but rather that we do not reject it. We will use the same point of view for model diagnostics whereby we eliminate model candidates that do not seem capable of reproducing the observed data, i.e., models for which we conclude that $\mathcal{M} \neq \mathcal{M}_0$.

Remarks: Running a statistical test only makes sense when we have doubts on the hypothesis of retaining a model. If it is clear, for example, from the beginning that the structural model is completely misspecified (e.g., we use a linear function of time even though curvature is clearly visible in the data), any basic goodness-of-fit plot (individual fits, observations vs predictions, residuals, etc.) will detect this misspecification without doubt and without the need to evaluate the probability of making a mistake.

To put statistical tests into practice, we usually construct a test statistic $T(\boldsymbol{y})$ which is a function of the observations for which we are able to calculate a distribution under the null hypothesis H_0. For a given significance level α, we then define a rejection region R_α such that:

$$\mathbb{P}_{H_0}(T(\boldsymbol{y}) \in R_\alpha) = \alpha.$$

Thus, α is the probability of incorrectly rejecting the null hypothesis H_0. The difficulty in creating and using such tests comes mainly from two areas:

- We need to be capable of calculating the distribution of the test statistic $T(\boldsymbol{y})$ under H_0 in order to carefully track the significance level, i.e., ensure that the probability of incorrectly rejecting H_0 is indeed α.
- Being able to control the type I error α is of no interest if the test has low power, i.e., the probability of correctly rejecting H_0 is low. Rejecting H_0 means that the model is found to be misspecified. The procedure needs to be able to detect different types of misspecification.

In the current context, the first point is clearly a problem. Due to the complexity of the models in which we are interested, it is impossible to analytically calculate the distribution of a function of the observations, even for something as simple as the empirical mean $\overline{\boldsymbol{y}} = \sum_{i,j} y_{ij} / \sum_i n_i$. Using limit theorems to approximate such distributions is also essentially hopeless. Perhaps the most powerful, general and precise solution we have available to us is Monte Carlo simulation:

- Generate independent replicates $\boldsymbol{y}^{(1)}, \boldsymbol{y}^{(2)}, \ldots, \boldsymbol{y}^{(L)}$ of the original data $\boldsymbol{y}$ under model $\mathcal{M}_0$ using the same design and covariates as in the original data.
- Calculate the L statistics $T(\boldsymbol{y}^{(1)}), T(\boldsymbol{y}^{(2)}), \ldots, T(\boldsymbol{y}^{(L)})$.
- Estimate the distribution of $T(\boldsymbol{y})$ under $\mathcal{M}_0$ with the empirical distribution of the $T(\boldsymbol{y}^{(\ell)})$.

The estimation error essentially depends on the number L of simulated data sets. We must therefore choose L large enough so that this error is negligible. This solves part of the problem. But it remains hard to define a rejection region R_α if the test statistic is multidimensional. We can of course calculate relevant prediction intervals for each component of $T(\boldsymbol{y})$ individually, but this does not really help us define a real multidimensional rejection region.

Consequently, diagnostic methods are essentially visual: we compare the observed statistic $T(\boldsymbol{y})$ with the expected distribution under $\mathcal{M}_0$ by graphically displaying (for example) 90% or 95% prediction intervals for each component of $T(\boldsymbol{y})$.

The second point mentioned is also problematic because we need to decide what $\mathcal{M} \neq \mathcal{M}_0$ means, i.e., H_0 being false. Does it mean that the structural model is misspecified? Or the distribution of the random effects, the residual error model, the covariate model? There are so many ways in which a model can be misspecified that we cannot realistically expect to be able to create one unique statistic sufficiently powerful to detect all of them at once. We therefore prefer to construct several different test statistics, i.e., several graphical diagnostics tools, each good at dealing with one particular type of misspecification. It is then the combination of all these tools that will make up our test; we can fairly reasonably hope that a misspecified model will not succeed in passing through this filter.

7.3.2.2 Some diagnostic plots based on observed data

Let us now look at several types of diagnostic plots based on the data, and apply them to our warfarin PK example.

Individual fits: In the continuous data model $y_{ij} = f(t_{ij}; \psi_i) + a\varepsilon_{ij}$, estimation of the population parameters ψ_{pop} and individual parameters ψ_i allows us to compute for each individual:

- $f(t; \hat{\psi}_{\text{pop}})$, the predicted profile given by the estimated population model.
- $f(t; \hat{\psi}_i)$, the predicted profile given by the estimated individual model where $\hat{\psi}_i$ is an estimate of ψ_i (see Section 7.2.5). We use the conditional mode in this example.

Figure 7.6 shows for several individuals these two curves for the predicted concentration. There is evidence of inter-individual variability in the kinetics, and clearly these plots do not allow us to reject the proposed PK model since the fits seem acceptable. The same types of fits are obtained for the rest of the 32 subjects (not shown here).

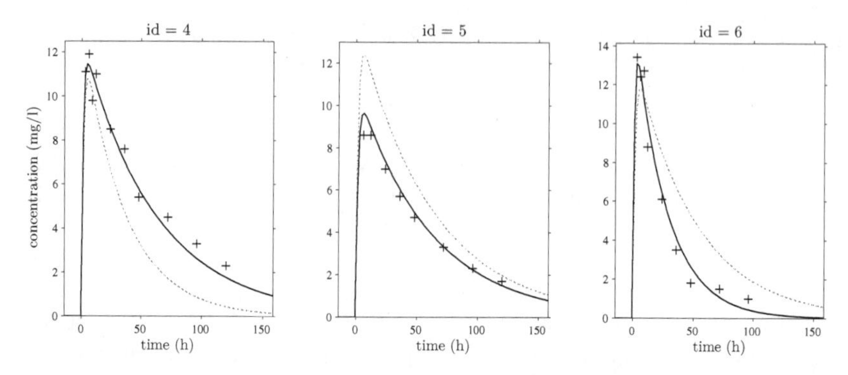

FIGURE 7.6: Individual fits for three patients obtained with the estimated individual parameters (solid line) and estimated population parameters (dotted line).

Observations vs predictions: The population and individual models also allow us to calculate predictions $f(t_{ij}; \hat{\psi}_{\text{pop}})$ and $f(t_{ij}; \hat{\psi}_i)$ for each individual at the observation times t_{ij}.

Figure 7.7 shows observations vs predictions and reveals no obvious misspecification. However, looking attentively at the right-hand plot, which compares observations with the individual predictions, we notice that some nonzero predictions correspond to concentrations of zero. We therefore suspect that there is a lag-time, i.e., a delay between administration and absorption of the drug, which would explain these concentrations. We also wonder whether the choice of a constant error model is correct because the amplitude of the residual errors seems to increase along with the predicted concentration.

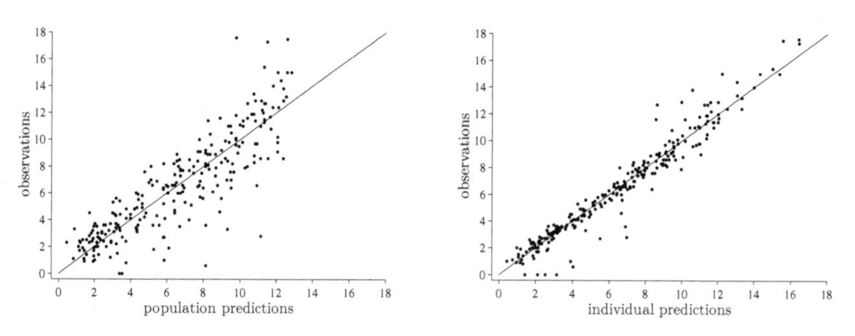

FIGURE 7.7: Observations versus predictions using the population model (left) and individual models (right).

We now need to see whether these suspicions concerning the structural and residual error models can be confirmed in other diagnostic plots.

Residuals: Several types of residuals can be defined.

1. *Individual weighted residuals* (IWRES_{ij}) are estimates of the standardized residual (ε_{ij}) based on individual predictions:

$$\text{IWRES}_{ij} = \frac{y_{ij} - f(t_{ij}; \hat{\psi}_i)}{g(t_{ij}; \hat{\psi}_i)}.$$

If the residual errors are assumed to be correlated, the individual weighted residuals can be decorrelated by multiplying each individual vector $\text{IWRES}_i = (\text{IWRES}_{ij}, 1 \leq j \leq n_i)$ by $\hat{R}_i^{-1/2}$, where $\hat{R}_i$ is the estimated correlation matrix of the vector of residuals $(\varepsilon_{ij}, 1 \leq j \leq n_i)$.

2. *Population weighted residuals* (PWRES_{ij}) are defined as the normalized difference between the observations and their mean. Let $y_i = (y_{ij}, 1 \leq j \leq n_i)$ be the vector of observations for subject i. The mean of y_i is the vector $\mathbb{E}(y_i) = (\mathbb{E}(f(t_{ij}; \psi_i), 1 \leq j \leq n_i)$. Let V_i be the $n_i \times n_i$ variance-covariance matrix of y_i. The ith vector of population weighted residuals $\text{PWRES}_i = (\text{PWRES}_{ij}, 1 \leq j \leq n_i)$ is therefore defined as

$$\text{PWRES}_i = V_i^{-1/2}(y_i - \mathbb{E}(y_i)).$$

$\mathbb{E}(y_i)$ and V_i are unknown in practice but can be estimated by Monte Carlo simulation.

3. *Normalized prediction distribution errors* (NPDE_{ij}) are a non-parametric version of PWRES_{ij} based on a rank statistic (Comets et al., 2008). For any (i, j), let $F_{ij} = F_{PWRES_{ij}}(\text{PWRES}_{ij})$ where $F_{PWRES_{ij}}$ is the cumulative distribution function (cdf) of PWRES_{ij}. The distribution of F_{ij} is by definition the uniform distribution on $[0, 1]$. The distribution of $\Phi^{-1}(F_{ij})$ is therefore the standard normal distribution.[1] NPDEs are defined as an empirical estimation of $\Phi^{-1}(F_{ij})$ where the F_{ij} are obtained through Monte Carlo simulation: a large number of replicates $\boldsymbol{y}^{(1)}, \boldsymbol{y}^{(2)}, \ldots, \boldsymbol{y}^{(K)}$ of the original data $\boldsymbol{y}^{obs}$ are drawn under model $\mathcal{M}_0$ and F_{ij} estimated by

$$\hat{F}_{ij} = \frac{1}{K} \sum_{k=1}^{K} \mathbb{I}_{y_{ij}^{(k)} \leq y_{ij}^{obs}}.$$

[1] Φ is the cdf of this standard normal distribution.

The NPDEs are then defined as $\text{NPDE}_{ij} = \Phi^{-1}(\hat{F}_{ij})$.

Under H_0, i.e., under model $\mathcal{M}_0$, these three sequences should behave as independent standardized normal random variables. We see in Figure 7.8 that both the IWRES and NPDEs suggest that the model is misspecified. In particular we see that the amplitudes of the residuals are particularly large around 5-10 h, i.e., when the concentration is at its largest. This tends to confirm that a proportional component needs to be added to the error model.

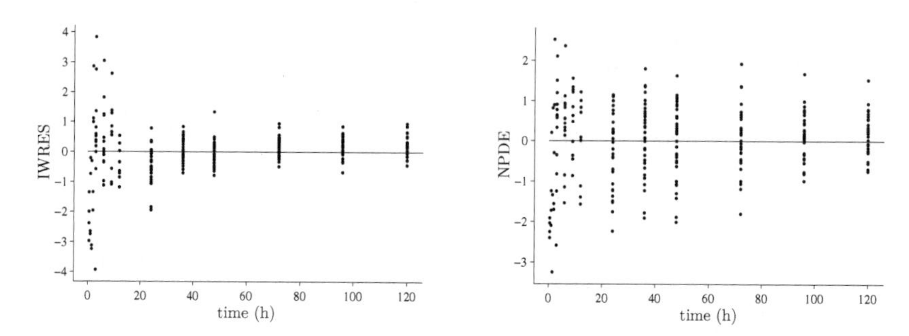

FIGURE 7.8: Individual weighted residuals (left) and normalized prediction distribution errors (right).

The distributions of these residuals can be summarized by computing empirical quantiles for successive time intervals. Figure 7.9 shows the order 10%, 50% and 90% quantiles of the IWRES and NPDE. The 90% prediction intervals given by the model for these quantiles are also displayed. These plots are more informative than the original residual plots; we can now reasonably conclude that the behavior of the three quantiles is not what is expected under $\mathcal{M}_0$. In particular, a proportional component in the residual error model appears not to have been taken into account.

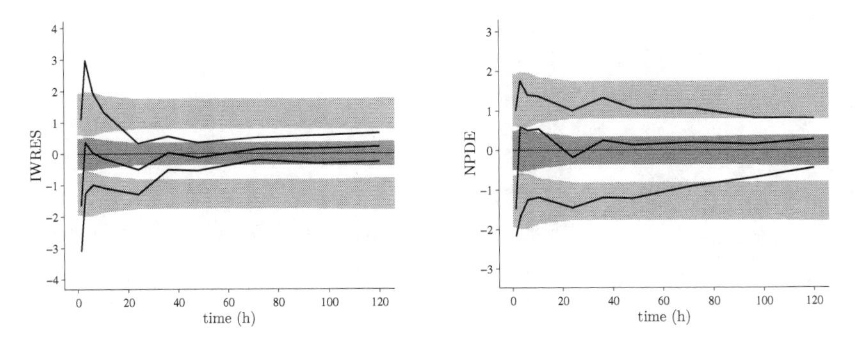

FIGURE 7.9: Individual weighted residuals (left) and normalized prediction distribution errors (right). The empirical quantiles of order 10%, 50% and 90% are displayed (solid lines) with their respective 90% prediction intervals.

Visual predictive checks: A visual predictive check (VPC) is a diagnostic tool well-suited to continuous data. It allows us to summarize in the same graphic the structural and statistical models by computing several quantiles of the empirical distribution of the data after having regrouped them into bins over successive intervals. Then, prediction intervals for these quantiles under $\mathcal{M}_0$ are estimated using Monte Carlo. The procedure for constructing basic VPCs is detailed in Section 9.7. It is of interest to note that several authors have proposed modifications in order to take into account large variability in dosage or covariates (Bergstrand et al., 2011; Post et al., 2008).

In our example, the structural model seems to be correct except slightly after $t = 0$ where the model overestimates the concentration. This is another sign that there may be a lag-time. The statistical model also exhibits some incoherencies when the concentration decreases after 60 hours. In particular, the three quantiles obtained using the observations appear much closer together than the model $\mathcal{M}_0$ would suggest. This adds weight to the suggestion that a proportional component should be added to the error model.

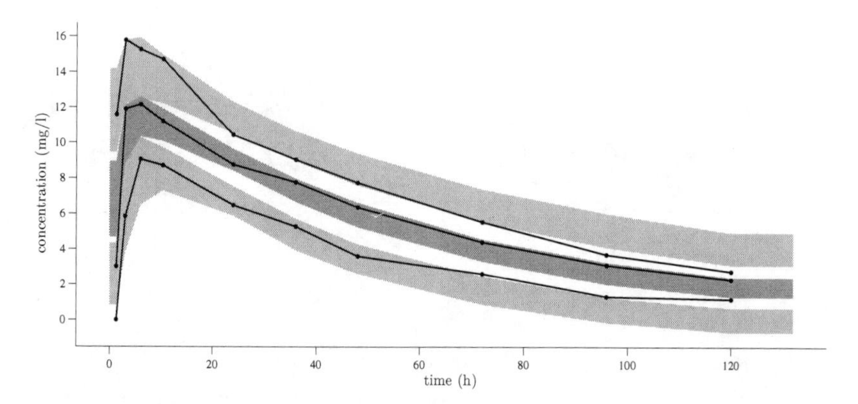

FIGURE 7.10: Visual predictive check. 90% prediction intervals and observed quantiles of order 10%, 50% and 90%.

7.3.2.3 Diagnostic plots based on the individual parameters

Diagnostic plots constructed using only the observations are useful for looking at the distribution p_y of the observations, but do not help with testing hypotheses made on the nonobserved individual parameters concerning their distributions, covariate models, etc. One possible solution is to estimate the individual parameters (using, for example, the conditional mode) and then use these estimates to create new diagnostic tools. This strategy is only useful when the individual parameters have been estimated well.

If instead the data does not contain enough information to estimate certain individual parameters well, individual estimates are all shrunk towards the same population value, which is the mode of the population distribution of the parameter if we are using the conditional mode. For a parameter ψ_i which is a function of a random effect η_i, we can quantify this phenomena by defining the so-called η-shrinkage as

$$\eta\text{-shrinkage} = 1 - \frac{\widehat{\mathrm{Var}}\,(\hat{\eta}_i)}{\mathrm{Var}\,(\eta_i)},$$

where $\widehat{\mathrm{Var}}\,(\hat{\eta}_i)$ is the empirical variance of the $\hat{\eta}_i$'s and $\hat{\eta}_i$ an estimate of η_i. This shrinkage phenomenon is simple to understand because the conditional distribution $p_{\eta_i|y_i}$ of η_i is defined by the product $p_{y_i|\eta_i}p_{\eta_i}$. Saying that the observations y_i provide little information about η_i means that the conditional distribution of y_i has reduced importance in the construction of $p_{\eta_i|y_i}$. The mode and the mean of $p_{\eta_i|y_i}$ will therefore be close to 0, which is both the mode and mean of p_{η_i}. This results is a high level of shrinkage (close to 1) whenever $\text{Var}(\hat{\eta}_i) \ll \text{Var}(\eta_i)$.

Estimates of the ψ_i are therefore biased because they do not correctly reflect the marginal distribution p_{ψ_i} (in particular, their variance is much reduced). A particularly effective solution is to simulate the individual parameters ψ_i with the conditional distribution $p_{\psi_i|y_i}$ rather than taking the mode. The resulting estimator is unbiased under H_0 in the following sense:

$$\begin{aligned} \text{p}(\psi_i) &= \int \text{p}(\psi_i|y_i)\text{p}(y_i)d\,y_i \\ &= \mathbb{E}_{y_i}\left(\text{p}(\psi_i|y_i)\right). \end{aligned} \tag{7.5}$$

This relationship is a fundamental one when considering inverse problems, incomplete data models, mixed effects models, etc. So what does it imply exactly? Well, if we randomly draw a vector y_i of observations for an individual in a population and then generate a vector ψ_i using the conditional distribution $p_{\psi_i|y_i}$, the distribution of ψ_i is the population distribution p_{ψ_i}. In other words, even if each ψ_i is simulated using its own conditional distribution, the fact of pooling them allows us to look at them as if they were a sample from p_{ψ_i}, i.e., the marginal distribution p_{ψ_i} is a mixture of conditional distributions $p_{\psi_i|y_i}$.

The procedure is therefore as follows: we generate several values from each conditional distribution $p_{\psi_i|y_i}$ using the MH algorithm described in Section 9.3, and use them in addition to the observations in order to build various diagnostic plots.

<u>The distributions of the individual parameters:</u> Hypotheses we make about the distributions of the individual parameters can be tested by visually comparing the pdf of the pre-selected distribution of each parameter with the empirical distribution of that parameter simulated with the conditional distribution $p_{\psi_i|y_i}$ for each individual.

Figure 7.11 shows for each model parameter ψ the pdf $p_{\psi}(\cdot;\hat{\theta})$ obtained from the estimated population parameters and the empirical distribution (presented as a histogram) of the individual parameters (ψ_i) where each ψ_i has been simulated with its own conditional distribution $p_{\psi_i|y_i}$. These graphics, which use the simulated individual parameter values, can be used as a diagnostic tool for testing the distributions of the individual parameters. Looking at the three of them, we cannot reject the hypothesis that the individual parameters come from the log-normal distributions defined in the model. Furthermore, we can show that under H_0, each η-shrinkage computed using the simulated parameters is a random variable with mean 0 and variance of approximately $1/N$. Here, the values of the η-shrinkages are not significantly different from 0.

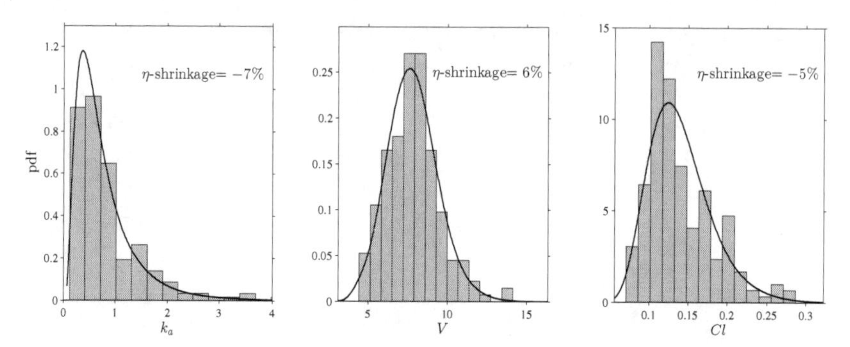

FIGURE 7.11: Estimated population distributions of the individual parameters of the model (solid line) and the empirical distributions of the individual parameters simulated with their conditional distributions (histograms).

The empirical distributions of the conditional modes of the individual parameters are displayed Figure 7.12. These plots are of very little interest as diagnostic plots. Indeed, the large η-shrinkage for ka does not mean that the model is misspecified, but that the data does not allow us to correctly recover the individual absorption rate constants.

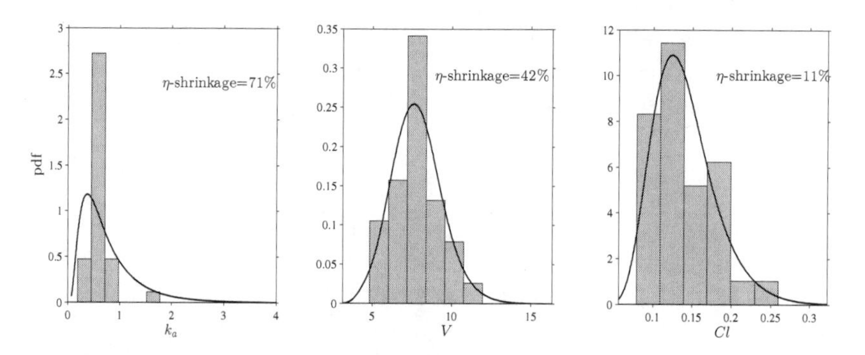

FIGURE 7.12: Estimated population distributions of the individual parameters of the model (solid line) and the empirical distributions of the individual parameters estimated as the mode of the conditional distributions (histograms).

<u>The covariate model</u>: The model assumes that the only relationship between the individual parameters and the covariates is a linear one between the log-weight and log-volume. We can then display the individual parameters simulated with the conditional distributions as a function of the various covariates in order to see whether this hypothesis is valid. Figure 7.13 clearly shows that the log-volume increases with weight. We

also see that the log-clearance seems to increase with weight. It is difficult to confirm absolutely categorically from these plots that the covariate model is misspecified. We can merely say that the statistical model "maybe" needs to take into account the fact that both predicted volume and clearance increase with weight and that this new model deserves to be compared with the current one.

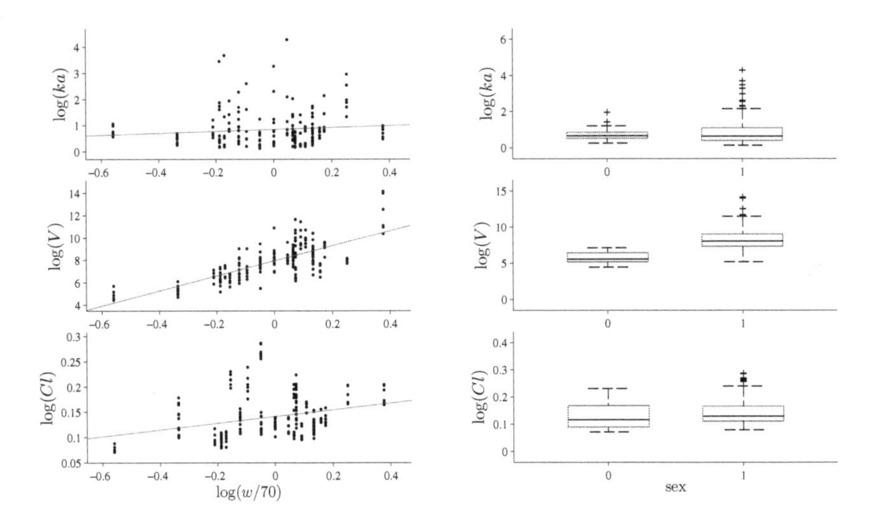

FIGURE 7.13: Relationships between the individual parameters and the covariates: transformed weight $\log(w_i/70)$ on the left and sex on the right. Each individual parameter has been drawn from its individual conditional distribution.

We also remark that V seems to have different distributions depending on gender. The weight being strongly related to gender, it is logical that this is the case, but it does not imply that gender brings extra information that can help explain variability in V and should therefore be included in the covariate model. Another plot that is useful for evaluating the covariate model is the one that shows the random effects, rather than the individual parameters, as a function of the covariates. In effect, under H_0 the distribution of the random effects does not depend on the covariates; they are i.i.d. normal variables with mean 0.

Figure 7.14 shows that the relationship between weight and volume has been well integrated into the model because the random effects $(\eta_{V,i})$ are no longer related to weight. They have no relationship with gender either; there is therefore no reason to reject the covariate model for V based on these plots. On the other hand, we see that there is a relationship between weight and $\eta_{Cl,i}$; a new covariate model for Cl should be investigated.

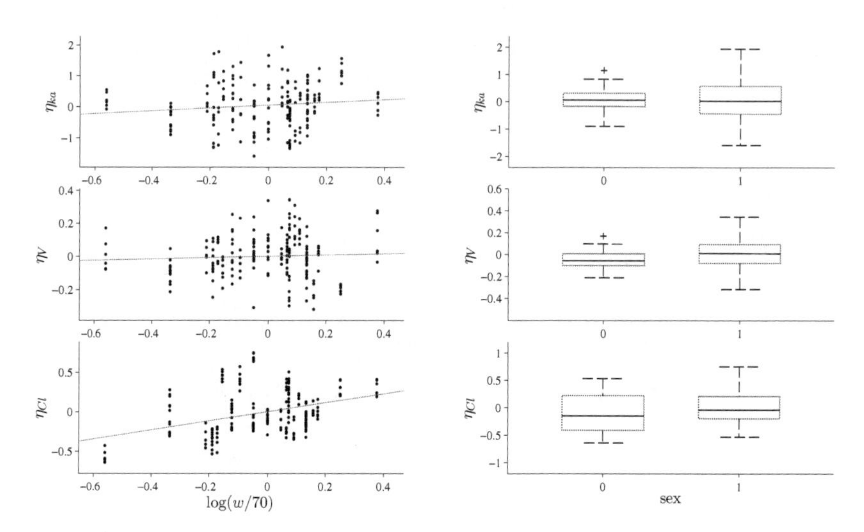

FIGURE 7.14: Relationships between the random effects and covariates: transformed weight $\log(w_i/70)$ on the left and sex on the right. Each random effect has been drawn from its individual conditional distribution.

<u>The model for the random effects</u>: This model assumes that for a given individual, the random effects associated with each individual parameter are independent and normally distributed. Figure 7.15 shows the empirical distributions of the standardized simulated random effects (the variances are normalized to 1) as box plots. The limits of the boxes are the first and third quartiles of these empirical distributions. When compared with the first and third quartiles of a standard normal distribution, there is no reason for rejecting the hypothesis that the random effects are normally distributed.

Figure 7.16 plots each pair of simulated random effects against each other. These plots show no correlation between random effects; there is therefore no reason for rejecting the hypothesis of a diagonal variance-covariance matrix.

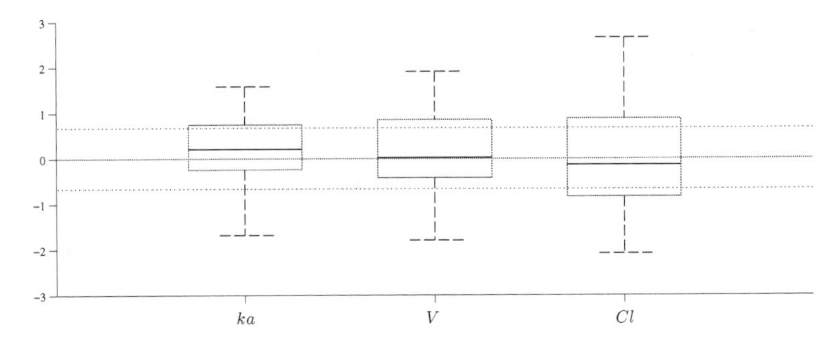

FIGURE 7.15: Empirical distributions of the random effects. Each random effect has been drawn from its individual conditional distribution. The horizontal line segments in the center of the boxes are the medians and the extremities the order 25% and 75% quantiles; the solid and dotted lines across the plot are respectively the 50%, 25% and 75% quantiles of the standard normal distribution.

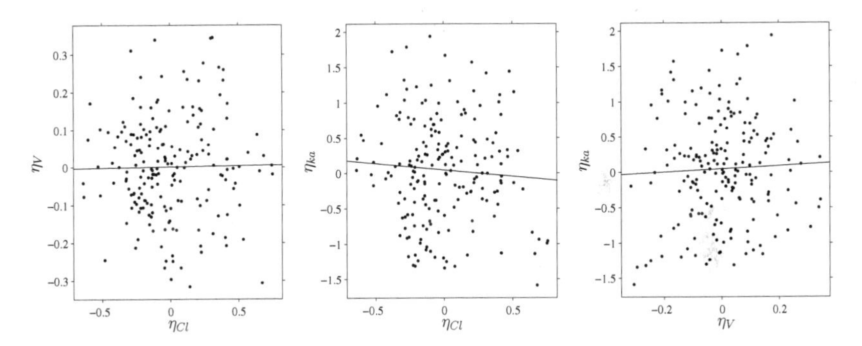

FIGURE 7.16: Joint distributions of the random effects. Each random effect has been drawn from its individual conditional distribution.

In summary, this ensemble of diagnostic plots suggests to us that model $\mathcal{M}_0$ can probably be improved. What is useful is that it not only suggests that the model can be improved, but also provides us with information on how to do so. In particular, a PK model which includes a lag-time, combined residual error model and statistical model for Cl which incorporates weight as a covariate, should be tested. Model selection tools can then be used to compare the different models.

7.3.3 Model selection

7.3.3.1 Statistical tools for model selection

Statistical tools for model selection include information criteria such as the Akaike information criterion (AIC) and Bayesian information criterion (BIC), and hypothesis tests such as the Wald test and likelihood ratio test (LRT).

AIC and BIC, both implemented in MONOLIX, are defined by

$$\text{AIC} = -2\mathcal{LL}_{\boldsymbol{y}}(\theta) + 2P \qquad (7.6)$$
$$\text{BIC} = -2\mathcal{LL}_{\boldsymbol{y}}(\theta) + \log(N)P, \qquad (7.7)$$

where P is the total number of parameters to be estimated and N the number of subjects. Models being compared using AIC or BIC need not be nested, unlike when using the Wald test or LRT.

Remarks:

- Surprisingly, the formula for calculating the BIC differs from software to software because the effective sample size is not clearly defined in the context of mixed effects models. The question is whether we should use the number of subjects N or the total number of observations n_{tot} in the penalty term. The penalty using n_{tot} is implemented in the R package nlme and SPSS procedure MIXED, while N is used in saemix, MONOLIX and SAS proc NLMIXED.

  An appropriate decomposition of the complete log-likelihood combined with the Laplace approximation can be used to derive the asymptotic BIC approximation. This leads to an optimal BIC penalty based on two terms proportional to $\log N$ and $\log n_{\text{tot}}$ that adapts to the mixed effects structure of a model (Delattre et al., 2014).

- The AIC and BIC methods are justified based on asymptotic criteria (Burnham and Anderson, 2002; Schwarz, 1978), i.e., when the number of individuals increases and the model dimension stays fixed. In the alternative, nonasymptotic approach, the model size can increase freely. The form of the penalty can differ from one model to the next in this framework. It can be shown for example that for certain Gaussian models, the penalty term has the form $c_1P + c_2P\log(N/P)$ (Birgé and Massart, 2001). The problem then becomes to calibrate coefficients c_1 and c_2 in order to obtain an optimal penalty, which is not necessarily a simple task, making it harder to use this approach in real-world applications.

- A conditional AIC (cAIC) has been proposed by Vaida and Blanchard (2005) for mixed effects models. This criterion has been used in several mixed model cases (Donohue et al., 2011; Lian, 2012; Liang et al., 2008) and its theoretical properties investigated (Greven and Kneib, 2010).

When comparing nested models $\mathcal{M}_0$ and $\mathcal{M}_1$ with dimensions P_0 and P_1 ($P_1 > P_0$), the LRT uses the test statistic

$$LRT = 2(\mathcal{LL}_{\boldsymbol{y}}(\widehat{\theta}_1) - \mathcal{LL}_{\boldsymbol{y}}(\widehat{\theta}_0)),$$

where $\widehat{\theta}_0$ and $\widehat{\theta}_1$ are the ML estimates of θ under $\mathcal{M}_0$ and $\mathcal{M}_1$. Depending on the hypotheses, the limit distribution of the LRT is either a χ^2 distribution or a mixture of χ^2 distributions and Dirac δ distributions (Stram and Lee, 1994). For example:

- Testing whether some fixed effects are null and assuming the same covariance structure under both hypotheses for the random effects implies that
$$LRT \underset{N\to\infty}{\longrightarrow} \chi^2(P_1 - P_0).$$
- Testing whether some correlations in the covariance matrix Ω are null and assuming the same covariate model under both hypotheses implies that
$$LRT \underset{N\to\infty}{\longrightarrow} \chi^2(P_1 - P_0).$$
- Testing whether the variance of one of the random effects is zero and assuming the same covariate model under both hypotheses implies that
$$LRT \underset{N\to\infty}{\longrightarrow} \frac{1}{2}\chi^2(1) + \frac{1}{2}\delta_0.$$

We have seen in Section 7.2.2 that the standard errors of the estimated parameters can be derived from the FIM. We can therefore use, for example, the Wald test to test whether a fixed effect β is null. The test statistic is $\hat{\beta}/\text{s.e.}(\hat{\beta})$; its distribution can be approximated by an $\mathcal{N}(0,1)$ when N is fairly large.

In order to better control the test's type I error (i.e., the probability of incorrectly concluding that $\beta \neq 0$) for small sample sizes, the distribution of the Wald statistic can be better approximated by a Student's t distribution or an F distribution (Bertrand et al., 2012). The issue here is to be able to derive appropriate degrees of freedom when the data is unbalanced (i.e., the number of observations are not the same for all individuals). Methods such as Satterthwaite's correction and others can be used, but the choice of method seems to have little impact in the longitudinal data case (Verbeke and Molenberghs, 2000).

7.3.3.2 Estimation of the log-likelihood

Performing likelihood ratio tests and computing information criteria for a given model requires computation of the log-likelihood

$$\mathcal{LL}_{\boldsymbol{y}}(\widehat{\theta}) = \log(\mathcal{L}_{\boldsymbol{y}}(\widehat{\theta})) \stackrel{\text{def}}{=} \log(\mathrm{p}(\boldsymbol{y};\widehat{\theta})),$$

where $\widehat{\theta}$ is the vector of population parameter estimates for the model being considered.

The log-likelihood cannot be computed in closed form for nonlinear mixed effects models. It can however be estimated in a general framework for all kinds of data and models using the importance sampling Monte Carlo method presented in Section 9.5. This method has the advantage of providing an unbiased estimate of the log-likelihood – even for nonlinear models – whose variance can be controlled by the Monte Carlo size.

In the case of continuous data, approximation of the model by a Gaussian linear one as in Section 7.2.2 for estimating the FIM also allows us to approximate the log-likelihood. The advantage of this method is that it provides a good and quick approximation of the likelihood, generally sufficient for discriminating between fairly different models. It can therefore be used during the first steps of model construction. Selection of the final model should instead use the unbiased estimator obtained by Monte Carlo.

The log-likelihoods (and therefore AIC and BIC) obtained with each method are quite similar for our PK example and for model $\mathcal{M}_0$ described in Section 7.1. The standard errors of the estimates obtained by importance sampling Monte Carlo are displayed in parentheses. By default, MONOLIX uses Student's t-distributions with 5 degrees of freedom as sampling distributions for the importance sampling method described in Section 9.5.

```
warfarinPK_M0

Log-likelihood Estimation by linearization

-2 x log-likelihood:                        877.97
Akaike Information Criteria    (AIC):       893.97
Bayesian Information Criteria  (BIC):       905.69
_______________________________________________________________

Log-likelihood Estimation by important sampling
Sampling distribution for the random effects: t with 5 d.f

-2 x log-likelihood:                        879.07 (0.078)
Akaike Information Criteria    (AIC):       895.07 (0.078)
Bayesian Information Criteria  (BIC):       906.80 (0.078)
```

7.3.3.3 Decision support vs decision making

This set of tools for model selection forms a decision support system to help modelers with their decision making process for model building. This does not mean that the system makes the decision to choose one model over another. In the end, the decision is always made by the modeler. For example, statistical tests and information criteria help modelers decide whether the difference between two models is statistically significant. Suppose that we want to test whether a fixed model parameter β is null:

$$H_0: \quad \text{“}\beta = 0\text{”} \qquad \text{vs} \qquad H_1: \quad \text{“}\beta \neq 0\text{”}.$$

We construct a statistical test T for which the distribution under H_0 allows us to calculate a p-value, i.e., the probability that T is at least as big as the value observed under H_0. A small p-value leads us to reject H_0 with high confidence. It is usual to use the arbitrary cutoff of 5% to make this decision; we frequently read statements such as “a decrease in the objective function of at least 3.84 was required to identify a significant covariate.” In the same way we can select models based on their BIC values under H_0 and H_1 by providing an arbitrary decision rule. It is sometimes suggested to choose H_1 if the difference $BIC_{H_1} - BIC_{H_0}$ is inferior to a certain arbitrary cutoff.

These approaches seem to simplify a modeler's life because they provide decision rules that can be applied systematically, and thus justify decisions. But a rule, whatever it is, should never stop us asking why we are applying it and whether it is applicable in the current situation. Remember that even a very small difference will be statistically significant if the sample size is large enough. The question is thus not to know whether a difference is statistically significant, but whether it is physically or biologically significant. We must therefore look carefully at the size of an effect and its real impact, for both understanding the model and the effect's impact on the model's predictive capacities.

7.3.4 Model building

We have now seen some graphical and diagnostic tools available for modelers to qualitatively evaluate a given model, and quantitative criteria for comparing potential models. These must now all be used effectively to build a model. Defining an optimal strategy for model building is far from easy because a model is the assembled product of numerous components that need to been evaluated and perhaps improved: the structural model, residual error model, covariate model, covariance model, etc. How to proceed so as to obtain the best possible combination of these components? Unfortunately there is no general answer to this question; it will depend on the context, the data, the modeler's previous experience, etc.

The strategy to take will mainly depend on the time we can dedicate to building the model and the time required for running it. For relatively simple models for which parameter estimation is fast, it is possible to fit many models and compare them. This can also be done if we have powerful computing facilities available (e.g., a cluster) allowing large numbers of simultaneous runs.

However, if we are working on a standard laptop or desktop computer, model building is a sequential process in which a new model is tested at each step. If the model is complex and requires significant computation time (e.g., when involving systems of ODEs), we are constrained to limit the number of models we can test in a reasonable time period. In this context, it also becomes important to carefully choose the tasks to run at each step.

- It is unnecessary to calculate the FIM and log-likelihood in the initial runs when we are only looking to check whether the chosen structural model fits the data reasonably well. We can limit ourselves to estimating the population parameters with only the first phase of SAEM and output a few basic goodness-of-fit plots (individual fits, observations vs predictions) using the individual parameters obtained during the final iterations of SAEM.

- The FIM and log-likelihood obtained by model linearization will generally be able to identify the main features of the model. More precise – and time-consuming – estimation procedures such as stochastic approximation and importance sampling will have very limited impact in terms of decisions for these most obvious features. A p-value of approximately 0.001 or differences in BIC of around 30 do not require more precise calculations when making decisions.

- Precise results are required for the final runs where it becomes more important to rigorously defend decisions made to choose the final model and provide precise estimates and diagnostic plots.

Let us illustrate this model building process by trying to improve model $\mathcal{M}_0$ taking into account the diagnostic plots shown in Sections 7.3.2.2 and 7.3.2.3. First, consider a model $\mathcal{M}_1$ defined like $\mathcal{M}_0$ but for which the PK model (7.1) now includes a lag-time:

$$C(t,\phi) = \begin{cases} \frac{D\,ka}{V\,ka - Cl}\left(e^{-Cl/V\,(t-Tlag)} - e^{-ka\,(t-Tlag)}\right) & \text{if } t \geq Tlag \\ 0, & \text{otherwise.} \end{cases}$$

There is now an additional individual PK parameter $Tlag_i > 0$ that can vary in the population. Suppose model $\mathcal{M}_1$ assumes a log-normal distribution for $Tlag_i$. We can now estimate the population parameters for $\mathcal{M}_1$ and compute information criteria using a linearization of the model:

```
warfarinPK_M1

              parameter      s.e. (lin)    r.s.e.(%)
Tlag_pop        0.838           0.2            24
omega_Tlag      0.603          0.18            30

-2 x log-likelihood:                        715.03
Akaike Information Criteria    (AIC):       735.03
Bayesian Information Criteria (BIC):        749.69
```

Improvements in the approximate AIC and BIC are extremely significant (< -150). We retain $\mathcal{M}_1$ over $\mathcal{M}_0$ without hesitation. We can then define a new model $\mathcal{M}_2$ starting with $\mathcal{M}_1$ but assuming a combined error model of the form $y = f + \sqrt{a^2 + b^2 f^2}\,\varepsilon$.

```
warfarinPK_M2

       parameter      s.e. (lin)   r.s.e.(%)
a        0.327          0.048         15
b        0.0782         0.0082        10

-2 x log-likelihood:                        657.56
Akaike Information Criteria    (AIC):       679.56
Bayesian Information Criteria (BIC):        695.68
```

The estimated values of a and b show that it is relevant to include these two components in the error model. Furthermore, the information criteria (still obtained by linearization of the model) indicates a clear preference for $\mathcal{M}_2$ over $\mathcal{M}_1$.

Lastly, the diagnostic plot for the covariate model shown in Figure 7.13 suggests a possible relationship between weight and clearance. We therefore define a new model $\mathcal{M}_3$ based on $\mathcal{M}_2$ but now supposing the following model for Cl_i:

$$\log(Cl_i) \sim \mathcal{N}(\log(Cl_{\text{pop}}) + \beta_{Cl}\log(w_i/70),\, \omega_{Cl}^2).$$

The following results are obtained with this new model:

```
warfarinPK_M3

              parameter      s.e. (lin)    r.s.e.(%)    p-value
Cl_pop          0.134          0.0065          5
beta_Cl         0.607          0.26           42         0.018


-2 x log-likelihood:                        652.24
Akaike Information Criteria    (AIC):       676.24
Bayesian Information Criteria (BIC):        693.83
```

The Wald test for testing $\beta_{Cl} = 0$ gives a p-value of about 0.018 and the difference in the information criteria for $\mathcal{M}_2$ and $\mathcal{M}_3$ is now quite small. It is therefore time to use more precise estimates if we really want to properly compare these models. Both log-likelihoods can now be computed using Monte Carlo importance sampling:

```
Log-likelihood Estimation by important sampling
Sampling distribution for the random effects: t with 5 d.f

                                              warfarinPK_M2     warfarinPK_M3

-2 x log-likelihood:                          660.48 (0.11)     655.26 (0.096)
Akaike Information Criteria    (AIC):         682.48 (0.11)     679.26 (0.096)
Bayesian Information Criteria (BIC):          698.60 (0.11)     696.84 (0.096)
```

The LRT statistic is $2(\mathcal{LL}_{\boldsymbol{y}}(\widehat{\theta}_3) - \mathcal{LL}_{\boldsymbol{y}}(\widehat{\theta}_2)) = 5.22$ and the associated p-value is 0.022. We see therefore that all these statistical criteria (AIC, BIC, LRT, Wald) choose $\mathcal{M}_3$ over $\mathcal{M}_2$. This model building process has therefore led to a new model $\mathcal{M}_3$ which we can consider to be the "best" among those examined with respect to the statistical criteria. However, the final decision is up to the modeler, including the final decision as to whether the final model should include the weight for partly explaining variability in the clearance.

As a final note, the modeler may very well come to the conclusion that there are no reasons left for rejecting model $\mathcal{M}_3$ after taking a look at the diagnostic plots shown in Figure 7.17.

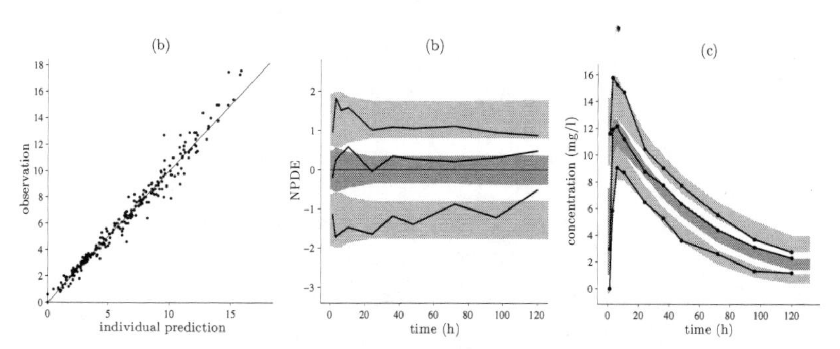

FIGURE 7.17: Diagnostic plots obtained with model $\mathcal{M}_3$; (a) observations vs predictions, (b) NPDEs, (c) VPC.

8

Examples

8.1 Body weight curves in a toxicity study

8.1.1 Introduction

Genetically modified (GM) organisms are living species whose genome has been altered, often by the addition of a gene, for specific reasons such as conferring protection against pests like corn rootworm or resistance to herbicides such as glyphosate. For example, Monsanto created the transgenic corn MON 863 by inserting DNA sequences that encode a modified *Bacillus thuringiensis* Cry3Bb1 protein that is selectively toxic to Coleoptera (beetles) such as corn rootworm larvae.

Global regulatory authorities require that food and animal feed derived from GM plants be as safe as food produced from conventionally bred plants. More precisely, the European Food Safety Authority (EFSA, 2008) recommends that "the safety assessment of GM plants and derived food and feed follows a comparative approach, i.e., the food and feed are compared with their non-GM counterparts in order to identify intended and unintended (unexpected) differences which subsequently are assessed with respect to their potential impact on the environment, safety for humans and animals, and nutritional quality."

Safety assessment usually means running a subchronic toxicity study on rats. For 90 days, groups of animals are put on different diets (GM or non-GM) and doses (e.g., 11% and 33% of the diet are from GM sources in the corn example). Each rat is weighted each week and a large number of measurements (blood and urine characteristics, organ weight, etc.) are taken at the end of the trial. These results are then subjected to statistical analyses in order to compare data from the test and control groups.

In the case of GM corn MON 863, Monsanto performed one such 90-day rat feeding study. The results of this study were first analyzed by Hammond et al. (2006). Let us first consider the evaluation of weekly body weight data. We note first that Hammond et al. did not account for the temporal structure of the data, instead performing a week-by-week analysis. This approach wasted potentially useful temporal information and led to complex multiple comparison problems due to the complex dependency structure of the data.

Séralini et al. (2007) reanalyzed the data by fitting a three-parameter Gompertz curve to the weight data of each treatment group:

$$f_0(t) = w_\infty \exp(-\exp(-\alpha\,(t-\tau))), \tag{8.1}$$

where w_∞ is the asymptotic weight. The fitting of a Gompertz curve to the weight data thus brings together measurements conducted each week into a single analysis rather than analyzing each week separately. Fitting a parametric curve to the weight data was an interesting idea, but their subsequent statistical analysis was erroneous because they did not take into account inter-rat variability in the statistical model. Instead they simply compared the average growth curves of each group considering the residual errors (between observed and mean weights) as independent and identically distributed (i.i.d.) random variables. This assumption is obviously incorrect since the sequence of residuals for a given animal are highly correlated (a rat being above the mean weight at week j is likely also to be above the mean weight at weeks $j-1$ and $j+1$). Ignoring the variability in rat weights within each group greatly inflated the probability of finding statistically significant differences, and led Séralini et al. to incorrectly infer that the observed differences ($\simeq 3\%$) were statistically significant (p-value < 0.01).

A detailed analysis of these results was performed by several institutes and authorities (EFSA, 2007). One of the main conclusions was that mixed models would be more suitable to analyze the weight data of this study because they are better able to take into account between-rat variability. The use of mixed effects models and other appropriate models for longitudinal data was also emphasized by the French Agency for Food, Environmental and Occupational Health and Safety (ANSES, 2011). A relevant approach is therefore to choose parametric growth models for each rat's weight curve, then consider the model parameters to be random variables.

8.1.2 Using mixed effects models

In the study, for each sex, two groups were fed with GM corn, one with 11% and the other with 33% of MON 863 in the overall diet, and two groups with the closest control line were fed non-GM corn in the same proportions. There were 20 rats per group, for a total of 160 animals.

The goal of the study is to look for evidence of a potential effect due to the GM diet. If we consider that this effect can be different for males and females, we should be careful to analyze these groups (each of 80 individuals) separately. An alternative approach is to use the same model for all 160 rats while considering gender to be a categorical covariate. In this way we gain statistical power due to the increase in number of individuals, but risk not correctly identifying possible GM effects if these effects are quite different for males and females. A preliminary study of the power is therefore necessary to work out what we can hope to realistically detect in either case.

A similar problem arises if we aim to detect different GM effects in the two groups fed 11% and 33% GM corn. Overall then, various scenarios are possible, from a global analysis of the 160 rats to four independent analyses by gender and diet on each group of 40 rats.

Looking at the graphs of Figure 8.1, we see clearly a gender effect but no obvious dose effect. Therefore, we decide to analyze separately the groups of 80 males and 80 females, forgetting the 11% and 33% dose differences. We will only present results obtained with the 80 males in the following. The goal of the statistical analysis is therefore to compare the 40 body weight curves from the control group (non-GM) with the 40 from the test group (GM).

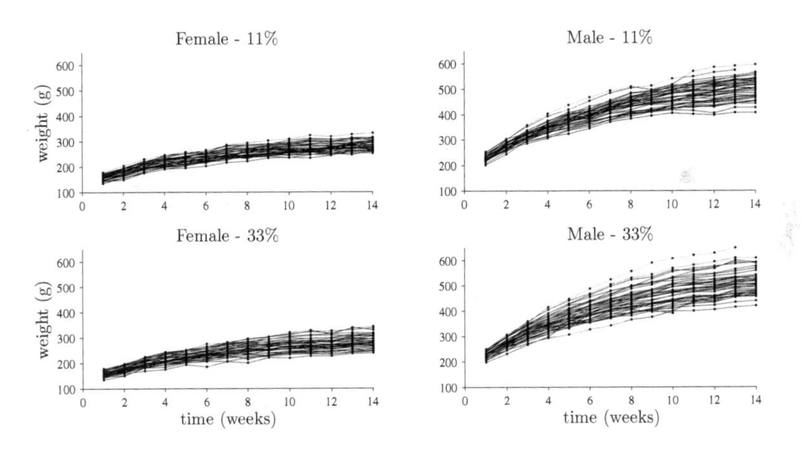

FIGURE 8.1: The 160 growth curves divided up into gender and dose (proportion of corn in the diet).

Let us start by reanalyzing the growth data of the 80 male rats using the Gompertz model (8.1) treated as a mixed effects model. The structural model can be immediately implemented using MLXTRAN for MONOLIX.

```
gompertz_model.txt

INPUT:
parameter={winf, alpha, tau}

EQUATION:
f0=winf*exp(-exp(-alpha*(t-tau)))

OUTPUT:
output=f0
```

Here, the vector of individual parameters of the structural model is $\phi_i = (w_{\infty,i}, \alpha_i, \tau_i)$. A log-normal distribution is used for α_i and normal ones for $w_{\infty,i}$ and τ_i. The only covariate is diet (1 if GM corn, 0 otherwise). Let ${w_\infty}^{(0)}$, $\alpha^{(0)}$ and $\tau^{(0)}$ be the population parameters in the control group (used as reference group). We assume that there exists β_w, β_α and β_τ such that the population parameters in the test group are

$$
\begin{aligned}
{w_\infty}^{(1)} &= {w_\infty}^{(0)} + \beta_w \\
\alpha^{(1)} &= \alpha^{(0)} e^{\beta_\alpha} \\
\tau^{(1)} &= \tau^{(0)} + \beta_\tau .
\end{aligned}
$$

We propose initially a constant error model. The population parameters can then be estimated using SAEM, implemented in MONOLIX:

	parameter	s.e. (lin)	r.s.e.(%)	p-value
winf	536	8.7	2	
beta_winf	-7.52	12	164	0.54
alpha	0.22	0.0048	2	
beta_alpha	-0.0316	0.031	99	0.31
tau	0.129	0.078	60	
beta_tau	-0.0676	0.11	163	0.54
omega_winf	54.4	4.4	8	
omega_alpha	0.122	0.012	10	
omega_tau	0.474	0.04	8	
a	6.47	0.16	2	

Here, none of the β values are significantly different from 0 statistically speaking (Wald test). By comparing the values of population parameters by group, we can also conclude that the differences are not biologically significant (asymptotic weight differs by only 1.3%).

	parameter	s.e. (lin)	r.s.e.(%)
winf_(gmo=0*)	536	8.7	2
winf_(gmo=1)	529	8.7	2
alpha_(gmo=0*)	0.22	0.0048	2
alpha_(gmo=1)	0.214	0.0047	2

```
tau_(gmo=0*)          0.129          0.078          60
tau_(gmo=1 )          0.0618         0.078          126
```

Before using these results for inference however, it is important to evaluate the quality of the model to ensure that it is itself capable of detecting possible differences in weight due to diet. Individual fits for the first four rats are given in Figure 8.2 and show that the structural model predicts well the observed rat weights.

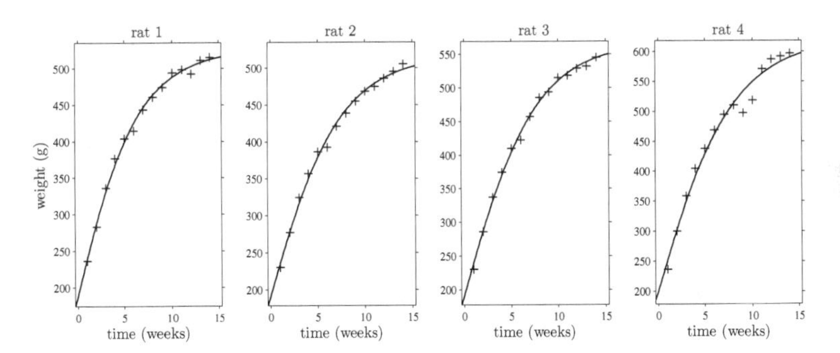

FIGURE 8.2: Individual fits obtained with the Gompertz model.

We also have to assure ourselves that the statistical model used to characterize the inter-individual variability is reasonable. The joint distributions of the random effects drawn from the conditional distributions, shown in Figure 8.3, lead us to believe that there is probably a linear correlation between the random effects $\eta_{w,i}$ and $\eta_{\tau,i}$.

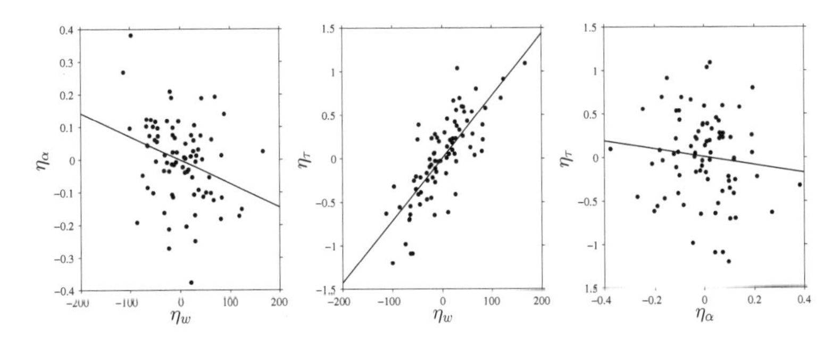

FIGURE 8.3: Joint distributions of the random effects.

The visual predictive checks (VPCs) displayed in Figure 8.4(a) confirm that the statistical model is misspecified. We therefore consider a new model that still uses the Gompertz structural model (8.1) but now assumes a linear correlation between $\eta_{w,i}$ and $\eta_{T,i}$. Looking at the resulting VPCs in Figure 8.4(b), we find no reason to reject the new model.

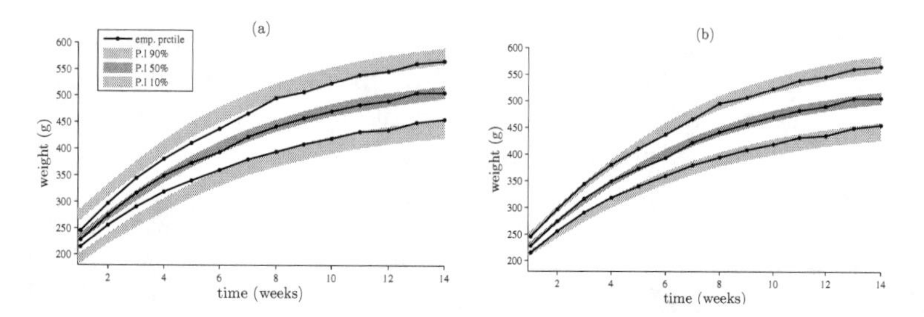

FIGURE 8.4: VPCs obtained with the Gompertz model. (a) Assuming that the individual parameters are independent; (b) assuming that $\eta_{w,i}$ and $\eta_{T,i}$ are correlated. The empirical quantiles of order 10%, 50% and 90% are displayed (solid lines) with their respective 90% prediction intervals

Except for the correlation between $\eta_{w,i}$ and $\eta_{T,i}$, the estimates of model parameters differ little from the original model:

	parameter	s.e. (lin)	r.s.e.(%)	p-value
winf	537	8.6	2	
beta_winf	-7.91	12	153	0.51
alpha	0.22	0.0047	2	
beta_alpha	-0.0295	0.03	103	0.33
tau	0.121	0.077	63	
beta_tau	-0.0643	0.11	169	0.55
omega_winf	53.5	4.3	8	
omega_alpha	0.117	0.012	10	
omega_tau	0.469	0.04	8	
corr(winf,tau)	0.878	0.031	4	
a	6.51	0.16	2	

We can add to the results of the three Wald tests above by performing a global test:

$$H_0: \text{“}\beta_w = \beta_\alpha = \beta_T = 0\text{”} \quad \text{vs} \quad H_1: \text{“}\beta_w \neq 0,\ \beta_\alpha \neq 0,\ \beta_T \neq 0\text{”}.$$

The deviances computed under H_0 and H_1 are, respectively, 7996 and 7995. The likelihood ratio test (LRT, p-value $= 0.76$), Bayesian information criterion (BIC, 8031 vs 8043) and Akaike information criterion (AIC, 8012 vs 8017) therefore all agree with the Wald tests, selecting H_0.

In conclusion, based on this data and our subsequent analyses, there is no reason to suspect a GM effect on rat weight. As a final remark however, we are not claiming that there is no health risk linked to GM corn MON 863, only that the data and analyses do not allow us to reject the hypothesis that there is no GM effect on weight.

8.1.3 Different parametrizations of the same structural model

We have seen that model choice is intimately linked to the usage of it that we have in mind. It is therefore not necessary to construct the "best" model for studying potential GM effects.

If we do want to characterize as well as possible the observed data, we could try to propose a model other than Gompertz (8.1) (traditionally used for modeling tumor and population growth). Instead, we could use an asymptotic regression model (Pinheiro and Bates, 2009) of the form:

$$f_1(t) = w_0 e^{-k\,t} + w_\infty(1 - e^{-k\,t}), \tag{8.2}$$

where w_0 is the weight at birth, w_∞ the asymptotic weight and k the growth rate constant. As usual, this model parametrization is not the only one possible. We should try to choose a parametrization that both allows interpretation of model parameters and satisfies reasonable statistical criteria.

Indeed, the parametrization in (8.2) involves an asymptotic weight that is not included in the time interval being studied. An alternative parametrization might therefore involve the weights w_0, w_7 and w_{14} at times $t = 0$, $t = 7$ and $t = 14$:

$$f_2(t) = w_0 + \frac{(w_7 - w_0)^2}{2w_7 - w_{14} - w_0}\left(1 - \left(\frac{w_7 - w_0}{w_{14} - w_7}\right)^{-t/7}\right). \tag{8.3}$$

A quick look at the data displayed in Figure 8.1 shows that the weights at times t_7 and t_{14} are strongly correlated. Therefore, we use for this new model Gaussian distributions for the three individual parameters $w_{0,i}$, $w_{7,i}$ and $w_{14,i}$, supposing moreover that $w_{7,i}$ and $w_{14,i}$ are correlated. Results obtained with this new model show that the differences in population weights between the GM and non-GM groups at 7 and 14 weeks are less than 10g and not statistically significant.

```
                parameter     s.e. (s.a.)   r.s.e.(%)   p-value
w0                 175            1.6            1
w7                 428            5.3            1
beta_w7          -9.25            7.5           81         0.21
```

```
w14                 513            7.7              1
beta_w14           -9.9             11            110        0.36

omega_w0             12            1.3             11
omega_w7           33.3            2.6              8
omega_w14          48.4            3.9              8
corr(w7,w14)       0.95          0.011              1

a                  5.96           0.14              2
```

The VPC displayed in Figure 8.5(a) shows that there is an extremely good fit between the model and the data. Furthermore, the BIC is much better for this model than the Gompertz one (7880 vs 8043). Nevertheless, a closer look at the correlation matrix of the estimators shows that $\hat{w}_{7,\text{pop}}$ and $\hat{w}_{14,\text{pop}}$ are strongly correlated, as well as $\hat{\omega}_{w_7}$ and $\hat{\omega}_{w_{14}}$:

```
Correlation matrix of the estimates (Stochastic Approximation):

w0        1
w7    -0.02        1
w14    0.01     0.95        1

Eigenvalues (min, max, max/min): 0.054  1.9  36

omega_w0          1
omega_w7         -0        1
omega_w14        -0     0.89        1
a             -0.08       -0       -0        1

Eigenvalues (min, max, max/min): 0.11  1.9  18
```

We could then suggest a new parametrization of the same model in which the estimates are much less correlated:

$$f_3(t) = w_0 + \frac{w_{14} - w_0}{1 - r^2}\left(1 - r^{t/7}\right), \tag{8.4}$$

where $0 < r < 1$ indicates the growth rate. The following results have been obtained using a logit-normal distribution for the individual parameter r_i:

```
               parameter     s.e. (s.a.)   r.s.e.(%)    p-value
w0                   176           1.5            1
r                  0.337         0.011            3
beta_r            0.0475         0.067          142       0.48
w14                  513           7.6            1
beta_w14           -9.83            11          109       0.36

omega_w0            11.8           1.2           10
omega_r             0.28         0.027           10
omega_w14           47.8           3.8            8

a                   6.01          0.14            2
```

It is not necessary with this model to introduce correlation between random effects to get a nice VPC, as can been seen in Figure 8.5(b).

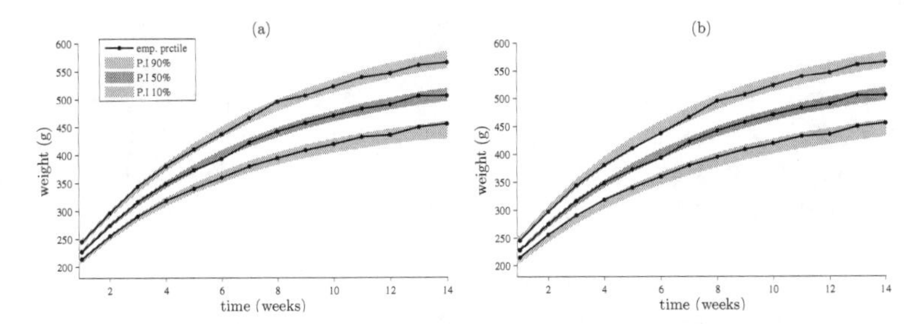

FIGURE 8.5: VPCs obtained with the asymptotic regression model and different parametrizations. (a) Parametrization (w_0, w_7, w_{14}) assuming that $w_{7,i}$ and $w_{14,i}$ are correlated; (b) parametrization (w_0, r, w_{14}) assuming that parameters are independent.

We see clearly that the estimates of model parameters have little correlation:

```
correlation matrix of the estimates(Stochastic Approximation)

w0        1
r      0.16        1
w14    0.01     0.02         1

Eigenvalues (min, max, max/min): 0.84  1.2  1.4

omega_w0         1
omega_r       0.01        1
omega_w14       -0     0.01        1
a             -0.1    -0.06       -0        1

Eigenvalues (min, max, max/min): 0.89  1.1  1.3
```

In conclusion, we prefer this model because it describes the observed data well, uses easily interpretable parameters, has independent individual parameters and ensures good statistical properties for the estimators of the model's population parameters.

8.1.4 Power analysis and equivalence testing

As emphasized by ANSES (2011), difference tests should be accompanied by a power analysis so as to evaluate the size of an effect we can hope to find for a given protocol. We see immediately the advantage of using a parametrization with easily interpretable parameters since the power analysis may directly weigh on one of these. For example, we might look at rat weights at 14 weeks and test the following hypothesis:

$$H_0 : \text{"}\beta_{w_{14}} = 0\text{"} \qquad \text{vs} \qquad H_1 : \text{"}\beta_{w_{14}} \neq 0\text{"}.$$

We might take a classical approach and consider only the data at time t_{14}, i.e., 39 observations in each group (there is one missing data point at time t_{14} in both groups). In this case, we can construct a t-test and calculate its power (see Figure 8.6) as the type I and II error probabilities are easily calculated.

It gets more complicated when we want to work with our nonlinear mixed effects model as it is now impossible to calculate these probabilities, either for the LRT or Wald test. We can however estimate them using Monte Carlo: for several values of $\beta_{w_{14}}$ between -50 and 50, we can draw several replicates of the data using our model under H_1 with the original design. Then, for each replicate, the population parameters can be estimated and the LRT and Wald tests performed. For each value of $\beta_{w_{14}}$, the estimated power of a given test is the proportion of tests which are statistically significant.

Each power displayed in Figure 8.6 was obtained using 100 replicates. We can see that in this example, the Wald test and LRT have very similar powers. Furthermore, these tests' powers are systematically close to the power of the basic t-test. Thus, our modeling provides no advantage in terms of power in this particular example. If little data is available at t_{14}, a test performed after modeling will now be much more powerful than a t-test on the t_{14} data because all individuals are used to construct the model, not just those with data at t_{14}. More generally, if we wish to construct a test on an unobserved parameter (weight at 21 weeks, for example), only modeling will allow us to create such a test.

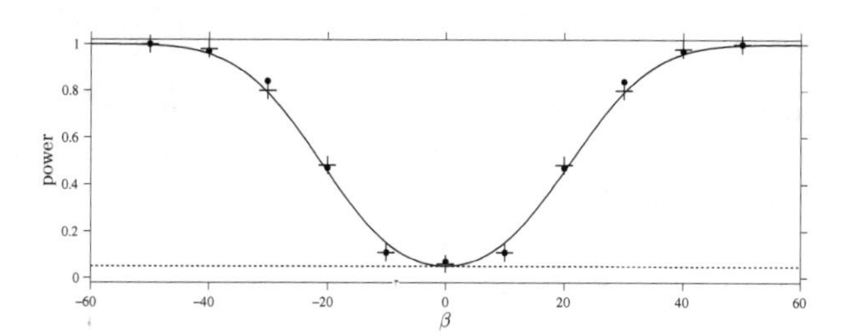

FIGURE 8.6: Power of the test $\beta_{w_{14}} = 0$ vs $\beta_{w_{14}} \neq 0$. Solid line: t-test, dots: LRT, crosses: Wald test.

Tests for making comparisons that aim to see whether a difference is statistically significant are of limited interest if we do not also look at the size of the difference, i.e., the magnitude of the GM effect on rat weight. It is highly probable that *any* change in diet will affect weight. Even if this effect is tiny, it will be statistically significant if we have the resources to run the study on a large number of rats. We may therefore end up rejecting the null hypothesis out of hand without much risk of being "wrong." This avoids the true question: is the effect biologically significant and furthermore, does it signal GM toxicity? This question deserves to be asked in terms of equivalence: can we, given the data, reject the hypothesis that the effect's size is greater than a certain value? Let us again take the weight data at 14 weeks as an example, and look to test:

$$H_0 : \text{``}|\beta_{w_{14}}| > \delta\text{''} \qquad \text{vs} \qquad H_1 : \text{``}|\beta_{w_{14}}| < \delta\text{''},$$

where δ is an arbitrary equivalence value given in grams, like w_{14} is. We will conclude that there is equivalence if H_0 is rejected.

Following Dubois et al. (2011), the null hypothesis H_0 can be divided into two one-sided hypotheses: $H_{0,-\delta}$: "$\beta_{w_{14}} < -\delta$" and $H_{0,\delta}$: "$\beta_{w_{14}} > \delta$". These are then tested separately with one-sided tests. Then, the global null hypothesis H_0 is rejected with type I error α if both one-sided tests are rejected with type I error α. The p-value of the test is the maximum of the p-values of the one-sided tests. An alternative way to run this equivalence test is to compute the $(1 - 2\alpha)$ confidence interval (CI) for $\hat{\beta}_{w_{14}}$. H_0 is then rejected if the equivalence interval $(-\delta, \delta)$ contains this confidence interval.

With the last model we looked at, we get the following 90% CI for $\hat{\beta}_{w_{14}}$: $\mathrm{CI}_{90\%} = [-27.9\mathrm{g}, 8.3\mathrm{g}]$. This means that if we define equivalence as a weight difference at 14 weeks of less than 30g, we do have equivalence here. If instead we restrict equivalence to mean difference less than 20g, we can no longer conclude that there is equivalence, based on this criterion.

The choice of the size of the equivalence interval is a delicate one, but not itself a statistical problem. It is up to toxicologists to decide what a meaningful inter-group variability is. More generally speaking, it is not statistics themselves that can decide whether or not GM products are safe for human health; they are merely tools for helping make decisions. Their role is to correctly evaluate uncertainties and the risk of making an error when concluding as to the presence or absence of negative effects resulting from GM products.

8.2 Joint PKPD modeling of warfarin data

Warfarin pharmacokinetic (PK) and pharmacodynamic (PD) data was introduced in Example 4.11 and shown in Figure 4.26. The pharmacokinetics of warfarin were used in Chapter 7 to illustrate various tasks and methods in the modeling context. We will now consider joint population modeling of warfarin PK and PD data.

The model proposed in Example 4.11 provided excellent individual fits (Figure 4.27) but was of limited interest because it did not invoke a relationship between dose and effect. PKPD modeling on the other hand aims to define the relationships between time, drug concentration, drug effect and clinically observable outcomes.

We have already constructed a PK model for warfarin data in Section 7.3.4:

- The structural PK model is a one-compartment model with a lag-time followed by a first-order absorption process and linear elimination. For a single dose administration at time $t = 0$, a mathematical representation of this structural model is, for $t > Tlag$,

$$C(t, \phi^{(1)}) = \frac{D\,ka}{V\,ka - Cl}\left(e^{-\frac{Cl}{V}\,(t-Tlag)} - e^{-ka\,(t-Tlag)}\right),$$

  where $C(t, \phi^{(1)})$ is the plasmatic concentration of warfarin at time t. Here, $\phi^{(1)} = (Tlag, ka, V, Cl)$ is the vector of PK parameters; $Tlag$ is the delay between administration and absorption, ka the absorption rate constant, V the volume of distribution and Cl the clearance.

- The statistical model assumes a combined residual error model $y = f + (a + bf)\varepsilon$, log-normal distributions for the PK parameters and linear relationships between log-volume and log-weight and between log-clearance and log-weight.

We will therefore use this PK model as a component of the joint PKPD model. Let $y_{ij}^{(1)}$ and $y_{ij}^{(2)}$ be, respectively, the measured plasmatic concentration and measured prothrombin complex activity (PCA) for patient i at times $t_{ij}^{(1)}$ and $t_{ij}^{(2)}$. Denoting $\phi_i^{(2)}$ the vector of individual PD parameters for patient i and assuming a constant error model for the PD data, the joint PKPD model has the form:

$$\begin{aligned} y_{ij}^{(1)} &= C(t_{ij}^{(1)}, \phi_i^{(1)}) + \left(a_1 + b_1 C(t_{ij}^{(1)}; \phi_i^{(1)})\right) \varepsilon_{ij}^{(1)} \\ y_{ij}^{(2)} &= R(t_{ij}^{(2)}, \phi_i^{(2)}) + a_2 \varepsilon_{ij}^{(2)}, \end{aligned}$$

where $R(t, \phi_i^{(2)})$ is the predicted PCA given by the PD model for patient i at time t, and where $(\varepsilon_{ij}^{(1)})$ and $(\varepsilon_{ij}^{(2)})$ are independent sequences of $\mathcal{N}(0,1)$ random variables.

8.2.1 Simultaneous PKPD modeling

In simultaneous modeling, both PK and PD modeling are done at the same time. As the PK model has already been selected, PK modeling reduces to estimating the population PK parameters, whereas PD modeling consists of both selecting a model for the observed PD data and estimating its parameters. Let us now take a look at some basic PD models for warfarin data.

8.2.1.1 Immediate response model

The relationship between dose and effect can be separated into two components: the dose-concentration relationship (PK) and concentration-effect relationship (PD). In other words, drug effect is directly determined by the plasmatic concentration defined in the PK model.

From a biological point of view, warfarin is known to reduce synthesis of prothrombin complex by inhibiting vitamin K epoxide reductase and vitamin K reductase (Holford, 1986). A maximal inhibition (Imax) model for characterizing this drug effect has the form:

$$E(t) = 1 - I_{max} \frac{C(t)}{IC_{50} + C(t)}, \tag{8.5}$$

where IC_{50} is the concentration producing 50% inhibition and I_{max} the maximal drug-induced effect. An immediate response model assumes that for a given time, the response R is proportional to the drug effect E:

$$R_1(t) = S_0 \, E(t),$$

where S_0 is the baseline PCA before warfarin is taken. This joint PKPD structural model can be implemented with MLXTRAN for MONOLIX as follows:

```
                     Immediate response model

INPUT:
parameter = {Tlag, ka, V, Cl, S0, Imax, IC50}

EQUATION:
C = pkmodel(Tlag, ka, V, Cl)
R  = S0*(1-Imax*C/(C+IC50))

OUTPUT:
output = {C, R}
```

We then use a logit-normal distribution for I_{max} and log-normal distributions for S_0 and IC_{50}. Figure 8.7 shows four individual fits obtained with this model. For each of these four patients, the maximum effect predicted by the model is reached when the concentration is maximal, but the maximum effect is observed approximately 50 hours after the peak concentration (minimum of the observed PCA). An immediate response model is therefore not appropriate for this data since it ignores the lag-time that exists between the plasmatic drug concentration and the time course of the pharmacodynamic response.

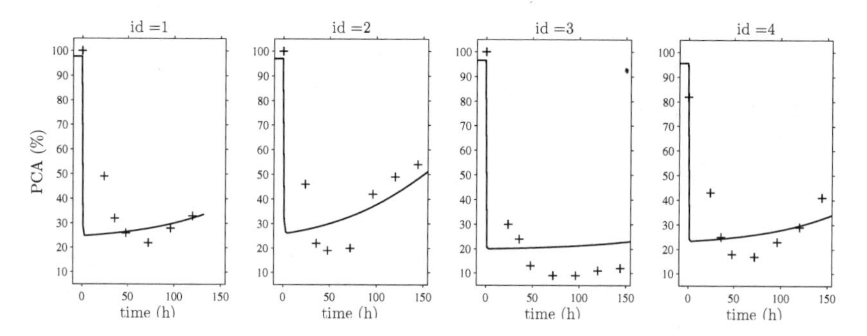

FIGURE 8.7: Individual fits for PD data of four patients obtained with an immediate response model.

When analyzing PKPD data, an important plot used to visualize data is a scatter plot with the PK concentration on the x-axis and the PD data on the y-axis. One such plot, produced here by DATXPLORE (see Appendix D.3) and shown in Figure 8.8, highlights a *hysteresis*[1] phenomenon which refers to the delay of the bioresponse time-course with respect to the exposure time-course.

[1]Hysteresis refers to systems and organisms that have memory. In such cases, consequences of an input are experienced with a certain lag-time, i.e., delay.

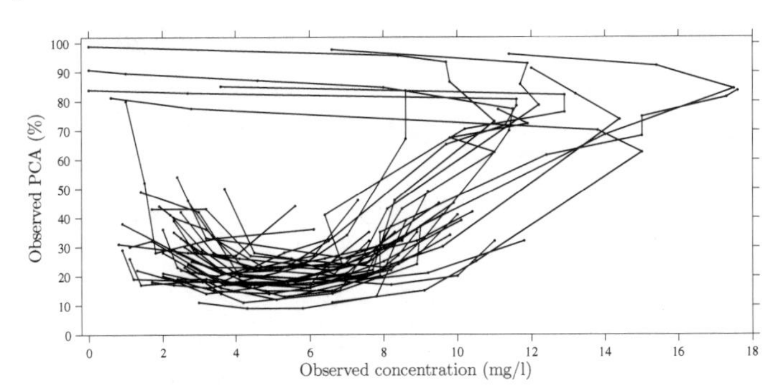

FIGURE 8.8: Warfarin PD data vs PK data for the 32 patients in the study.

These hysteresis loops mean that the observed effect is indirectly affected by the concentration. To properly model this relationship, we would be better served to use effect compartment or indirect PKPD models, which we will now describe.

8.2.1.2 Effect compartment models

For some drugs, a delay may occur between the value of the plasmatic concentration and the effect it has on the observed effect, because the effect site is not the central compartment and hence time is required for drug delivery to it. The idea of effect compartments has been introduced to help explain this time delay (Holford and Sheiner, 1981). We suppose that the virtual concentration C_e of this virtual compartment is the solution to the following ODE:

$$\dot{C_e}(t) = k_{e0}(C(t) - C_e(t)). \tag{8.6}$$

The drug effect is then determined by the concentration in the effect compartment instead of the central compartment:

$$E_e(t) = 1 - I_{max}\frac{C_e(t)}{IC_{50} + C_e(t)}.$$

The response R is now proportional to E_e:

$$R_2(t) = S_0\, E_e(t).$$

The MLXTRAN script for this new structural model is slightly modified from the previous one. The `pkmodel` function is now used for computing the concentration in the central and effect compartments.

```
                    Effect compartment model
INPUT:
parameter = {Tlag, ka, V, Cl, ke0, S0, Imax, IC50}

EQUATION:
{C, Ce} = pkmodel(Tlag, ka, V, Cl, ke0)
R = S0*(1-Imax*Ce/(Ce+IC50))

OUTPUT:
output = {C, R}
```

Using the same statistical model as for the immediate response model and a log-normal distribution for the rate constant k_{e0_i}, Figure 8.9 shows the four individual fits obtained with the new overall model.

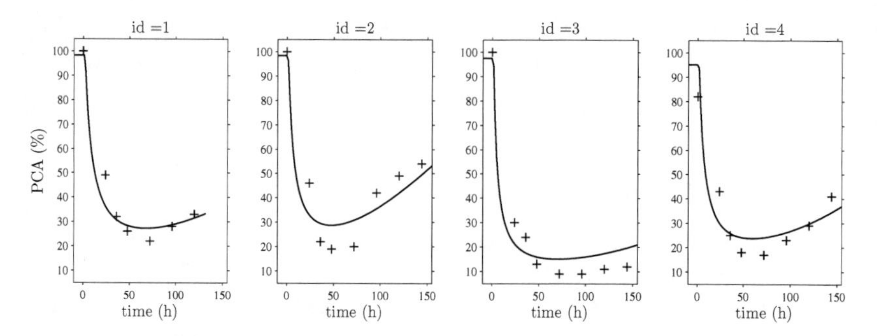

FIGURE 8.9: Individual fits for the PD data of four patients obtained with an effect compartment model.

While these individual fits appear better than the previous ones and indeed acceptable, more informative diagnostic plots such as individual weighted residuals and VPCs displayed in Figure 8.10 show that the delay is still not properly described with the effect compartment model.

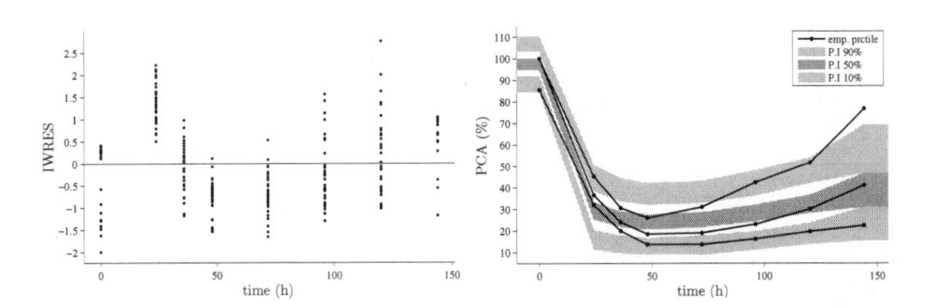

FIGURE 8.10: Diagnostic plots for the PD model when an effect compartment is used. Left: individual weighted residuals (IWRES), right: visual predictive check.

8.2.1.3 Indirect response model

The pharmacology of warfarin cannot be simply broken down into a dose-concentration relationship and a concentration-effect relationship because the clinically observable response, anticoagulation, is not the same as the drug effect, inhibition of vitamin K synthesis. A physiological effect relationship is therefore required to describe the link between the drug effect and prothrombin complex activity (Holford, 1986).

Before a patient receives the drug, the concentration of prothrombin complex is determined by a balance between synthesis and degradation:

$$\dot{R_3}(t) = k_{in} - k_{out}\, R_3(t).$$

At steady-state, the concentration of PCA is therefore $S_0 = k_{in}/k_{out}$. The arrival of warfarin then inhibits the production process (Holford, 1986; Sharma and Jusko, 1998):

$$\dot{R_3}(t) = k_{in}\, E(t) - k_{out}\, R_3(t),$$

where $E(t)$ is the drug effect defined in (8.5).

This new model is implemented in MLXTRAN using an ODE and defining the initial condition $R_3(t)$ for $t \leq 0$ (the dose is administered to each patient at $t = 0$).

```
                    Indirect response model

INPUT:
parameter = {Tlag, ka, V, Cl, Imax, IC50, kin, kout}

EQUATION:
C = pkmodel(Tlag, ka, V, Cl)
E = 1-Imax*C/(C+IC50)
R_0 = kin/kout
ddt_R = kin*E - kout*R

OUTPUT:
output = {C, R}
```

The diagnostic plots shown in Figure 8.11 show that this model describes well the observed data.

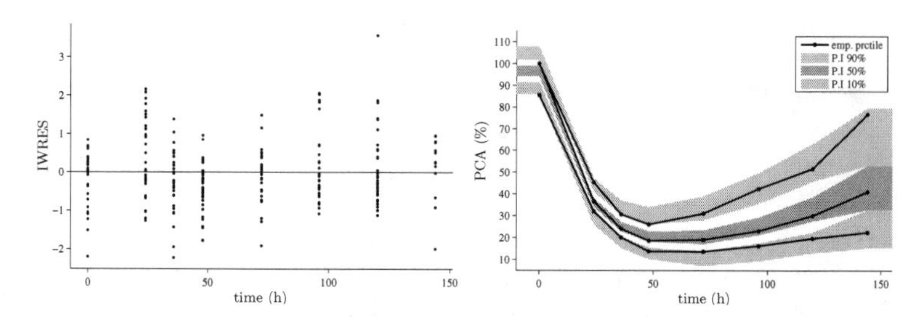

FIGURE 8.11: Diagnostic plots for the PD indirect response model. Left: individual weighted residuals, right: visual predictive check.

The estimated value of $Imax_{\text{pop}}$ is 0.999 for this model. We can therefore consider that inhibition is maximal and set $I_{max} = 1$ in (8.5). Following Sharma and Jusko (1998), we can also try to improve the drug effect model by introducing a Hill coefficient, i.e., replacing $E(t)$ with $E_h(t)$, defined by

$$E_h(t) = 1 - I_{max}\frac{C^h(t)}{IC_{50}{}^h + C^h(t)},$$

where $h > 0$ is assumed to be fixed across the population. All the parameters are well estimated with this PKPD model:

	parameter	s.e. (lin)	r.s.e.(%)	p-value
Tlag	0.869	0.19	21	
ka	1.61	0.46	29	
V	8.06	0.23	3	
beta_V	0.844	0.14	17	3.5e-09
Cl	0.134	0.0063	5	
beta_Cl	0.616	0.25	41	0.014
Imax	0.943	0.018	2	

```
IC50              1.3         0.13        10
kin                 5         0.19         4
kout           0.0522       0.0019         4
h                1.47        0.078         5

omega_Tlag      0.553         0.16        29
omega_ka        0.753         0.24        32
omega_V          0.14        0.022        16
omega_Cl         0.26        0.034        13
omega_Imax      0.411         0.22        54
omega_IC50      0.443        0.064        15
omega_kin      0.0451        0.019        41
omega_kout     0.0305         0.02        66
omega_h             0            -         -

a_1              0.34        0.047        14
b_1            0.0758       0.0081        11
a_2              3.73         0.22         6
```

We conclude from these results that h is significantly different from 1. Furthermore, the BIC is better when h is estimated (BIC=2161) than when it is fixed at 1 (BIC=2177). On the other hand, the VPCs and other diagnostic plots obtained with $h = 1.47$ and $h = 1$ are almost indistinguishable. We can therefore consider this model as our "final" one. The population distributions of the PKPD parameters are shown in Figure 8.12.

These probability distributions and the joint PKPD model can now, for instance, be used for simulating virtual patients in a virtual trial in order to find the optimal dose regimen, i.e., the one that optimizes therapeutic effect (efficacy) while minimizing undesirable side-effects such as bleeding (safety).

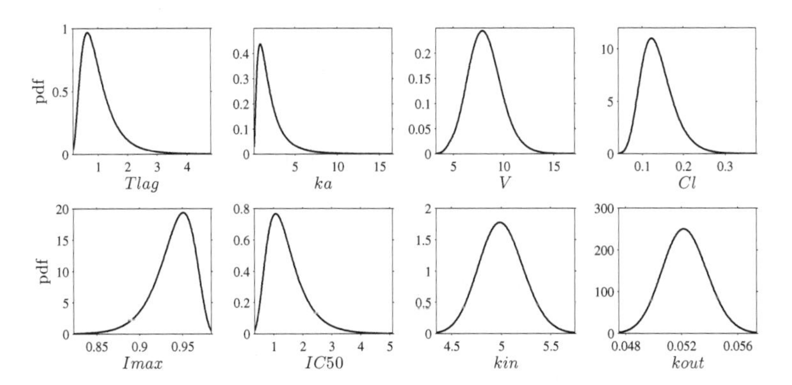

FIGURE 8.12: Population distributions of the PKPD parameters of the indirect response model with a Hill coefficient.

8.2.2 Sequential PKPD modeling

In the sequential approach, a PK model is developed and parameters estimated in the first step. For a given PD model, different strategies are then possible for the second step, i.e., for estimating the population PD parameters:

1. Population PK parameters are set to their estimated values but individual PK parameters are not assumed to be known and sampled from their conditional distributions at each SAEM iteration. In MONOLIX, this simply means changing the status of the population PK parameter values so that they are no longer used as initial estimates for SAEM but considered fixed.

2. Individual PK parameters are set to their estimated values and used as constants in the model. In this case, additional columns with the individual PK parameters need to be added in the dataset and defined as *regression variables* in MONOLIX. The PK data is then ignored. Lastly, we have to modify the status of the PK parameters in the structural model and define R as the only output.

```
Sequential PKPD modeling

INPUT:
parameter = {Imax, IC50, kin, kout, h}
regressor = {Tlag, ka, V, Cl}

EQUATION:
C = pkmodel(Tlag, ka, V, Cl)
R_0 = kin/kout
ddt_R = kin*(1-Imax*C^h/(C^h+IC50^h)) - kout*R

OUTPUT:
output = {R}
```

Estimation results for the population PD parameters for the simultaneous and two sequential approaches are summarized in Table 8.1. We see that there is very little difference between the simultaneous method and the sequential one which uses the estimated population PK parameters. This means that the PD data provides practically no information for population PK parameter estimation. However, there are several slight differences with the sequential method which uses the estimated individual parameters. We conclude therefore that the PD data does provide a small amount of information when estimating the individual PK parameters.

Remark: The sequential approach is justified when the joint model is a complex one with many parameters to estimate and simultaneous

TABLE 8.1: Estimation of the population PD parameters and their standard errors.

	Simultaneous	Sequential (1)	Sequential (2)
I_{max}	0.943 (0.018)	0.943 (0.017)	0.918 (0.015)
IC_{50}	1.30 (0.13)	1.33 (0.13)	1.22 (0.12)
k_{in}	5.00 (0.19)	4.97 (0.18)	5.21 (0.18)
k_{out}	0.052 (0.002)	0.052 (0.002)	0.054 (0.002)
h	1.47 (0.078)	1.51 (0.064)	1.56 (0.088)

Left: simultaneous approach; center: sequential approach using estimated population PK parameters; right: sequential approach using estimated individual PK parameters.

estimation of the whole set of parameters has a large computational cost. One possible strategy is to use a sequential approach to construct the PD model, then a simultaneous one for the final run, using the results of the sequential approach as initial estimates.

The sequential approach is not necessary in the case of the warfarin example as no particular problems come up with SAEM's parameter estimation.

8.2.3 Joint modeling of continuous PK and categorical PD data

International Normalized Ratio (INR) values are commonly used in clinical practice to target optimal warfarin therapy. Low INR values (<2) are associated with high blood clot risk and high ones (>3) with high risk of bleeding, so the targeted value of INR, corresponding to optimal therapy, is between 2 and 3.

Prothrombin complex activity is inversely proportional to the INR. We can therefore associate the three ordered categories for the INR to three ordered categories for PCA: Low PCA values if PCA is less than 33% (corresponding to INR$>$3), medium if PCA is between 33% and 50% ($2 \leq$INR≤ 3) and high if PCA is more than 50% (INR$<$2).

Instead of modeling the original continuous PD data, we can model the probabilities of each of these categories, which have direct clinical interpretations. The model is still a joint PKPD model since this probability distribution is expected to depend on exposure, i.e., the plasmatic concentration predicted by the PK model. We introduce an effect compartment to mimic the effect delay.

Let us first recode the three PCA levels as 1 (Low), 2 (Medium) and 3 (High). Let $y_{ij}^{(2)}$ be the PCA level for patient i at time $t_{ij}^{(2)}$. We can then used the proportional odds model proposed by Savic et al. (2011)

for modeling this categorical data:

$$\begin{aligned}
\text{logit}\left(\mathbb{P}\left(y_{ij}^{(2)} \leq 1|\psi_i\right)\right) &= \alpha_i + \beta_i\, Ce(t_{ij}^{(2)}, \phi_i^{(1)}) \\
\text{logit}\left(\mathbb{P}\left(y_{ij}^{(2)} \leq 2|\psi_i\right)\right) &= \alpha_i + \gamma_i + \beta_i\, Ce(t_{ij}^{(2)}, \phi_i^{(1)}) \\
\text{logit}\left(\mathbb{P}\left(y_{ij}^{(2)} \leq 3|\psi_i\right)\right) &= 1,
\end{aligned}$$

where $Ce(t, \phi_i^{(1)})$ is the predicted concentration of warfarin in the effect compartment at time t for patient i with PK parameters $\phi_i^{(1)}$. This model defines a probability distribution for y_{ij} if $\gamma_i \geq 0$. If $\beta_i > 0$, the probability of low PCA at time $t_{ij}^{(2)}$ ($y_{ij}^{(2)} = 1$) increases along with the predicted concentration $Ce(t_{ij}^{(2)}, \phi_i^{(1)})$.

The distribution of the categorical data is defined in a `DEFINITION` block of MLXTRAN. As in the previous examples, the predicted concentration is defined in the MLXTRAN script and the residual error model in the MONOLIX GUI.

```
Continuous and categorical data model

INPUT:
parameter = {Tlag, ka, V, Cl, ke0, alpha, beta, gamma}

EQUATION:
{C,Ce}= pkmodel(Tlag,ka,V,Cl,ke0)

DEFINITION:
Level = {type=categorical, categories={1,2,3},
         logit(P(Level<=1)) = alpha + beta*Ce,
         logit(P(Level<=2)) = alpha + beta*Ce + gamma}

OUTPUT:
output = {C, Level}
```

We use in this example a very simple statistical model for the individual PD parameters: a normal distribution for α_i, no inter-individual variability for β and γ, and γ constrained to take nonnegative values.

The visual predictive checks shown in Figure 8.13 compare the empirical proportions of the PCA categories as functions of time with their associated prediction intervals given by the model. We can conclude from these plots that the proposed model provides a fairly good prediction of the probability of having a low, medium and high PCA level.

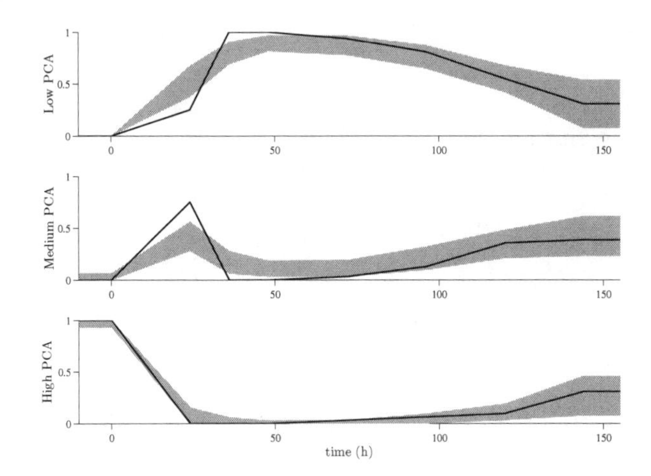

FIGURE 8.13: Visual predictive checks for categorical data. Solid line: observed proportions of low, medium and high PCA level as a function of time; shaded area: 90% prediction intervals given by the model for these proportions.

8.3 Gene expression in single cells

The population approach may also be relevant for building predictive computational models of intracellular processes. For example, consider as a case study the experiments performed in Uhlendorf et al. (2012) looking at the high-osmolarity glycerol (HOG) pathway in budding yeast. Yeast cells are exposed to osmotic shocks, i.e., sudden changes in the solute concentration of their surroundings. Signal transduction pathways, most notably the HOG pathway, provide information to the cell about the osmolarity of its environment and activate responses to deal with these stress conditions. In particular, a large set of genes is turned on and corresponding stress-responsive proteins are produced. This protein production process can be quantified by replacing one target protein, for example STL1, by a fluorescent protein such as yECitrine. This can be done by genetically modifying the yeast genome.

Thanks to time-lapse microscopy and cell tracking algorithms, single cell responses can be measured over time (Uhlendorf et al., 2012). Significant inter-cell variability is often observed.

We are now going to take a closer look at the data and models presented in Uhlendorf et al. (2012) and Gonzalez et al. (2013). The observed data y_{ij} is the measured fluorescence of yECitrine in cell i at time t_{ij}. The measure is taken every 6 minutes for each cell, so $t_{ij} = t_j = 6j$. Preprocessing of the data consists of removing cells considered outliers and correcting for tracking errors. Furthermore, only forty cells that were successfully tracked for more than 90 minutes are retained by the study's authors. Figure 8.14 shows the osmotic shocks applied to them and their observed fluorescent responses. Periods of 5 to 8 minutes of exposure to the hyperosmotic environment (*valve on*) alternated with periods of normal osmotic conditions (*valve off*).

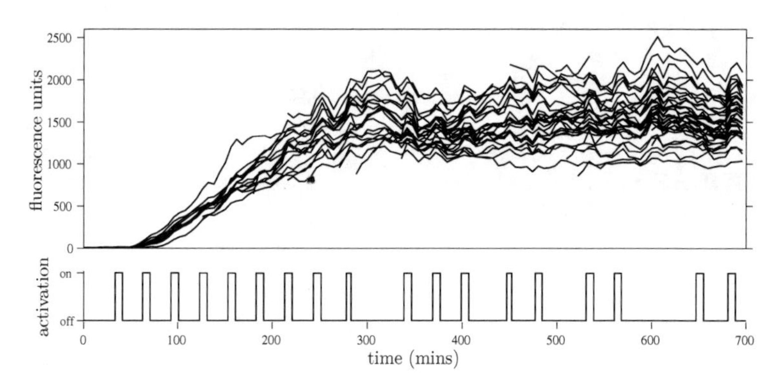

FIGURE 8.14: Experimental data. Top: fluorescent response of 40 yeast cells to repeated osmotic shocks; bottom: osmotic shocks applied to the system.

The related Hog1-induced gene expression model is given by a reaction network described in Zechner et al. (2012) and adapted in Gonzalez et al. (2013). We will now work with the mathematical representation of this model proposed by Gonzalez et al.. Let x_1, x_2 and x_4 be the proportions of promoters that are in the *off* state, in the *on* state or bound to chromatin remodeling factors. Let x_3, x_5 and x_6 be the concentrations of remodeling factors, messenger RNA and fluorescent yECitrine proteins. Then, the system can be described by the following set of reaction rate equations:

$$\begin{aligned}
\dot{x_1}(t) &= c_2x_2(t) - c_1u(t-\tau)x_1(t) \\
\dot{x_2}(t) &= c_1u(t-\tau)x_1(t) - c_2x_2(t) + c_4x_4(t) - c_3x_2(t)x_3(t) \\
\dot{x_3}(t) &= c_4x_4(t) - c_3x_2(t)x_3(t) \\
\dot{x_4}(t) &= c_3x_2(t)x_3(t) - c_4x_4(t) \\
\dot{x_5}(t) &= c_5x_4(t) - c_8x_5(t) \\
\dot{x_6}(t) &= c_6x_5(t) - c_7x_6(t),
\end{aligned} \tag{8.7}$$

where $u(t-\tau)$ is the delayed gene activation rate caused by an osmotic shock. The initial conditions at $t = t_0$ are $x_1(t_0) = 1$, $x_2(t_0) = x_4(t_0) = x_5(t_0) = x_6(t_0) = 0$ and $x_3(t_0) = x_{3,0}$.

We see in Figure 8.15 that the promoter activation rate $u(t)$ is directly related to the valve status $v(t)$ (on or off) displayed in Figure 8.14. For modeling, we need first to take into account the lag between change in valve status and change of osmolarity $h(t)$ of the cell environment. We assume that the medium needs one minute to change from normal to hyperosmotic when the valve is turned on and four minutes to return to normal when turned off. Then, the extracted nuclear Hog1 function $s(t)$ for a given salt concentration is a solution to the following ODE:

$$\dot{s}(t) = \kappa\, h(t) - \gamma\, s(t). \tag{8.8}$$

Lastly, the corresponding time-varying gene activation intensity $u(t)$ is obtained by transforming the Hog1 abundance using a Hill function:

$$u(t) = \frac{(s(t) + s_0)^{n_H}}{K_d^{n_H} + (s(t) + s_0)^{n_H}}. \tag{8.9}$$

Parameters κ, γ, n_H, K_d and s_0 are assumed known, taking the estimated values obtained in Zechner et al. (2012).

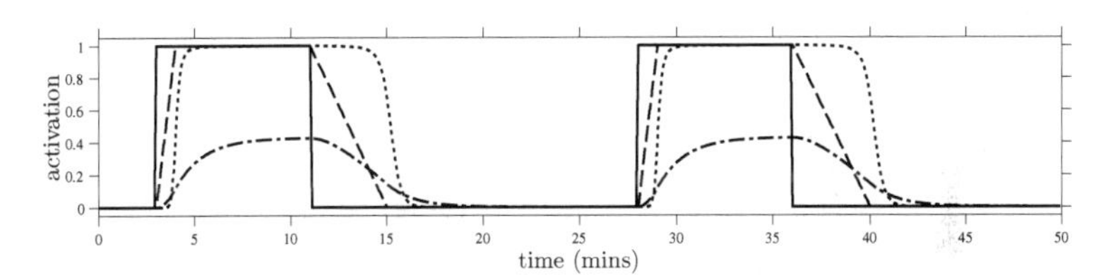

FIGURE 8.15: Input functions. Solid line: temporal evolution of the status of the microfluidic valve $v(t)$, 0: normal media (off), 1: hyperosmotic media (on); dashed line: osmolarity $h(t)$ of the cell environment; dotted line: nuclear Hog1 enrichment $s(t)$; dash-dot line: gene activation rate $u(t)$.

Here, the structural model combines the model for the activation intensity described by equations (8.8) and (8.9) and the dynamical system in (8.7). This model can easily be implemented using MLXTRAN:

```
reactionRate_mlxt.txt
[LONGITUDINAL]
input={c1,c2,c3,c4,c5,c6,c7,c8,x30,tau}

PK:
depot(target=h,Tlag=tau)

EQUATION:
kappa = 0.7
gamma = 0.3
nH = 6.13
Kd = 0.1418
s0 = 0.0158

ddt_h = 0
ddt_s = kappa*h - gamma*s
sh = (s+s0)^nH
u = sh/(Kd^nH+sh)

x1_0 = 1
x3_0 = x30
ddt_x1 = c2*x2 - c1*u*x1
ddt_x2 = c1*u*x1 - c2*x2 + c4*x4 - c3*x2*x3
ddt_x3 = c4*x4 - c3*x2*x3
ddt_x4 = c3*x2*x3 - c4*x4
ddt_x5 = c5*x4 - c8*x5
ddt_x6 = c6*x5 - c7*x6
```

The function h can then be defined by introducing inputs of value 1 at times $(t_k^{on}, 1 \leq k \leq K)$ with a rate of 1, and inputs with value -1 at times $(t_k^{off}, 1 \leq k \leq K)$ with rate 0.25. Here, $t_k^{off} - t_k^{on}$ is the duration of the kth shock.

We could then use MLXPLORE to visualize, for example, the signals shown in Figure 8.15. Source terms are considered as "infusions" with positive and negative amounts in the MLXPLORE script:

```
reactionRate1_mlxplore.txt
<MODEL>
file = 'reactionRate_mlxt.txt'

<DESIGN>
[ADMINISTRATION]
adm = {time={3,11,28,36}, amount={1,-1,1,-1},
       rate={1,0.25,1,0.25}}

<OUTPUT>
list = {h,s,u}
grid = 0:0.1:50
```

We could also use the experimental design for exploring properties of the structural model, i.e., by representing graphically one or several of the components of the system (8.7). Figure 8.16 displays predicted fluorescence x_6 using the parameter estimates obtained by Gonzalez et al. (2013).

```
                                    reactionRate2_mlxplore.txt
<MODEL>
file='reactionRate_mlxt.txt'

<DESIGN>
[ADMINISTRATION]
adm1={time={35,65,95,125,155,185,215,245,280,341,
            371,401,449,479,533,563,649,683},
      amount= 1, rate=1}
adm2={time={43,73,103,133,163,193,223,253,285,349,
            379,409,454,486,541,570,657,691},
      amount=-1, rate=0.25}

[TREATMENT]
trt={adm1,adm2}

;--------------------------------
<PARAMETER>
c1=73
c2=2500
c3=0.000019
c4=0.037
c5=1.3
c6=860
c7=0.0048
c8=0.1
x30=140
tau=14

<OUTPUT>
list={x6}
grid=0:1:800
```

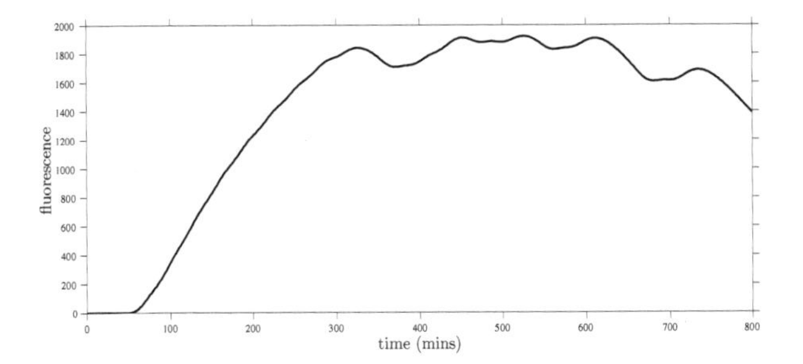

FIGURE 8.16: Predicted fluorescence defined as x_6 in model (8.7) using the given experimental design and $c_1 = 73$, $c_2 = 2500$, $c_3 = 1.9\,10^{-5}$, $c_4 = 3.7\,10^{-2}$, $c_5 = 1.3$, $c_6 = 860$, $c_7 = 4.8\,10^{-3}$, $c_8 = 0.1$, $x_{3,0} = 140$ and $\tau = 14$.

We can then use MONOLIX to estimate the model parameters using the data given in Figure 8.14. Here, source terms are included as part of the data. We therefore need columns with the "amounts" $(+1, -1, +1, -1, \ldots)$ and rates $(1, 0.25, 1, 0.25, \ldots)$.

id	time	amt	rate	y
1	0	.	.	4.2749
1	6	.	.	2.1614
1	12	.	.	0
1	18	.	.	1.8142
1	24	.	.	5.6618
1	30	.	.	2.3194
1	35	1	1	.
1	36	.	.	6.9808
1	42	.	.	6.2517
1	43	-1	0.25	.
1	48	.	.	2.9795
1	54	.	.	7.6437
1	60	.	.	20.149
1	65	1	1	.
1	66	.	.	41.159
1	72	.	.	65.205
1	73	-1	0.25	.
1	78	.	.	74.724
1	84	.	.	103.92
1	90	.	.	161.35

We also need to define a preliminary statistical model $\mathcal{M}_1$ for the data. Let us assume a combined error model for the observations: $y = x_6 + (a + bx_6)\varepsilon$, where x_6 is the predicted fluorescence defined in model (8.7). The individual parameters of the model are the reaction rates c_1 through c_8, delay τ and initial condition $x_{3,0}$. We use log-normal distributions for these ten parameters, considering for this first model that they are mutually independent.

All population parameters for $\mathcal{M}_1$ and their respective standard errors can then be estimated by MONOLIX:

	parameter	s.e. (s.a.)	r.s.e.(%)
c1	70.2	7.5	11
c2	2.48e+03	2e+02	8
c3	1.45e-05	1.3e-06	9
c4	0.0365	0.002	6
c5	1.12	0.08	7
c6	756	79	10
c7	0.00325	0.00047	14
c8	0.087	0.0092	11
x30	141	11	7
tau	8.15	1.4	18
omega_c1	0.629	0.09	14
omega_c2	0.482	0.056	12
omega_c3	0.548	0.085	16
omega_c4	0.324	0.033	10
omega_c5	0.429	0.059	14
omega_c6	0.645	0.077	12
omega_c7	0.893	0.11	12
omega_c8	0.654	0.077	12
omega_x30	0.46	0.052	11
omega_tau	0.832	0.13	15
a	8.98	0.72	8
b	0.0694	0.0013	2

The correlation matrix of the estimators is almost diagonal. There is therefore no reason, based on these results, to suspect over-parametrization of the structural model.

```
c1       1
c2    0.03      1
c3   -0.03   0.01      1
c4   -0.04  -0.02      0      1
c5   -0.02   0.02   0.03   0.01      1
c6   -0.01  -0.01  -0.04   0.02  -0.03      1
c7   -0.01  -0.01      0      0  -0.01   0.01      1
c8    0.02      0   0.01  -0.02   0.03  -0.01  -0.02      1
x30  -0.03     -0  -0.01   0.02  -0.02   0.01   0.01  -0.01      1
tau   0.02  -0.02   0.01   0.01     -0  -0.01   0.01   0.01  -0.02      1

Eigenvalues (min, max, max/min): 0.93  1.1  1.2
```

Furthermore, Figure 8.17 shows individual fits obtained with the MAP estimate for four cells under model $\mathcal{M}_1$. We can see that the structural model is capable of capturing quite different kinetics for different cells with different individual parameters.

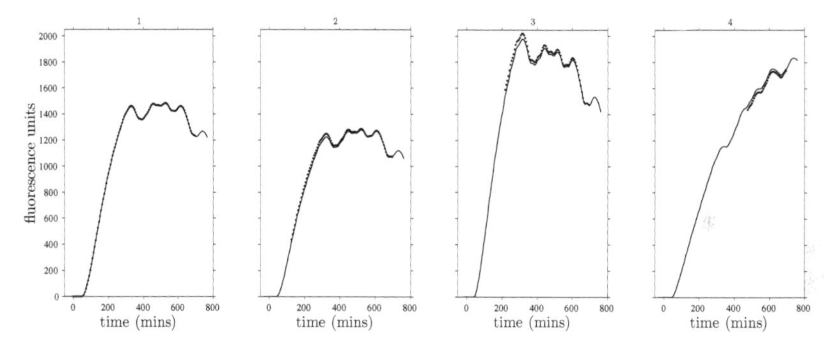

FIGURE 8.17: Individual fits obtained for four cells with model $\mathcal{M}_1$ assuming a diagonal variance-covariance matrix for the random effects. The dots are the observed fluorescence and the solid lines the predicted fluorescence.

However, kinetics simulated with this model may be quite different from those observed. The VPC obtained with model $\mathcal{M}_1$ (see Figure 8.18, left) shows unrealistic prediction intervals for the 10%, 50% and 90% quantiles. As the parametrization of the structural model is unlikely to be at fault, it is very likely the statistical model that is misspecified. In effect, the only constraints on its parameters are positivity ones because they are considered independent. It is nevertheless extremely probable that certain combinations of values are not realistic, producing entirely different kinetics to those observed. Let us instead define a joint distribution for these parameters, essentially meaning that we introduce the possibility of linear correlation between random effects. This means defining a new statistical model $\mathcal{M}_2$ in which we assume a full variance-covariance matrix for the random effects (i.e., none of the correlations between random effects are set to 0). After again performing parameter estimation with MONOLIX, we see in Figure 8.18 (right) that the VPC obtained with model $\mathcal{M}_2$ are significantly better than with model $\mathcal{M}_1$; indeed, they are quite acceptable.

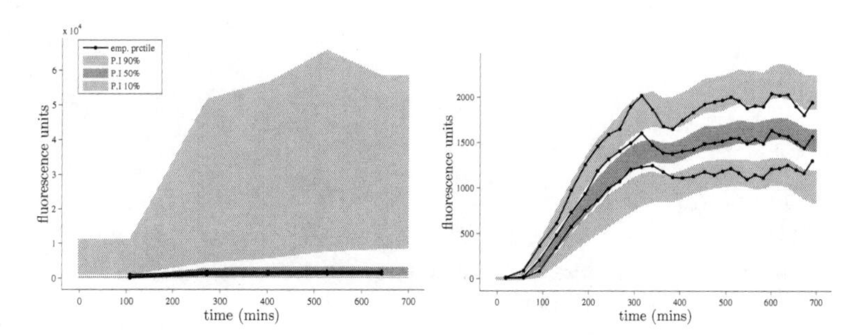

FIGURE 8.18: Visual predictive checks obtained with model $\mathcal{M}_1$ (left) and $\mathcal{M}_2$ (right).

9

Algorithms

9.1 Introduction

In this chapter we are going to present a number of algorithms for various tasks such as maximum likelihood estimation of population parameters θ, estimation of the Fisher information matrix, sampling the conditional distribution of the individual parameters (ψ_i) and estimation of the observed log-likelihood $\mathcal{LL}_{\boldsymbol{y}}(\theta)$. We will also present a very efficient method for automatic data binning.

The chapter can be approached in different ways. If the goal is only to get a general impression of the methods and how they work without necessarily understanding all the technical details, readers can take a brief look at each method. This does not mean we recommend using them like a "black box," but rather that this will give the reader access to criteria that help evaluate the quality of the results, and avoid using them unwisely.

If instead the reader has the goal of implementing these methods, a certain number of technical details are provided. For example, in Section 9.6 we give explicit calculations of the log-likelihood and its first and second derivatives. These can be ignored by anyone who is not aiming to implement the methods.

Neither is it our aim to give an exhaustive list of all possible methods for all possible models. We restrict ourselves to the Gaussian model for individual parameters presented in Section 5.3.3, making the hypothesis that there exists a monotone transform $h : \mathbb{R}^d \to \mathbb{R}^d$ such that

$$h(\psi_i) = \mu(\beta, c_i) + \eta_i, \tag{9.1}$$

where $\eta_i \sim_{\text{i.i.d.}} \mathcal{N}(0, 1)$ and c_i is a vector of individual covariates. In particular we are going to focus on the linear covariate model described in Section 5.3.2. The model proposed in (5.15) supposes that there exists a matrix C_i and vector β such that

$$h(\psi_i) = C_i \, \beta + \eta_i.$$

The most theoretical aspects of the algorithms will not be presented here. Nevertheless, these aspects and in particular convergence results (for EM, SAEM, MCMC, etc.) can be found in some of the works cited in the text.

9.1.1 Notation

We assume that the set of population parameters θ takes its values in Θ, an open subset of $\mathbb{R}^m$.

Let $f : \Theta \to \mathbb{R}$ be a twice differentiable function of θ. For $\zeta \in \Theta$, we will denote:

- $\partial_{\theta_j} f = \partial f / \partial \theta_j$ the partial derivative of f with respect to θ_j and $\partial_\theta f(\zeta) = (\partial_{\theta_j} f(\zeta), 1 \leq j \leq m)$ the gradient of f at ζ (i.e., the vector of partial derivatives of f evaluated at ζ).
- $\partial^2_{\theta_j \theta_k} f = \partial^2 f / \partial \theta_j \partial \theta_k^t$ the second-order partial derivatives of f with respect to θ_j and θ_k, and $\partial^2_\theta f(\zeta) = (\partial^2_{\theta_j \theta_k^t} f(\zeta), 1 \leq j, k \leq m)$ the Hessian of f at ζ (i.e., the square matrix of second-order partial derivatives of f evaluated at ζ).

The symbol $\simeq$ means *approximately equal to* and is used when dealing with numbers (for example, $x \simeq 3$). The symbol $\approx$ means *approximately distributed as* and is used for dealing with distributions of random variables (for example, $\varepsilon \approx \mathcal{N}(0, 1)$).

9.1.2 Different representations of the same model

Describing a model requires variables such as observations (y_i), individual parameters (ψ_i), covariates (c_i) and population parameters θ. Tasks to be performed (estimation, simulation, likelihood calculation, etc.) involve these variables. Algorithms used to perform these tasks can use different parametrizations, i.e., different mathematical representations of the same model. We will see that depending on the task, some mathematical representations are more suitable than others.

It is important to thoroughly understand how the various methods presented here can be implemented. In effect, all these methods (SAEM, MCMC, importance sampling, etc.) are based on the use of the joint probability distribution of all variables of the model. It is therefore critical to be able to correctly write out this distribution and all the conditional and marginal distributions that result from it. With this in mind, let us look at some possible mathematical representations.

- *ψ-representation*: There exists for modelers the natural parametrization involving a vector of individual parameters ψ_i which have a physical or biological meaning (rate, volume, bioavailability, etc.). The joint distribution of y_i and ψ_i is then associated with this representation:

$$\mathrm{p}(y_i, \psi_i; \theta, c_i) = \mathrm{p}(y_i|\psi_i)\mathrm{p}(\psi_i; \theta, c_i). \tag{9.2}$$

It is therefore this representation that modelers will typically use to represent their model.

EXAMPLE 9.1 Consider the following model for the observations:

$$y_{ij} = A_i\, e^{-k_i\, t_{ij}} \;+\; a_i \varepsilon_{ij}, \tag{9.3}$$

where $\varepsilon_{ij} \sim_{\text{i.i.d.}} \mathcal{N}(0,1)$. This model defines the conditional distribution of $y_i = (y_{ij}, 1 \leq j \leq n_i)$ given $\psi_i = (A_i, k_i, a_i)$:

$$y_{ij}\;|\psi_i \;\sim\; \mathcal{N}\left(A_i\, e^{-k_i\, t_{ij}}, a_i^2\right).$$

If there are no covariates in the model and if we use, respectively, logit-normal, log-normal and normal distributions for A_i, k_i and a_i, then the following statistical model $\mathrm{p}(\psi_i; \beta, \Omega)$ is assumed for the individual parameters:

$$\begin{pmatrix} \mathrm{logit}(A_i) \\ \log(k_i) \\ a_i \end{pmatrix} \sim \mathcal{N}(\beta,\; \Omega),$$

where $\beta = (\mathrm{logit}(A_{\text{pop}}), \log(k_{\text{pop}}), a_{\text{pop}})$. The model can therefore be decomposed as

$$\mathrm{p}(y_i, \psi_i; \beta, \Omega) = \mathrm{p}(y_i|\psi_i)\mathrm{p}(\psi_i; \beta, \Omega).$$

- *z-representation*: If there exists a transformation h such that $z_i = h(\psi_i)$ is a Gaussian vector, it is equivalent to use the representation which involves the transformed parameters (log-rate, log-volume, logit-bioavailability, etc.) and now represent the joint distribution of y_i and z_i:

$$\mathrm{p}(y_i, z_i; \theta, c_i) = \mathrm{p}(y_i|z_i)\mathrm{p}(z_i; \theta, c_i),$$

where $z_i \sim \mathcal{N}(\mu(\beta, c_i), \Omega)$ and $\theta = (\beta, \Omega)$. We will see that this representation turns out to be well adapted to the various tasks that interest us. For this reason, many of the algorithms we present will use this representation.

EXAMPLE 9.2 By defining $z_{A,i} = \text{logit}(A_i)$, $z_{k,i} = \log(k_i)$ and $z_{a,i} = a_i$, we can rewrite (9.3) as

$$y_{ij} = \frac{e^{-(e^{z_{k,i}})t_{ij}}}{1+e^{-z_{A,i}}} + z_{a,i}\varepsilon_{ij}. \tag{9.4}$$

Now, (9.4) defines the conditional distribution of y_i given $z_i = (z_{A,i}, z_{k,i}, z_{a,i})$. Here, z_i is normally distributed:

$$z_i \sim \mathcal{N}(\beta,\ \Omega).$$

The model can be decomposed as $\mathrm{p}(y_i, z_i; \beta, \Omega) = \mathrm{p}(y_i|z_i)\mathrm{p}(z_i; \beta, \Omega)$.

- *η-representation*: There is yet another mathematical representation to represent the individual parameter model which uses the vector of random effects η_i introduced in (9.1). This representation leads to the joint distribution of y_i and η_i:

$$\mathrm{p}(y_i, \eta_i; \theta, c_i) = \mathrm{p}(y_i|\eta_i; \beta, c_i)\mathrm{p}(\eta_i; \Omega).$$

We can see that using the η-representation, the fixed effects β now appear in the conditional distribution of the observations. This will have a strong impact on tasks such as estimation of population parameters since a sufficient statistic for estimating β derived from this representation will be a function of the observations (y_i), as opposed to the other representations where the sufficient statistic is a function of the individual parameters (ψ_i) (or equivalently, (z_i)). It will therefore sometimes be useful to use the z-representation for algorithmic reasons.

Certain tasks such as estimation require the use of regular statistical models. Furthermore, we will see in Section 9.1.3 that only the η-representation can be used in certain situations.

EXAMPLE 9.3

By supposing now that

$$\begin{aligned} z_{A,i} &= \text{logit}(A_{\text{pop}}) + \eta_{A,i} \\ z_{k,i} &= \log(k_{\text{pop}}) + \eta_{k,i} \\ z_{a,i} &= a_{\text{pop}} + \eta_{a,i}, \end{aligned}$$

we can rewrite (9.4) as

$$y_{ij} = \frac{A_{\text{pop}}e^{-(k_{\text{pop}}\,e^{\eta_{k,i}})\,t_{ij}}}{A_{\text{pop}} + (1 - A_{\text{pop}})e^{-\eta_{A,i}}} + (a_{\text{pop}} + \eta_{a,i})\varepsilon_{ij}. \tag{9.5}$$

Equation (9.5) defines the conditional distribution $p(y_i \,|\, \eta_i; \beta)$ where $(\eta_{A,i}, \eta_{k,i}, \eta_{a,i})$ is normally distributed: Here, $\eta_i \sim \mathcal{N}(0, \Omega)$. Our model can thus be decomposed as

$$p(y_i, \eta_i; \beta, \Omega) = p(y_i|\eta_i; \beta)p(\eta_i; \Omega).$$

9.1.3 Using nondegenerate statistical models

We will say that the probability distribution of the Gaussian vector z_i is *degenerate* if the variance-covariance matrix of z_i is not positive-definite. This can happen, for example, if one of the components of z_i is nonrandom and constant, or when certain components are linearly related.

A mathematical representation of a model using nondegenerate distributions will turn out to be particularly necessary for being able to define sufficient statistics for estimating its parameters. Let us look at several examples.

1. Consider the following model for continuous data with a constant error model, using the z-representation:

$$\begin{aligned} y_{ij} &\sim \mathcal{N}(f(t_{ij}, z_i), a_i^2) \\ z_i &\sim \mathcal{N}(\mu(\beta, c_i), \Omega) \\ a_i &\sim p_a(\,\cdot\,; \theta_a). \end{aligned}$$

   Here, the standard deviation of the residual error is a random variable and $\theta = (\beta, \Omega, \theta_a)$. Assuming that z_i and a_i are independent and Ω is positive-definite, the joint model of y_i, z_i and a_i can be decomposed into a product of three regular models:

$$p(y_i, z_i, a_i; \theta) = p(y_i|z_i, a_i)p(z_i; \beta, \Omega)p(a_i; \theta_a).$$

EXAMPLE 9.4 Let us go back to Example 9.2 introduced in Section 9.1.2. Let $z_i = (z_{A,i}, z_{k,i})$ and assume that a_i is independent of z_i. We can then decompose the joint distribution of (y_i, z_i, a_i) into a product of three regular models:

- The conditional distribution of y_i given (z_i, a_i), still defined by (9.4).
- Let $\beta = (\text{logit}A_{\text{pop}}, \log k_{\text{pop}})$ and Ω be the variance-covariance matrix of z_i. Then, $z_i \sim \mathcal{N}(\beta,\ \Omega)$.
- Let ω_a^2 be the variance of a_i. Then, $\theta_a = (a_{\text{pop}}, \omega_a^2)$ and $a_i \sim \mathcal{N}(a_{\text{pop}}, \omega_a^2)$.

2. Assume instead that the variance of the residual error is the same for the whole population:

$$y_{ij} \sim \mathcal{N}(f(t_{ij}, z_i), a^2).$$

The vector of population parameters is now $\theta = (\beta, \Omega, a)$ and the joint model of y_i and z_i can be decomposed as

$$\mathrm{p}(y_i, z_i; \theta) = \mathrm{p}(y_i | z_i; a)\mathrm{p}(z_i; \beta, \Omega).$$

EXAMPLE 9.5 If $a_i = a$ is no longer random, the conditional distribution $\mathrm{p}(y_i|z_i; a)$ is now defined by the model

$$y_{ij} = \frac{e^{-(e^{z_{k,i}})t_{ij}}}{1 + e^{-z_{A,i}}} + a\varepsilon_{ij}.$$

The distribution of $z_i = (z_{A,i}, z_{k,i})$ remains unchanged.

3. Suppose that some components of z_i have no inter-individual variability. More precisely, let $z_i = (z_i^{(1)}, z_i^{(0)})$ and $\beta = (\beta_1, \beta_0)$ such that

$$z_i^{(1)} \sim \mathcal{N}(\mu_1(\beta_1, c_i), \Omega_1)$$
$$z_i^{(0)} = \mu_0(\beta_0, c_i),$$

where Ω_1 is positive definite. Here, $\theta = (\beta_1, \beta_0, \Omega_1, a)$ and

$$\mathrm{p}(y_i, z_i; \theta, c_i) = \mathrm{p}(y_i | z_i^{(1)}; \beta_0, a, c_i)\mathrm{p}(z_i^{(1)}; \beta_1, \Omega_1, c_i).$$

EXAMPLE 9.6 Assume that $A_i = A$ is fixed. Then, the conditional distribution $\mathrm{p}(y_i|z_{k,i}; A, a)$ is now defined by the model:

$$y_{ij} = A\, e^{-e^{z_{k,i}} t_{ij}} + a\varepsilon_{ij},$$

where $z_{k,i} = \log(k_i)$ is normally distributed with mean $\log(k_{\mathrm{pop}})$ and variance ω_k^2. The joint model can then be decomposed as

$$\mathrm{p}(y_i, z_{k,i}; A, k_{\mathrm{pop}}, \omega_k^2, a) = \mathrm{p}(y_i | z_{k,i}; A, a)\mathrm{p}(z_{k,i}; k_{\mathrm{pop}}, \omega_k^2).$$

4. Assume instead that $z_i = (z_{1,i}, z_{2,i})$, where

$$z_{1,i} = \beta_1 + \eta_i$$
$$z_{2,i} = \beta_2 + B\eta_i,$$

and $\eta_i \sim \mathcal{N}(0, \Omega)$. Here, $\theta = (\beta_1, \beta_2, \Omega, B, a)$. We can no longer use the z-representation for this model since the variance-covariance matrix of z_i is not positive-definite. In this example, the most useful model is the joint distribution of y_i and η_i. We should therefore use the following η-representation:

$$\mathrm{p}(y_i, \eta_i; \theta) = \mathrm{p}(y_i|\eta_i; \beta_1, \beta_2, B, a)\mathrm{p}(\eta_i; \Omega).$$

EXAMPLE 9.7 Assume that

$$z_{A,i} = \mathrm{logit}(A_{\mathrm{pop}}) + \eta_i$$
$$z_{k,i} = \log(k_{\mathrm{pop}}) + b\eta_i,$$

where $\eta_i \sim \mathcal{N}(0, \omega^2)$. It is not possible here to construct a sufficient statistic that is a function of $z_{A,i}$ and $z_{k,i}$ for estimating $(A_{\mathrm{pop}}, k_{\mathrm{pop}}, b)$. We will therefore use the following η-representation:

$$\mathrm{p}(y_i, \eta_i; A_{\mathrm{pop}}, k_{\mathrm{pop}}, b, a, \omega) = \mathrm{p}(y_i|\eta_i; A_{\mathrm{pop}}, k_{\mathrm{pop}}, b, a)\mathrm{p}(\eta_i; \omega),$$

where the conditional distribution $\mathrm{p}(y_i|\eta_i; A_{\mathrm{pop}}, k_{\mathrm{pop}}, b, a)$ is defined by the model

$$y_{ij} = \frac{A_{\mathrm{pop}} e^{-(k_{\mathrm{pop}} e^{\eta_i})\, t_{ij}}}{A_{\mathrm{pop}} + (1 - A_{\mathrm{pop}})e^{-\eta_i}} + a\varepsilon_{ij}.$$

9.2 The SAEM algorithm for estimating population parameters

9.2.1 Introduction

The SAEM (stochastic approximation of EM) algorithm is a stochastic algorithm for computing the maximum likelihood (ML) estimate in the general setting of incomplete data models. SAEM has been shown to be a very powerful tool in the population context (see, for example, Chan et al., 2011; Delattre et al., 2012; Makowski and Lavielle, 2006), known to accurately estimate population parameters as well as have good theoretical properties. In fact, it converges to the ML estimate under quite general hypotheses (Allassonnière et al., 2010; Delyon et al., 1999; Kuhn and Lavielle, 2004).

The SAEM algorithm was originally implemented in the MONOLIX software. It has subsequently been implemented in NONMEM, the R package `saemix` and the MATLAB statistics toolbox as the function `nlmefitsa`.

In this section, we will consider a model that includes observations $\boldsymbol{y} = (y_i, 1 \leq i \leq N)$, unobserved individual parameters $\boldsymbol{\psi} = (\psi_i, 1 \leq i \leq N)$ and a vector of parameters θ. By definition, the maximum likelihood estimator of θ maximizes

$$\mathcal{L}_{\boldsymbol{y}}(\theta) = \mathrm{p}(\boldsymbol{y};\theta) = \int \mathrm{p}(\boldsymbol{y},\boldsymbol{\psi};\theta)\, d\boldsymbol{\psi} = \int \mathrm{p}(\boldsymbol{y},\boldsymbol{z};\theta)\, d\boldsymbol{z}.$$

We can then use interchangeably the ψ-representation or z-representation for defining the objective function to maximize; however, the use of normal distributions simplifies the calculations. We will therefore use the z-representation here.

We are going to give a general description of the algorithm highlighting the connection with the EM algorithm, and present by way of a simple example how to implement SAEM and use it in practice. Also, we will look at some extensions of the original algorithm that allow us to improve its convergence properties. For instance, it is possible to stabilize its convergence by using several Markov chains per individual. Also, a simulated annealing variant allows us to improve the chances of converging to the global maximum of the likelihood rather than to a local one. Lastly, a version using parameter expansion can accelerate SAEM's convergence.

9.2.2 The EM algorithm

We first remark that if the individual parameters $\boldsymbol{z}$ could be observed, estimation would not be held up by any particular problem because an estimator could be found by directly maximizing the joint distribution $\mathrm{p}(\boldsymbol{y},\boldsymbol{z};\theta)$. However, since they are not observed, the EM algorithm replaces $\boldsymbol{z}$ by its conditional expectation (Dempster et al., 1977). Then, given some initial value θ_0, iteration k updates θ_{k-1}^{EM} to θ_k^{EM} with the following two steps:

- **E-step:** Evaluate the quantity

$$Q_k^{EM}(\theta) = \mathbb{E}\left(\log \mathrm{p}(\boldsymbol{y},\boldsymbol{z};\theta)|\boldsymbol{y};\theta_{k-1}^{EM}\right). \tag{9.6}$$

- **M-step:** Update the estimation of θ:

$$\theta_k^{EM} = \arg\max_\theta Q_k^{EM}(\theta).$$

It can be proved that each EM iteration increases the likelihood of the observations and that the EM sequence (θ_k^{EM}) converges to a stationary point of the observed likelihood under mild regularity conditions (Wu, 1983).

Unfortunately, in the framework of nonlinear mixed effects models, there is no explicit expression for the E-step since the relationship between observations $\boldsymbol{y}$ and individual parameters $\boldsymbol{z}$ is nonlinear. However, even though this expectation cannot be computed in closed-form, it can be approximated by simulation. For instance, the Monte Carlo EM (MCEM) algorithm replaces the E-step by a Monte Carlo approximation based on a large number of independent simulations of the nonobserved individual parameters $\boldsymbol{z}$ (Wei and Tanner, 1990). Alternatively, the SAEM algorithm replaces the E-step by a stochastic approximation based on a single simulation of $\boldsymbol{z}$ (Delyon et al., 1999).

9.2.3 The SAEM algorithm

SAEM is an iterative algorithm which requires an initial guess θ_0. Then, iteration k of SAEM consists of three steps:

- **Simulation step**: For $i = 1, 2, \ldots, N$, draw $z_i^{(k)}$ from the conditional distribution $\mathrm{p}(z_i|y_i; \theta_{k-1})$.
- **Stochastic approximation**: Update $Q_{k-1}(\theta)$ according to

$$Q_k(\theta) = Q_{k-1}(\theta) + \gamma_k \left(\log \mathrm{p}(\boldsymbol{y}, \boldsymbol{z}^{(k)}; \theta) - Q_{k-1}(\theta) \right),$$

  where (γ_k) is a decreasing sequence of positive numbers such that $\gamma_1 = 1$.

- **Maximization step**: Update θ_{k-1} according to

$$\theta_k = \arg\max_\theta Q_k(\theta).$$

Remarks:

1. Convergence of SAEM requires that $\sum_{k=1}^{\infty} \gamma_k = \infty$ and $\sum_{k=1}^{\infty} \gamma_k^2 < \infty$ (Delyon et al., 1999). This condition is satisfied if, for instance, (γ_k) decreases as $1/k$.

2. Setting $\gamma_k = 1$ for all k means that there is no memory in the stochastic approximation:

$$Q_k(\theta) = \log \mathrm{p}(\boldsymbol{y}, \boldsymbol{z}^{(k)}; \theta).$$

   This algorithm, also known as Stochastic EM (SEM, see Celeux and Diebolt, 1985 for an application to mixtures), thus consists of successively simulating $\boldsymbol{z}^{(k)}$ with the conditional distribution $\mathrm{p}(\boldsymbol{z}^{(k)}|\boldsymbol{y}; \theta_{k-1})$, then computing θ_k by maximizing the joint distribution $\mathrm{p}(\boldsymbol{y}, \boldsymbol{z}^{(k)}; \theta)$.

3. When the number N of subjects is small, convergence of SAEM can be improved by running L Markov chains for each individual instead of one. The simulation step at iteration k therefore involves drawing L sequences $z_i^{(k,1)}, \ldots, z_i^{(k,L)}$ for each individual i and combining stochastic approximation and Monte Carlo in the approximation step:

$$Q_k(\theta) = Q_{k-1}(\theta) + \gamma_k \left(\frac{1}{L} \sum_{\ell=1}^{L} \log \mathrm{p}(\boldsymbol{y}, \boldsymbol{z}^{(k,\ell)}; \theta) - Q_{k-1}(\theta) \right). \quad (9.7)$$

   Note that by default, MONOLIX selects L so that $N \times L \geq 50$.

4. When $\gamma_k = 1$ and $L \gg 1$ for all k, $Q_k(\theta)$ defined in (9.7) is a Monte Carlo approximation of the expectation $Q_k^{EM}(\theta)$ defined in (9.6). This algorithm is known as MCEM (Wei and Tanner, 1990). Convergence of MCEM requires that L increases at each iteration (Fort and Moulines, 2003), which can be computationally expensive in practice.

Implementation of SAEM is simplified when the complete model $\mathrm{p}(\boldsymbol{y}, \boldsymbol{z}; \theta)$ belongs to a regular (curved) exponential family:

$$\mathrm{p}(\boldsymbol{y}, \boldsymbol{z}; \theta) = \exp\left\{ -\zeta(\theta) + \tilde{S}(\boldsymbol{y}, \boldsymbol{z}) \cdot \varphi(\theta) \right\},$$

where $\tilde{S}(\boldsymbol{y}, \boldsymbol{z})$ is a sufficient statistic[1] of the complete model which takes its values in an open subset $\mathcal{S}$ of $\mathbb{R}^m$. Then, there exists a function $\tilde{\theta}$ such that for any $s \in \mathcal{S}$,

$$\tilde{\theta}(s) = \arg\max_{\theta} \left\{ -\zeta(\theta) + s \cdot \varphi(\theta) \right\}. \quad (9.8)$$

The approximation step in SAEM simplifies to a general Robbins-Monro-type scheme for approximating this conditional expectation:

[1]That is, whose value contains all the information needed to compute any estimate of θ.

- **Stochastic approximation**: Update s_k according to

$$s_k = s_{k-1} + \gamma_k(\tilde{S}(\boldsymbol{y}, \boldsymbol{z}^{(k)}) - s_{k-1}).$$

Then, SAEM uses (9.8) for the M-step: $\theta_k = \tilde{\theta}(s_k)$. Note that the EM E-step simplifies to computing $s_k^{EM} = \mathbb{E}\left(\tilde{S}(\boldsymbol{y}, \boldsymbol{z})|\boldsymbol{y}; \theta_{k-1}^{EM}\right)$ and $\theta_k^{EM} = \tilde{\theta}(s_k^{EM})$.

Precise results for the convergence of SAEM were obtained by Delyon et al. (1999) in the case where $\mathrm{p}(\boldsymbol{y}, \boldsymbol{z}; \theta)$ belongs to a regular curved exponential family. This first version of SAEM and these initial theoretical results assume that the individual parameters are simulated exactly under the conditional distribution at each iteration. Unfortunately, for most nonlinear models and non-Gaussian models, the unobserved data cannot be simulated exactly under this conditional distribution. A well-known alternative consists in using the Metropolis-Hastings (MH) algorithm: introduce a transition probability which has as unique invariant distribution the conditional distribution we want to simulate.

In other words, the procedure consists of replacing SAEM's simulation step at iteration k by m iterations of the MH algorithm described in Section 9.3. When the individual parameters z_i are assumed to take their values in a compact set, it has been shown by Kuhn and Lavielle (2004) that SAEM still converges under general conditions when coupled with a Markov chain Monte Carlo (MCMC) procedure. Extensions of this result to distributions defined on noncompact sets have been obtained by Allassonnière et al. (2010).

Remark: Convergence of the Markov chains $(z_i^{(k)})$ is not necessary at each SAEM iteration. It suffices to run a few MH iterations with various transition kernels before resetting θ_{k-1}. In MONOLIX, by default the three transition kernels described in Section 9.3 are used twice each, successively, in each SAEM iteration.

9.2.4 Implementing SAEM

Implementation of SAEM can be difficult to describe when looking at complex statistical models such as mixture models, hidden Markov models or models with inter-occasion variability. We are therefore going to limit ourselves to looking at some basic models in order to illustrate how SAEM can be implemented in practice.

9.2.4.1 SAEM for general hierarchical models

Consider first a very general model for any type (continuous, categorical, survival, etc.) of data:

$$\begin{aligned} y_i|z_i &\sim \mathrm{p}(y_i|z_i) \\ z_i &\sim \mathcal{N}(\beta, \Omega), \end{aligned}$$

where $z_i = (z_{i,1}, z_{i,2}, \dots, z_{i,d})^t$ is a d-vector of (transformed) individual parameters, β a d-vector of fixed effects and Ω a $d \times d$ variance-covariance matrix assumed to be positive-definite. Then, a sufficient statistic for the complete model $\mathrm{p}(\boldsymbol{y}, \boldsymbol{z}; \theta)$ is $\tilde{S}(\boldsymbol{z}) = (\tilde{S}_1(\boldsymbol{z}), \tilde{S}_2(\boldsymbol{z}))$, where

$$\begin{aligned} \tilde{S}_1(\boldsymbol{z}) &= \sum_{i=1}^{N} z_i \\ \tilde{S}_2(\boldsymbol{z}) &= \sum_{i=1}^{N} z_i z_i^t. \end{aligned}$$

At iteration k of SAEM, we have the following:

- **Simulation step**: For $i = 1, 2, \dots, N$, draw $z_i^{(k)}$ from m iterations of the MH algorithm described in Section 9.3 with $\mathrm{p}(z_i|y_i; \mu_{k-1}, \Omega_{k-1})$ as the limiting distribution.
- **Stochastic approximation**: Update $s_k = (s_{k,1}, s_{k,2})$ according to

$$\begin{aligned} s_{k,1} &= s_{k-1,1} + \gamma_k \left(\sum_{i=1}^{N} z_i^{(k)} - s_{k-1,1} \right) \\ s_{k,2} &= s_{k-1,2} + \gamma_k \left(\sum_{i=1}^{N} z_i^{(k)} (z_i^{(k)})^t - s_{k-1,2} \right). \end{aligned}$$

- **Maximization step**: Update $(\mu_{k-1}, \Omega_{k-1})$ according to

$$\begin{aligned} \mu_k &= \frac{s_{k,1}}{N} \\ \Omega_k &= \frac{s_{k,2}}{N} - \mu_k \mu_k^t. \end{aligned}$$

What is remarkable is that it suffices to be able to calculate $\mathrm{p}(y_i|z_i)$ (i.e., $\mathrm{p}(y_i|\psi_i)$) for all z_i and y_i in order to be able to run SAEM. In effect, this calculation allows the simulation step to be run using MH since the acceptance probabilities can be calculated.

9.2.4.2 SAEM for continuous data models

Consider now a continuous data model in which the residual error variance is constant:

$$\begin{aligned} y_{ij} &= f(t_{ij}, z_i) + a\varepsilon_{ij} \\ z_i &\sim \mathcal{N}(\beta, \Omega). \end{aligned} \tag{9.9}$$

If we suppose that the variance-covariance matrix Ω is positive-definite, then noting $\theta = (\beta, \Omega, a)$, a natural decomposition of the model is

$$\mathrm{p}(\boldsymbol{y}, \boldsymbol{z}; \theta) = \mathrm{p}(\boldsymbol{y}|\boldsymbol{z}; a)\mathrm{p}(\boldsymbol{z}; \beta, \Omega).$$

The previous statistic $\tilde{S}(\boldsymbol{z}) = (\tilde{S}_1(\boldsymbol{z}), \tilde{S}_2(\boldsymbol{z}))$ is not sufficient for estimating a. In fact, we need an additional component which is a function of both $\boldsymbol{y}$ and $\boldsymbol{z}$:

$$\tilde{S}_3(\boldsymbol{y}, \boldsymbol{z}) = \sum_{i=1}^{N} \sum_{j=1}^{n_i} (y_{ij} - f(t_{ij}, z_i))^2.$$

Then,

$$\begin{aligned} s_{k,3} &= s_{k-1,3} + \gamma_k(\tilde{S}_3(\boldsymbol{y}, \boldsymbol{z}) - s_{k-1,3}) \\ a_k^2 &= \frac{s_{k,3}}{\sum_{i=1}^{N} n_i} . \end{aligned}$$

9.2.4.3 Choosing SAEM parameters

The choice of step-size (γ_k) is extremely important for ensuring convergence of SAEM. The sequence (γ_k) used in MONOLIX decreases like $k^{-\alpha}$. We recommend using $\alpha = 0$ (that is, $\gamma_k = 1$) during the first K_1 iterations in order to converge quickly to a neighborhood of a maximum of the likelihood, and $\alpha = 1$ during the next K_2 iterations. Indeed, the initial guess θ_0 may be far from the maximum likelihood value we are seeking, and the first iterations with $\gamma_k = 1$ allow SAEM to converge quickly to a neighborhood of this value. Following this, smaller step-sizes ensure the almost sure convergence of the algorithm to the maximum likelihood estimator.

EXAMPLE 9.8 Consider a simple model for continuous data:

$$\begin{aligned} y_{ij} &\sim \mathcal{N}(A_i\, e^{-k_i\, t_{ij}}, a^2) \\ \log(A_i) &\sim \mathcal{N}(\log(A_{\text{pop}}), \omega_A^2) \\ \log(k_i) &\sim \mathcal{N}(\log(k_{\text{pop}}), \omega_k^2), \end{aligned}$$

where $A_{\text{pop}} = 6$, $k_{\text{pop}} = 0.25$, $\omega_A = 1$, $\omega_k = 0.3$ and $a = 0.2$. Using simulated data with $N = 40$ subjects and $(t_{ij}) = (2, 4, 12, 20)$ for all i, let us look at the effect of different settings for (γ_k) and L when estimating the population parameters of the model with SAEM. We use the same initial guess $\theta_0 = (1, 0.5, 3, 1, 1)$ for the different runs shown below.

1. For all k, $\gamma_k = 1$, the sequence (θ_k) converges very quickly (fewer than 20 iterations in this example) to a neighborhood of the "solution" (Figure 9.1). The sequence (θ_k) does not converge to a fixed limit; it is a homogeneous Markov Chain that converges in distribution.

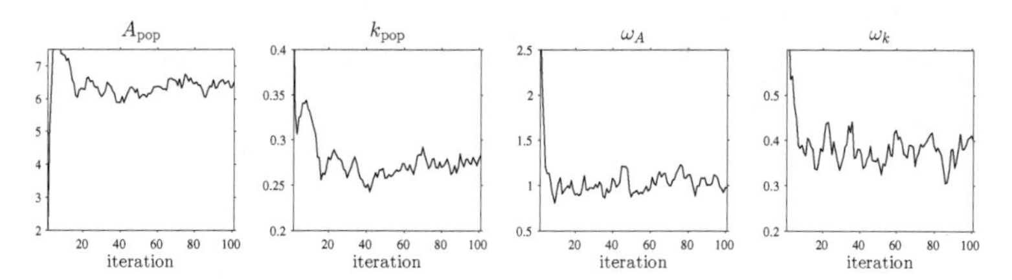

FIGURE 9.1: Sequence of SAEM estimates (θ_k) obtained with $\gamma_k = 1$.

2. For all k, $\gamma_k = 1/k$, the sequence (θ_k) converges *almost surely* (i.e., with probability 1) to the maximum likelihood estimate of θ, but very slowly; more than 500 iterations are required here (Figure 9.2).

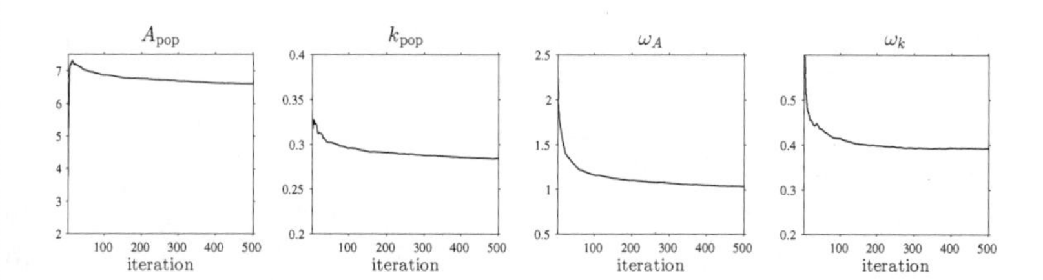

FIGURE 9.2: Sequence of SAEM estimates (θ_k) obtained with $\gamma_k = 1/k$.

3. We can instead combine these two strategies, first using $\gamma_k = 1$ for $k = 1, \ldots, K_1$ to quickly converge to a neighborhood of the solution, then $\gamma_k = 1/(k - K_1)$ for $k > K_1$ to ensure almost sure convergence of the sequence (θ_k) to the maximum likelihood estimate of θ (Figure 9.3). Here, $K_1 = 50$.

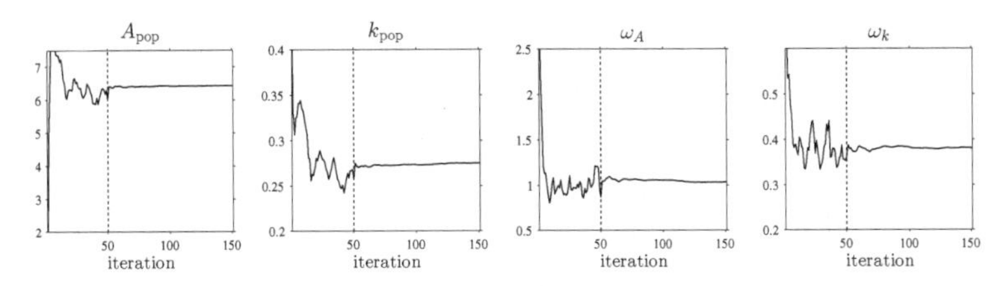

FIGURE 9.3: Sequence of SAEM estimates (θ_k) obtained with $\gamma_k = 1$ for $k = 1, \ldots, 50$ and $\gamma_k = 1/(k-50)$ for $k > 50$.

4. Using the same sequence (γ_k), we can reduce the simulation variance by simulating $L = 40$ chains per individual. In this case, SAEM behaves like EM (Figure 9.4).

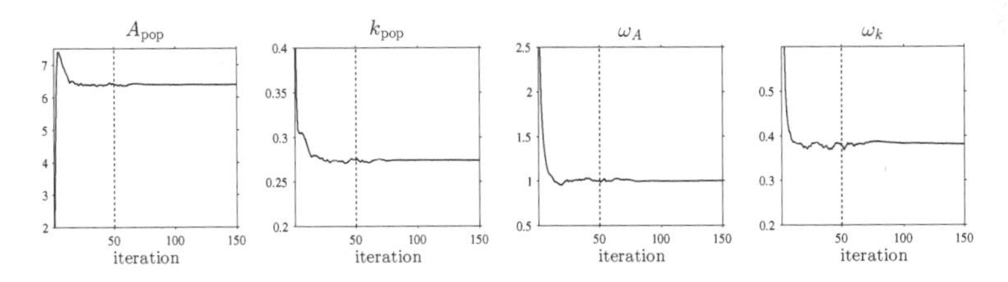

FIGURE 9.4: Sequence of SAEM estimates (θ_k) obtained with $L = 40$ chains, $\gamma_k = 1$ for $k = 1, \ldots, 50$ and $\gamma_k = 1/(k-50)$ for $k > 50$.

9.2.5 A simple example to understand why SAEM converges in practice

Convergence of SAEM means that the sequence (θ_k) tends to move closer to the ML estimator $\hat{\theta}$ when k increases. This type of convergence is difficult to precisely quantify in general. Practically speaking, we can "look" at the behavior of the sequence (θ_k) from iteration to iteration and verify that it tends towards an acceptable solution. From a theoretical point of view, under fairly general hypotheses, it can be shown that $\theta_k \to \hat{\theta}$ with probability 1 when $k \to \infty$, but this is an asymptotic result which does not allow us to characterize the behavior of (θ_k) for all k. In consequence, we are going to present here an extremely simple model that will allow us to explicitly characterize SAEM's behavior and thus understand clearly why, in this example, it converges both theoretically and in practice.

Consider, thus, a very simple Gaussian model with only one observation per individual:

$$\begin{aligned} y_i|\psi_i &\sim \mathcal{N}(\psi_i, \sigma^2), \quad 1 \leq i \leq N \\ \psi_i &\sim \mathcal{N}(\theta, \omega^2). \end{aligned}$$

We will also assume that both ω^2 and σ^2 are known. Here, the maximum likelihood estimate $\hat{\theta}$ of θ is easy to compute since $y_i \sim_{i.i.d.} \mathcal{N}(\theta, \omega^2 + \sigma^2)$. We find that

$$\hat{\theta} = \frac{1}{N} \sum_{i=1}^{N} y_i = \bar{y}.$$

We now propose to use SAEM for computing $\hat{\theta}$. The simulation step is straightforward since the conditional distribution of ψ_i is normal:

$$\psi_i | y_i; \theta \ \sim \ \mathcal{N}(\alpha\theta + (1-\alpha) y_i, \gamma^2),$$

where

$$\begin{aligned} \alpha &= \frac{\sigma^2}{\sigma^2 + \omega^2} \\ \gamma^2 &= \left(\frac{1}{\sigma^2} + \frac{1}{\omega^2} \right)^{-1}. \end{aligned}$$

The maximization step is also straightforward. Indeed, a sufficient statistic for estimating θ is

$$\mathcal{S}(\boldsymbol{\psi}) = \sum_{i=1}^{N} \psi_i.$$

Then,

$$\begin{aligned} \tilde{\theta}(\mathcal{S}(\boldsymbol{\psi})) &= \arg\max_{\theta} \mathrm{p}(y_1, \ldots, y_N, \psi_1, \ldots, \psi_N; \theta) \\ &= \arg\max_{\theta} \mathrm{p}(\psi_1, \ldots, \psi_N; \theta) \\ &= \frac{\mathcal{S}(\boldsymbol{\psi})}{N}. \end{aligned}$$

Let us now look at the behavior of SAEM when $\gamma_k = 1$. The algorithm is very simple in this case since it consists of alternately drawing the $\psi_i^{(k)}$ and computing their empirical mean:

- Simulation step: For $i = 1, 2, \ldots, N$, let $\psi_i^{(k)} \sim \mathcal{N}(\alpha\theta_{k-1} + (1 - \alpha) y_i, \gamma^2)$.
- Maximization step: $\theta_k = \mathcal{S}(\boldsymbol{\psi}^{(k)})/N = \sum_{i=1}^{N} \psi_i^{(k)}/N$.

Figure 9.5 illustrates one such SAEM iteration. $N = 5$ data have been simulated with $\theta = 6$, $\omega = 0.3$ and $\sigma = 0.3$, and the algorithm has been initialized with $\theta_0 = 2$. In Figure 9.5(b) we see that the conditional distributions are all different, but since for each i, $\mathrm{p}(\psi_i^{(1)}|y_i;\theta_0) \propto \mathrm{p}(\psi_i^{(1)};\theta_0)\mathrm{p}(y_i|\psi_i^{(1)})$, they combine simultaneously the incorrect prior and the correct information provided by the data. The result of this is that the five conditional distributions are centered around five different values between θ_0 and y_i. Then, the maximization step consists of pooling these simulated $(\psi_i^{(1)})$ by assuming that all of them are drawn from the same distribution $\mathrm{p}(\psi_i^{(1)};\theta)$. The new estimate θ_1 based on $(\psi_i^{(1)})$ is therefore somewhere "in between" θ_0 and $\hat{\theta} = \bar{y}$.

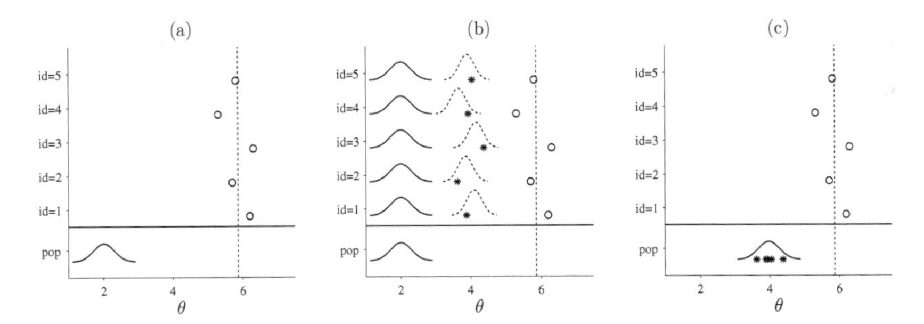

FIGURE 9.5: SAEM in practice. (a) the observations (circles), the empirical mean $\bar{y}$ (dashed line) and the initialization $\mathrm{p}(\psi_i;\theta_0)$ (solid curve), (b) the initialization $\mathrm{p}(\psi_i;\theta_0)$, the conditional distributions $\mathrm{p}(\psi_i|y_i;\theta_0)$ (dotted curves) and the simulated individual parameters $(\psi_i^{(1)})$ (asterisks), (c) the $(\psi_i^{(1)})$ pooled and the updated distribution $\mathrm{p}(\psi_i, \theta_1)$.

It is possible with this example to precisely determine the behavior of the sequence (θ_k). It is easy to show that

$$\theta_k - \hat{\theta} = \alpha(\theta_{k-1} - \hat{\theta}) + e_k, \tag{9.10}$$

where $e_k \sim \mathcal{N}(0, \gamma^2/N)$ is independent of θ_{k-1}. Thus,

$$\theta_k - \hat{\theta} \sim \mathcal{N}\left(\alpha^k(\theta_0 - \hat{\theta}), \frac{\gamma^2(1-\alpha^{2k})}{N(1-\alpha^2)}\right).$$

We see therefore that the difference $\theta_k - \hat{\theta}$ tends to decrease exponentially in the first iterations with a speed that is faster when α is smaller, i.e., when σ^2 is small or ω^2 large. We also remark that after a few iterations, the sequence (θ_k) behaves as a stationary autoregressive process of order 1 (AR(1)); this means that we can approximate the distribution of θ_k by a normal one with mean $\hat{\theta}$ and variance $\gamma^2/(N(1-\alpha^2))$. This variance is small when N is large and/or σ^2 is small.

Figure 9.6(a) illustrates this behavior: ten runs of the algorithm have been performed with the same simulated dataset and different initial values. The runs converge in a few iterations to a neighborhood of $\hat{\theta}$ (in this example, the ML estimate of θ is $\hat{\theta} = 5.86$) and from then on perform a random walk with constant variance around $\hat{\theta}$ following (9.10).

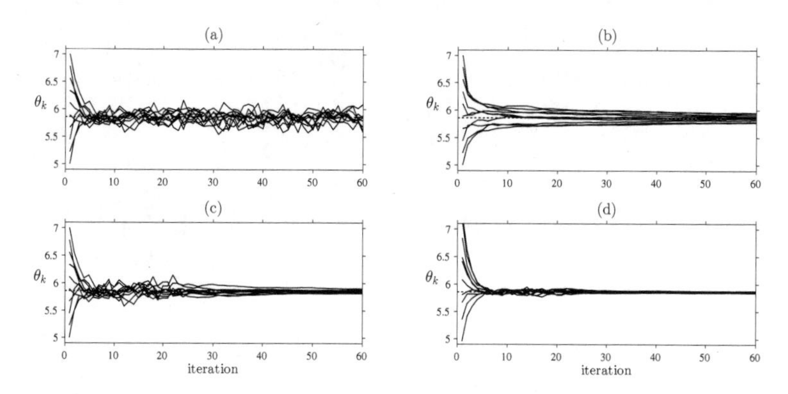

FIGURE 9.6: Each plot displays ten sequences (θ_k) obtained with different initial values and using different settings: (a) $L = 1$ and $\gamma_k = 1$ for $k \geq 1$, (b) $L = 1$ and $\gamma_k = 1/k$ for $k \geq 1$, (c) $L = 1$, $\gamma_k = 1$ for $k \leq 20$ and $\gamma_k = 1/(k-20)$ for $k \geq 21$, (d) $L = 10$, $\gamma_k = 1$ for $k \leq 20$ and $\gamma_k = 1/(k-20)$ for $k \geq 21$.

Now, let us see what happens instead when γ_k decreases as $1/k$. At iteration k, the simulation step remains the same but the maximization step becomes

$$\begin{aligned}\theta_k &= \theta_{k-1} + \frac{1}{k}\left(\frac{1}{N}\sum_{i=1}^{N}\psi_i^{(k)} - \theta_{k-1}\right) \\ &= \frac{1}{Nk}\sum_{j=1}^{k}\sum_{i=1}^{N}\psi_i^{(j)}.\end{aligned}$$

We no longer update θ_k using only the simulations from interation k, but combine all simulations performed in earlier iterations. This type of update leads to convergence of the sequence (θ_k). Again it is possible to study precisely the behavior of (θ_k). We find that

$$\theta_k - \hat{\theta} = \frac{k-a}{k}(\theta_{k-1} - \hat{\theta}) + \frac{e_k}{k}, \tag{9.11}$$

where $e_k \sim \mathcal{N}(0, \gamma^2/N)$. It can be shown that the sequence (θ_k) defined in (9.11) converges almost surely to $\hat{\theta}$. Figure 9.6(b) illustrates this version of SAEM, again using the same dataset.

We see in Figure 9.6(c) that by combining the two strategies, the sequence (θ_k) is a Markov chain that converges to a random walk around $\hat{\theta}$ during the first $K_1 = 20$ iterations, then converges almost surely to $\hat{\theta}$ during the next $K_2 = 40$ iterations.

If we now use L simulations per subject as suggested in (9.7), the sequence (θ_k) is still characterized by (9.10) for $k = 1, \ldots, K_1$ and by (9.11) for $k = K_1+1, \ldots, K_1+K_2$, but now $e_k \sim \mathcal{N}(0, \gamma^2/(N\,L))$. We see in Figure 9.6(d) that both types of convergence (in distribution during the first stage, almost sure during the second stage) are not accelerated when $L = 10$, but the variance in the simulations is reduced by a factor of 10.

9.2.6 A simulated annealing version of SAEM

Convergence of SAEM can strongly depend on the initial guess when the likelihood $\mathcal{L}$ has several local maxima. Simulated annealing is a probabilistic method proposed by Kirkpatrick (1984) for finding the global maximum of an objective function that may possess several local maxima. A simulated annealing version of SAEM may therefore improve convergence of the algorithm toward the global maximum of $\mathcal{L}$. To explain, let us first rewrite the joint pdf of $(\boldsymbol{y}, \boldsymbol{z})$ as follows:

$$\mathrm{p}(\boldsymbol{y}, \boldsymbol{z}; \theta) = C(\theta)\, \exp\left\{-U(\boldsymbol{y}, \boldsymbol{z}; \theta)\right\},$$

where $C(\theta)$ is a normalizing constant that depends only on θ. Then, for any "temperature" $T \geq 0$, we consider the complete model

$$\mathrm{p}_T(\boldsymbol{y}, \boldsymbol{z}; \theta) = C_T(\theta)\, \exp\left\{-\frac{1}{T} U(\boldsymbol{y}, \boldsymbol{z}; \theta)\right\},$$

where $C_T(\theta)$ is still a normalizing constant. We then introduce a decreasing temperature sequence $(T_k, 1 \leq k \leq K)$ and use the SAEM algorithm on the complete model $\mathrm{p}_{T_k}(\boldsymbol{y}, \boldsymbol{z}; \theta)$ at iteration k (the usual version of SAEM uses $T_k = 1$ at each iteration). The sequence (T_k) is chosen to have large positive values during the first iterations, then decrease with an exponential rate to 1, i.e., $T_k = \max(1, \tau\, T_{k-1})$ where $0 < \tau < 1$.

Consider for example the following model for continuous data defined in (9.9) with $\theta = (\beta, \Omega, a^2)$. We can easily show that for $T > 0$,

$$p_T(\boldsymbol{y}, \boldsymbol{z}; \theta) = C_T(\theta) \exp\left\{ -\frac{1}{2Ta^2} \sum_{i=1}^{N} \sum_{j=1}^{n_i} (y_{ij} - f(t_{ij}; z_i))^2 \right.$$
$$\left. - \frac{1}{2T} \sum_{i=1}^{N} (z_i - \beta)^t \Omega^{-1} (z_i - \beta) \right\},$$

where $C_T(\theta)$ is a normalizing constant that depends only on a, Ω and T. We see that $p_T(\boldsymbol{y}, \boldsymbol{z}; \theta)$ is defined as a transformation of the original distribution $p(\boldsymbol{y}, \boldsymbol{z}; \theta)$ obtained by replacing the residual error variance a^2 by Ta^2 and the variance-covariance matrix Ω for the random effects by $T\Omega$. In other words, a model with a "large temperature" is a model with large variances.

The algorithm therefore consists of choosing large initial variances Ω_0 and a_0^2 (that include the initial temperature T_0 implicitly) and setting $a_k^2 = \max(\tau\, a_{k-1}^2, \hat{a}(\boldsymbol{y}, \boldsymbol{z}^{(k)}))$ and $\Omega_k = \max(\tau\, \Omega_{k-1}, \hat{\Omega}(\boldsymbol{z}^{(k)}))$ during the first iterations. Here, $0 \leq \tau \leq 1$. These large values of the variance make the conditional distributions $p_T(z_i|y_i; \theta)$ less concentrated around their modes and thus allow the sequence (θ_k) to "escape" from local maxima of the likelihood during the first iterations of SAEM and converge to a neighborhood of the global maximum. After these initial iterations, the usual SAEM algorithm is used to estimate the variances at each iteration.

Remark: We can use two different coefficients τ_1 and τ_2 for Ω and a^2 in MONOLIX. It is possible for example to choose $\tau_1 < 1$ and $\tau_2 > 1$, with large initial inter-subject variances Ω_0 and small initial residual variance a_0^2. In this case, SAEM tries to obtain the best possible fit during the first iterations allowing for a large inter-subject variability. During the next iterations, this variability is reduced and the residual variance increases until reaching the best possible trade-off between the two criteria.

EXAMPLE 9.9 Consider a simple one-compartment model for oral administration:

$$f(t; ka, V, ke) = \frac{D\, ka}{V(ka - ke)} \left(e^{-ke\, t} - e^{-ka\, t} \right). \tag{9.12}$$

Let us simulate PK data from 80 patients using the following population PK parameters:

$$ka_{\text{pop}} = 1, \quad V_{\text{pop}} = 8, \quad ke_{\text{pop}} = 0.25.$$

We can see that the following parametrization gives the same prediction as in (9.12):

$$\tilde{ka} = ke, \quad \tilde{V} = V(ke/ka), \quad \tilde{ke} = ka.$$

We can then expect a (global) maximum of the likelihood around $(ka_{\text{pop}}, V_{\text{pop}}, ke_{\text{pop}}) = (1,\ 8,\ 0.25)$ and a (local) maximum around $(ka_{\text{pop}}, V_{\text{pop}}, ke_{\text{pop}}) = (0.25,\ 2,\ 1)$.

Figure 9.7 displays two SAEM runs without simulated annealing, with $ka_{\text{pop},0} = ke_{\text{pop},0} = 1$ and with different initial values of V_{pop}. We see that when $V_{\text{pop},0} = 10$ (solid line), SAEM converges to a solution which is the global maximum of the likelihood (log-likelihood = -366.8). When $V_{\text{pop},0} = 2$ (dotted line), SAEM converges to the other solution, a local maximum (log-likelihood = -408.4).

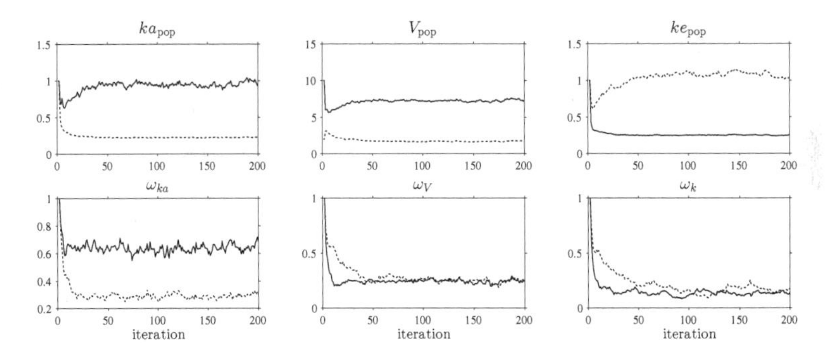

FIGURE 9.7: Two SAEM runs without simulated annealing with two different initial values of V_{pop}.

Figure 9.8 displays three SAEM runs with simulated annealing. The same initial values $ka_{\text{pop},0} = 1$, $V_{\text{pop},0} = 2$ and $ke_{\text{pop},0} = 1$ are used for each run.

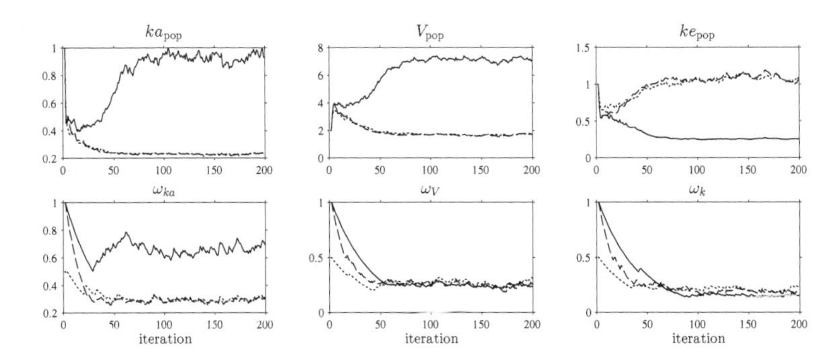

FIGURE 9.8: Three SAEM runs with simulated annealing and the same initial values. Solid line: $\Omega_0 = \text{diag}(1, 1, 1)$ and $\tau = 0.95$; dashed line: $\Omega_0 = \text{diag}(1, 1, 1)$ and $\tau = 0.9$; dotted line: $\Omega_0 = \text{diag}(0.5, 0.5, 0.5)$ and $\tau = 0.95$.

We see with this example that different temperature schemes give different results. When the initial variances of the random effects are large enough ($\Omega_0 = \text{diag}(1, 1, 1)$) and the temperature decreases slowly ($\tau = 0.95$), SAEM manages to "escape" the local maximum and successfully converge to the global maximum (solid line). On the other hand, if the initial variances (i.e., the initial temperature) are not large enough (dotted line) and/or the temperature decreases too quickly (dashed line), SAEM is no longer able to escape this local minimum.

The above example shows that there is no magic method leading to SAEM converging with probability 1 to the maximum of the likelihood in a given number of iterations independent of the initial parameter values. Certain settings will work well in some cases but not in others. MONOLIX uses by default $\tau_1 = \tau_2 = 0.98$ and initial variances set to 1 (corresponding to a level of variability of around 100% for log-normal distributions). Even though these settings generally give good results, it may be wise in some complex modeling situations to use a different strategy and to try different initial values.

9.2.7 A parameter expansion version of SAEM

A parameter expansion method PX-EM has been proposed by Liu et al. (1998) to speed up EM. The idea is to introduce an expanded complete-data model with a larger set of parameters in the E-step and a reduction function to return to the original model in the M-step.

Lavielle and Meza (2007) have shown that it is possible to adapt the PX-EM algorithm to SAEM in order to improve its convergence. Indeed, PX-SAEM substantially improves convergence speed (in terms of number of iterations) towards the maximum likelihood estimate. Furthermore, PX-SAEM helps to avoid local maxima of the likelihood.

The resulting PX-SAEM algorithm is a parameter expansion version of SAEM. The original complete-data model parameterized by θ is expanded to a larger model parameterized by $\zeta = (\theta, \alpha)$ where α is a kind of working parameter. There also exists a reduction function $R: \zeta \to R(\zeta)$ which preserves the original observed-data model, and a value α_0 of α that preserves the original complete-data model (see Liu et al., 1998, for more details).

This expanded version is used only during the first iterations of the algorithm when $\gamma_k = 1$. Each iteration of PX-SAEM is broken up into three steps: simulation, stochastic approximation using the expanded model, and PX-Maximization. Thus, at iteration k:

- **PX–Simulation**: For $i = 1, 2, \ldots, N$, draw $z_i^{(k)}$ from the conditional distribution $\mathrm{p}(z_i|y_i; \zeta_{k-1})$, where $\zeta_{k-1} = (\theta_{k-1}, \alpha_0)$.
- **PX–Stochastic approximation**: Compute $Q_k(\zeta) = \log \mathrm{p}(\boldsymbol{y}, \boldsymbol{z}^{(k)}; \zeta)$.

- **PX–Maximization**: Compute the $\hat{\zeta}_k$ that maximizes $Q_k(\zeta)$ and apply the reduction function to obtain $\theta_k = R(\hat{\zeta}_k)$ and $\zeta_k = (\theta_k, \alpha_0)$.

A quite general expansion for mixed effects models consists of replacing z_i in the observations model with $\Gamma_\alpha z_i + \mu_\alpha$, where Γ_α is a $d \times d$ diagonal matrix and μ_α a $d \times 1$ vector. Then, α is a $2d$-vector formed by μ_α and the main diagonal $(\gamma_1, \ldots, \gamma_d)$ of Γ_α while α_0 is the $2d$-vector $(0, 0, \ldots, 0, 1, 1, \ldots, 1)$.

Consider for example the following model for continuous data:

$$y_{ij} = f(t_{ij}, z_i) + a\varepsilon_{ij} \tag{9.13a}$$

$$z_i \sim \mathcal{N}(\beta, \Omega), \tag{9.13b}$$

where β is a d-vector and Ω a $d \times d$ variance-covariance matrix. Expansion consists of replacing (9.13a) with

$$y_{ij} = f(t_{ij}, \Gamma_\alpha z_i + \mu_\alpha) + a\varepsilon_{ij}.$$

Let p_{α, y_i} be the pdf of y_i under this expanded model. Then, for any i and any vector y of length $n - i$,

$$\begin{aligned}
p_{\alpha,y_i}(y; \beta, \Omega, a, \alpha) &= \int p_{y_i|z_i}(y|\Gamma_\alpha z + \mu_\alpha; a) p_{z_i}(z; \beta, \Omega) dz \\
&= \int p_{y_i|z_i}(y|u; a) p_{z_i}(\Gamma_\alpha^{-1}(u - \mu_\alpha); \beta, \Omega) \frac{du}{\gamma_1, \ldots, \gamma_d} \\
&= \int p_{y_i|z_i}(y|u; a) p_{\Gamma_\alpha z_i + \mu_\alpha}(u; \beta, \Omega) du \\
&= \int p_{y_i|z_i}(y|u; a) p_{z_i}(u; \Gamma_\alpha \beta + \mu_\alpha, \Gamma_\alpha \Omega \Gamma_\alpha) du \\
&= p_{y_i}(y; \Gamma_\alpha \beta + \mu_\alpha, \Gamma_\alpha \Omega \Gamma_\alpha, a).
\end{aligned}$$

We conclude therefore that the reduction function is

$$R(\beta, \Omega, a, \alpha) = (\Gamma_\alpha \beta + \mu_\alpha, \Gamma_\alpha \Omega \Gamma_\alpha, a).$$

Then, at iteration k, the PX-Simulation step consists of drawing $z_i^{(k)}$ from the conditional distribution $\mathrm{p}(z_i|y_i; \beta_{k-1}, \Omega_{k-1}, a_{k-1})$ using the original model (9.13), and the PX-Maximization step of computing

$$\alpha_k = \arg\min_{\alpha} \sum_{i=1}^{N} \sum_{j=1}^{n_i} (y_{ij} - f(t_{ij}, \Gamma_\alpha z_i^{(k)} + \mu_\alpha))^2$$

$$a_k = \frac{1}{\sum_{i=1}^{N} n_i} \sum_{i=1}^{N} \sum_{j=1}^{n_i} (y_{ij} - f(t_{ij}, D_{\alpha_k} z_i^{(k)} + \mu_\alpha))^2$$

$$\beta_k = \Gamma_{\alpha_k} \left(\frac{1}{N} \sum_{i=1}^{N} z_i^{(k)} \right) + \mu_{\alpha_k}$$

$$\Omega_k = \Gamma_{\alpha_k} \left(\frac{1}{N} \sum_{i=1}^{N} (z_i^{(k)} - \beta_k)(z_i^{(k)} - \beta_k)^t \right) \Gamma_{\alpha_k}.$$

EXAMPLE 9.10 We are going to use the same example as in Section 9.2.6 with initial values $ka_{\text{pop},0} = 1$, $V_{\text{pop},0} = 2.5$ and $k_{\text{pop},0} = 1$. We can see in Figure 9.9 that around 70 SAEM iterations are required for convergence to a neighborhood of the ML estimate. On the other hand, the PX-SAEM version converges in fewer than 10 iterations.

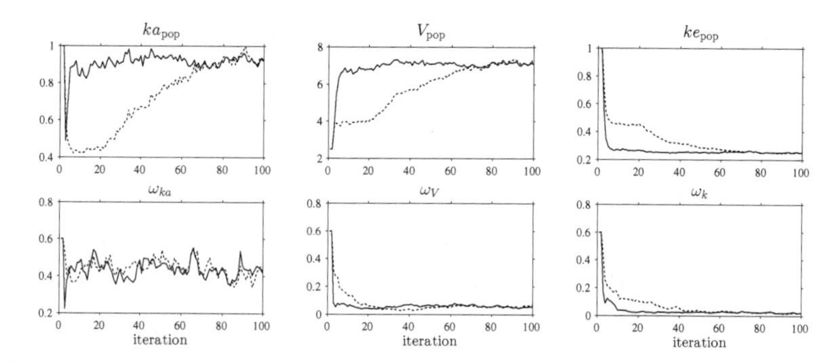

FIGURE 9.9: Convergence of SAEM and PX-SAEM. Dotted line: SAEM; solid line: PX-SAEM.

Remarks:

1. One of the advantages of this method is that it requires no tuning parameters; the transformation parameters α self-adjust automatically at each iteration.

2. PX-SAEM typically converges in a small number of iterations to a maximum of the likelihood, five or ten being usually sufficient. We can then use the basic SAEM algorithm in order to avoid the unnecessary optimization step for calculating α.

3. Just as for the simulated annealing version of SAEM, it should not be expected that PX-SAEM always provides a miraculous performance that leads to quick convergence to the global maximum of the likelihood. As for most optimization methods, this one has its limits and will not always provide results as spectacular as those shown here and in Lavielle and Meza (2007). In particular, it loses any advantage it has if good initial parameter guesses are given.

9.3 The Metropolis-Hastings algorithm for simulating the individual parameters

We consider a joint model for the observations and individual parameters for individual i:

$$\mathrm{p}(y_i, \psi_i) = \mathrm{p}(y_i|\psi_i)\mathrm{p}(\psi_i),$$

where $\mathrm{p}(y_i|\psi_i)$ is the conditional distribution of the observations of individual i (see Chapter 4) and $\mathrm{p}(\psi_i)$ the distribution of their individual parameters (see Chapter 5).

Remark: This distribution depends on a vector of population parameters θ and possibly covariates c_i, regression variables x_i and inputs u_i. We suppose that all of these components of the model are given, so it is not necessary to explicitly write them each time.

Our goal is to generate values for the individual parameters from the conditional distribution

$$\mathrm{p}(\psi_i|y_i) = \frac{\mathrm{p}(y_i, \psi_i)}{\mathrm{p}(y_i)}.$$

This distribution cannot usually be computed in closed-form when the model is not a linear Gaussian one.

Markov chain Monte Carlo (MCMC) methods are a class of algorithms for sampling from probability distributions for which direct sampling is difficult (Gilks et al., 1996; Robert and Casella, 2004). They consist of constructing a Markov chain that has the desired distribution as its stationary distribution. The states of the chain after a large number of steps are then used as a sample from the desired distribution.

The Metropolis-Hastings (MH) algorithm can draw samples from any probability distribution p that can be computed up to a constant (Robert and Casella, 2004). More precisely, the MH algorithm allows us to draw a sequence $(\psi_i^{(\ell)}, \ell = 1, 2, \ldots)$ which converges in distribution to the target distribution $p_{\psi_i|y_i}$.

We will consider a very general model for the individual parameters that involves random effects:

$$\psi_i = M(\beta, c_i, \eta_i), \tag{9.14}$$

where β is a vector of fixed effects, c_i a vector of (observed) individual covariates and η_i a vector of random effects whose probability distribution is denoted p_{η_i}.

The MH algorithm is used to simulate a sequence of random effects $(\eta_i^{(\ell)}, \ell = 1, 2, \ldots)$ with the target distribution being the conditional distribution $p_{\eta_i|y_i}$ of the random effects η_i. We can then obtain the sequence $(\psi_i^{(\ell)}, \ell = 1, 2, \ldots)$ using (9.14). The MH algorithm is iterative and requires an initial value $\eta_i^{(0)}$. Then, at iteration ℓ, we:

1. Draw a new value $\tilde{\eta}_i^{(\ell)}$ with some *proposal distribution* $q_\ell(\cdot\,; \eta_i^{(\ell-1)})$.

2. Compute $\tilde{\psi}_i^{(\ell)} = M(\beta, c_i, \tilde{\eta}_i^{(\ell)})$.

3. Accept this new value; that is, let $\eta_i^{(\ell)} = \tilde{\eta}_i^{(\ell)}$, with probability $\max(1, \alpha(\tilde{\eta}_i^{(\ell)}; \eta_i^{(\ell-1)}))$, where

$$\begin{aligned} \alpha(\tilde{\eta}_i^{(\ell)}; \eta_i^{(\ell-1)}) &= \frac{q_\ell(\eta_i^{(\ell-1)}; \tilde{\eta}_i^{(\ell)}) p_{\eta_i|y_i}(\tilde{\eta}_i^{(\ell)}|y_i)}{q_\ell(\tilde{\eta}_i^{(\ell)}; \eta_i^{(\ell-1)}) p_{\eta_i|y_i}(\eta_i^{(\ell-1)}|y_i)} \\ &= \frac{q_\ell(\eta_i^{(\ell-1)}; \tilde{\eta}_i^{(\ell)}) p_{\eta_i}(\tilde{\eta}_i^{(\ell)}) p_{y_i|\psi_i}(y_i|\tilde{\psi}_i^{(\ell)})}{q_\ell(\tilde{\eta}_i^{(\ell)}; \eta_i^{(\ell-1)}) p_{\eta_i}(\eta_i^{(\ell-1)}) p_{y_i|\psi_i}(y_i|\psi_i^{(\ell-1)})}. \end{aligned}$$

Remark: In order to run this algorithm, we need to be able to calculate the transition density $q_\ell(\tilde{\eta}_i; \eta_i)$, the random effects density $\mathrm{p}(\eta_i)$ (which poses no problem if η_i is a Gaussian vector, for example) and, in particular, the conditional distribution $\mathrm{p}(y_i|\psi_i)$. This is why this calculation is explicitly performed in the various examples provided in Chapter 4.

We denote q_ℓ the proposal distribution used at iteration ℓ of the algorithm because different proposals can be used at different iterations. Several proposal distributions are used in MONOLIX:

1. $q^{(1)} = p_{\eta_i}$ is the marginal distribution of η_i, that is, the normal distribution $\mathcal{N}(0, \Omega)$. The acceptance probability for this kernel is

$$\alpha(\tilde{\eta}_i^{(\ell)}; \eta_i^{(\ell-1)}) = \frac{p_{y_i|\psi_i}(y_i|\tilde{\psi}_i^{(\ell)})}{p_{y_i|\psi_i}(y_i|\psi_i^{(\ell-1)})}.$$

2. $q^{(2,m)}$, for $m = 1, 2, \ldots, d$, is the unidimensional Gaussian random walk for component m of η_i:

$$\tilde{\eta}_{i,m}^{(\ell)} = \eta_{i,m}^{(\ell-1)} + \xi_{i,m}^{(\ell)},$$

where $\xi_{i,m}^{(\ell)} \sim \mathcal{N}(0, \upsilon_m^{(\ell)})$. The variance $\upsilon_m^{(\ell)}$ of this random walk is calibrated in order to reach an optimal acceptance rate α^* (MONOLIX uses $\alpha^* = 0.3$ as default). Here, the transition kernel is symmetrical and

$$\alpha(\tilde{\eta}_i^{(\ell)}; \eta_i^{(\ell-1)}) = \frac{p_{\eta_i}(\tilde{\eta}_i^{(\ell)}) p_{y_i|\psi_i}(y_i|\tilde{\psi}_i^{(\ell)})}{p_{\eta_i}(\eta_i^{(\ell-1)}) p_{y_i|\psi_i}(y_i|\psi_i^{(\ell-1)})}.$$

3. $q^{(3,M)}$, for $M \subset \{1, 2, \ldots, d\}$, is the multidimensional Gaussian random walk for the vector $\eta_M = (\eta_m, m \in M)$:

$$\tilde{\eta}_{i,M}^{(\ell)} = \eta_i^{(\ell-1)} + \xi_{i,M}^{(\ell)},$$

where $\xi_{i,M}^{(\ell)} = (\xi_{i,m}^{(\ell)}, m \in M)$ is a Gaussian vector with diagonal variance-covariance matrix $\Upsilon_M^{(\ell)}$. Here as well, $\Upsilon_M^{(\ell)}$ is adjusted in order to reach the optimal acceptation rate α^*. Different subsets M are randomly chosen at each iteration.

The MH algorithm then consists of successively using these different proposals for $i = 1, 2, \ldots, N$. The variances $(\upsilon_m, m = 1, 2, \ldots, d)$ for proposal $q^{(2,m)}$ are updated at iteration ℓ as follows:

$$\upsilon_m^{(\ell)} = \upsilon_m^{(\ell-1)}(1 + \delta(\overline{\alpha}_m^{(\ell-1)} - \alpha^*)),$$

where $0 < \delta < 1$ is a constant and $\overline{\alpha}_m^{(\ell)}$ the empirical acceptance rate at iteration ℓ:

$$\overline{\alpha}_m^{(\ell)} = \frac{1}{N} \sum_{i=1}^{N} \mathbb{1}_{\eta_i^{(\ell)} = \tilde{\eta}_i^{(\ell)}}.$$

An overly small (resp. large) variance for the random walk leads to an overly large (resp. small) acceptance probability. The strategy proposed here therefore allows us to adaptively correct the variance for a given acceptance probability α^*. A small value of a allows us to smooth out the sequence $(\upsilon_m^{(\ell)})$. MONOLIX uses $a = 0.4$ as default value. We can use the same strategy for updating the diagonal variance-covariance matrices Υ_M, $M \subset \{1, 2, , \ldots, d\}$ for the kernel $q^{(3,M)}$.

The simulated sequence $(\psi_i^{(\ell)}, \ell = 1, 2, \ldots)$ can then be used for empirically estimating the conditional distribution $p_{\psi_i|y_i}$ and the conditional mean $\mathbb{E}\left(F(\psi_i)|y_i\right)$ of any function F such that $\mathbb{E}\left(F^2(\psi_i)|y_i\right) <$

$+\infty$. The accuracy of the estimation obviously depends on the length K of the sequence $(\psi_i^{(\ell)})$ used for the estimation, since the variance of the estimator merely decreases as $1/K$.

The stopping rule implemented in MONOLIX for deciding that convergence is satisfactory is based on the estimates of the conditional means $\mathbb{E}(\psi_i|y_i;\hat{\theta})$ and conditional standard deviations $\mathrm{sd}(\psi_i|y_i;\hat{\theta})$ updated at each iteration of the MH algorithm and averaged over the N individuals. The algorithm stops when these sequences remain in an interval of a given amplitude for a certain number of iterations. This procedure is illustrated in Figure 9.10 where intervals have an amplitude of 2% and the required number of iterations is 100.

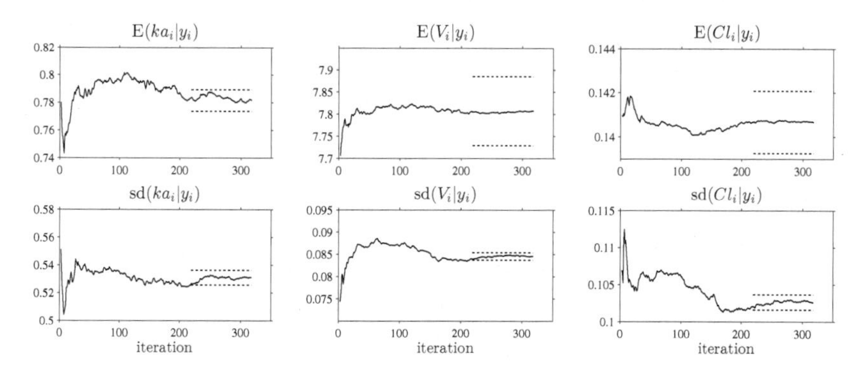

FIGURE 9.10: Estimation of the conditional means and conditional standard deviations of three individual parameters; stopping rule for the Metropolis-Hastings algorithm.

Estimation is also improved if the sequence starts from a point which is representative of the equilibrium distribution (burn-in is one method of finding a good starting point) or is known to have reasonably high probability (the conditional mode or the last value obtained with SAEM, for instance).

9.4 Estimation of the observed Fisher information matrix

9.4.1 Estimation using stochastic approximation

The *observed Fisher information matrix* (FIM) is a function of θ defined as

$$I_{\boldsymbol{y}}(\theta) = -\partial_\theta^2 \mathcal{LL}_{\boldsymbol{y}}(\theta),$$

where $\mathcal{LL} = \log \mathcal{L}$ is the log-likelihood:

$$\mathcal{LL}_{\boldsymbol{y}}(\theta) = \ell(\boldsymbol{y};\theta) = \log(\mathrm{p}(\boldsymbol{y};\theta)).$$

Due to the likelihood often being quite complex, $I_{\boldsymbol{y}}(\theta)$ usually has no closed-form expression. Following Kuhn and Lavielle (2005), it is however possible to estimate it using a Monte Carlo procedure based on Louis' formula (Louis, 1982):

$$\partial_\theta^2 \ell(\boldsymbol{y};\theta)) = \mathbb{E}\left(\partial_\theta^2 \ell(\boldsymbol{y},\boldsymbol{z};\theta)|\boldsymbol{y};\theta\right) + \mathrm{Cov}\left(\partial_\theta \ell(\boldsymbol{y},\boldsymbol{z};\theta)|\boldsymbol{y};\theta\right), \qquad (9.15)$$

where

$$\begin{aligned}\mathrm{Cov}\left(\partial_\theta \ell(\boldsymbol{y},\boldsymbol{z};\theta)|\boldsymbol{y};\theta\right) &= \mathbb{E}\left(\left(\partial_\theta \ell(\boldsymbol{y},\boldsymbol{z};\theta)\right)\left(\partial_\theta \ell(\boldsymbol{y},\boldsymbol{z};\theta)\right)^t|\boldsymbol{y};\theta\right) \\ &\quad - \mathbb{E}\left(\partial_\theta \ell(\boldsymbol{y},\boldsymbol{z};\theta)|\boldsymbol{y};\theta\right)\mathbb{E}\left(\partial_\theta \ell(\boldsymbol{y},\boldsymbol{z};\theta)|\boldsymbol{y};\theta\right)^t.\end{aligned}$$

Remark: The decomposition in (9.15) involves $\boldsymbol{z}$, but we could equally rewrite it using the original parameters $\boldsymbol{\psi}$ because the quantity of interest $I_{\boldsymbol{y}}(\theta)$ remains the same in either case. In this section we will use the z-representation of the model because calculations are much simpler than with the ψ-representation.

$\partial_\theta^2 \ell(\boldsymbol{y};\theta)$ is defined as a combination of conditional expectations that cannot be computed in closed-form for nonlinear models. However, each of these conditional expectations can be estimated by Monte Carlo:

1. For $i = 1,\ldots,N$, draw a sequence $(z_i^{(k)}, 1 \le k \le K)$ using the MH algorithm described in Section 9.3.
2. Compute:

$$\begin{aligned}\Delta_K &= \frac{1}{K}\sum_{k=1}^{K} \partial_\theta \ell(\boldsymbol{y},\boldsymbol{z}^{(k)};\theta) \\ D_K &= \frac{1}{K}\sum_{k=1}^{K} \partial_\theta^2 \ell(\boldsymbol{y},\boldsymbol{z}^{(k)};\theta) \\ G_K &= \frac{1}{K}\sum_{k=1}^{K} (\partial_\theta \ell(\boldsymbol{y},\boldsymbol{z}^{(k)};\theta))(\partial_\theta \ell(\boldsymbol{y},\boldsymbol{z}^{(k)};\theta))^t.\end{aligned}$$

3. Compute an estimate H_K of the FIM using

$$H_K = -(D_K + G_K - \Delta_K \Delta_K^t).$$

Implementing this algorithm therefore requires computing the first and second derivatives of

$$\ell(\boldsymbol{y}, \boldsymbol{z}; \theta) = \sum_{i=1}^{N} \ell(y_i, z_i; \theta).$$

To do this, assume first that the joint distribution of $\boldsymbol{y}$ and $\boldsymbol{z}$ can be decomposed as

$$\mathrm{p}(\boldsymbol{y}, \boldsymbol{z}; \theta) = \mathrm{p}(\boldsymbol{y}|\boldsymbol{z})\mathrm{p}(\boldsymbol{z}; \theta). \tag{9.16}$$

This assumption means that the statistical model for $\boldsymbol{z}$ is not degenerate and there exists a sufficient statistic $\mathcal{S}(\boldsymbol{z})$ for the estimation of θ. It is then enough to compute the first and second derivatives of $\ell(\boldsymbol{z}; \theta)$ in order to estimate the FIM. This can be done relatively simply in a closed-form way when the individual parameters are normally distributed, justifying the use of the z-representation here.

If some component of z_i has no variability, (9.16) no longer holds, but we can split θ into (θ_y, θ_z) so that

$$\mathrm{p}(\boldsymbol{y}, \boldsymbol{z}; \theta) = \mathrm{p}(\boldsymbol{y}|\boldsymbol{z}; \theta_y)\mathrm{p}(\boldsymbol{z}; \theta_z).$$

We then need to compute the first and second derivatives of $\ell(\boldsymbol{y}|\boldsymbol{z}; \theta_y)$ and $\ell(\boldsymbol{z}; \theta_z)$. Some examples of such computation are given Section 9.6. Derivatives of $\ell(\boldsymbol{y}|\boldsymbol{z}; \theta_y)$ that do not have a closed-form expression can be obtained using central differences.

Remarks:

1. This approach is used for computing the FIM $I_{\boldsymbol{y}}(\hat{\theta})$ in practice, where $\hat{\theta}$ is the maximum likelihood estimate of θ computed with the SAEM algorithm. The only difference with the MH used for SAEM is that the sequence of population parameter estimates (θ_k) is no longer updated and remains fixed at $\hat{\theta}$.

2. We normally use the whole sequence $(\boldsymbol{z}^{(k)}, 1 \leq k \leq K)$ for an *offline* estimation of the FIM. We could also make an *online* estimate of the FIM by replacing the Monte Carlo procedure with a stochastic approximation one. For instance,

$$\Delta_k = \Delta_{k-1} + \frac{1}{k}\left(\partial_\theta \ell(\boldsymbol{y}, \boldsymbol{z}^{(k)}; \theta) - \Delta_{k-1}\right).$$

Updating Δ_k, D_k and G_k at each iteration avoids having to store all simulated sequences $(\boldsymbol{z}^{(k)}, 1 \leq k \leq K)$ when computing Δ_K. This method also allows us to easily compute H_k at each iteration of the MH algorithm and perhaps derive a stopping rule based on this sequence.

3. We may be led to use an η-representation (completely or partially) if some of the components of z_i are linearly related.

9.4.2 Estimation using model linearization

Consider here the following model for continuous data (still using the z-parametrization):

$$\begin{aligned} y_{ij} &= f(t_{ij}, z_i) + g(t_{ij}, z_i)\varepsilon_{ij} \\ z_i &= z_{\text{pop}} + \eta_i. \end{aligned}$$

Let $\tilde{z}_i$ be some predicted value of z_i such as, for instance, the estimated mean or estimated mode of the conditional distribution $\mathrm{p}(z_i|y_i;\hat{\theta})$. We can then choose to linearize the model for the observations $(y_{ij},\ 1 \leq j \leq n_i)$ of individual i around the vector of predicted individual parameters $\tilde{z}_i$. Let $\partial_z f(t,z)$ be the row vector of derivatives of $f(t,z)$ with respect to z. Then,

$$\begin{aligned} y_{ij} &\simeq f(t_{ij}, \tilde{z}_i) + \partial_z f(t_{ij}, \tilde{z}_i)\,(z_i - \tilde{z}_i) + g(t_{ij}, \tilde{z}_i)\varepsilon_{ij} \\ &\simeq f(t_{ij}, \tilde{z}_i) + \partial_z f(t_{ij}, \tilde{z}_i)\,(z_{\text{pop}} - \tilde{z}_i) + \partial_z f(t_{ij}, \tilde{z}_i)\,\eta_i + g(t_{ij}, \tilde{z}_i)\varepsilon_{ij}. \end{aligned}$$

Following this, we can approximate the marginal distribution of the vector y_i by a normal one:

$$y_i \approx \mathcal{N}\left(\mu_i\,,\,\Gamma_i\right),$$

where

$$\mu_i = f(t_i, \tilde{z}_i) + \partial_z f(t_i, \tilde{z}_i)(z_{\text{pop}} - \tilde{z}_i) \tag{9.17a}$$

$$\Gamma_i = \partial_z f(t_i, \tilde{z}_i)\Omega\partial_z f(t_i, \tilde{z}_i)^t + g(t_i, \tilde{z}_i)\Sigma_i g(t_{ij}, \tilde{z}_i)^t, \tag{9.17b}$$

where Σ_i is the $n_i \times n_i$ variance-covariance matrix of $\varepsilon_{i,1}, \ldots, \varepsilon_{i,n_i}$. If the ε_{ij} are i.i.d., then Σ_i is the identity matrix.

Remark: The structural model f is usually defined using the original ψ-representation. We can instead use this original parametrization and the fact that $\tilde{z}_i = h(\tilde{\psi}_i)$ for computing

$$\partial_z f(t_i, \tilde{z}_i) = \partial_\psi f(t_i, \tilde{\psi}_i) J_h(\tilde{\psi}_i)^t,$$

where J_h is the Jacobian of h.

We can then approximate the observed log-likelihood $\mathcal{LL}_{\boldsymbol{y}}(\theta) = \sum_{i=1}^{N} \log(\mathrm{p}(y_i;\theta))$ using the normal approximation and derive the FIM by computing the matrix of second-order partial derivatives of $\mathcal{LL}_{\boldsymbol{y}}(\theta)$. Except for very simple models, computing these in closed-form is not straightforward. In such cases, finite differences can be used for numerically approximating them. We can use for instance a central difference approximation of the second derivative of $\mathcal{LL}_{\boldsymbol{y}}(\theta)$. To do this, first let $\nu > 0$. Then, for $j = 1, 2, \ldots, m$, let $\nu^{(j)} = (\nu_k^{(j)}, 1 \leq k \leq m)$ be the m-vector such that

$$\nu_k^{(j)} = \begin{cases} \nu & \text{if } j = k \\ 0 & \text{otherwise.} \end{cases}$$

Then, for ν small enough,

$$\begin{aligned} \partial_{\theta_j} \mathcal{LL}_{\boldsymbol{y}}(\theta) &\simeq \frac{\mathcal{LL}_{\boldsymbol{y}}(\theta + \nu^{(j)})) - \mathcal{LL}_{\boldsymbol{y}}(\theta - \nu^{(j)}))}{2\nu} \\ \partial^2_{\theta_j,\theta_k} \mathcal{LL}_{\boldsymbol{y}}(\theta)) &\simeq \frac{\mathcal{LL}_{\boldsymbol{y}}(\theta + \nu^{(j)} + \nu^{(k)})) + \mathcal{LL}_{\boldsymbol{y}}(\theta - \nu^{(j)} - \nu^{(k)}))}{4\nu^2} \\ &\quad - \frac{\mathcal{LL}_{\boldsymbol{y}}(\theta + \nu^{(j)} - \nu^{(k)})) + \mathcal{LL}_{\boldsymbol{y}}(\theta - \nu^{(j)} + \nu^{(k)}))}{4\nu^2}. \end{aligned}$$

9.5 Estimation of the log-likelihood

9.5.1 Estimation using importance sampling

For any $\theta \in \Theta$, the observed log-likelihood $\mathcal{LL}_{\boldsymbol{y}}(\theta) = \log(\mathcal{L}_{\boldsymbol{y}}(\theta))$ can be estimated without requiring approximation of the model, using a Monte Carlo approach. Since $\mathcal{LL}_{\boldsymbol{y}}(\theta) = \sum_{i=1}^{N} \log(\mathrm{p}(y_i;\theta))$, we can estimate $\log(\mathrm{p}(y_i;\theta))$ for each individual and derive an estimate of the log-likelihood as the sum of these individual log-likelihoods. Let us now explain how to estimate $\log(\mathrm{p}(y_i;\theta))$ for any individual i. Using the z-representation of the model, notice first that $\mathrm{p}(y_i;\theta)$ can be developed as follows:

$$\begin{aligned} \mathrm{p}(y_i;\theta) &= \int \mathrm{p}(y_i, z_i;\theta)\, dz_i \\ &= \int \mathrm{p}(y_i|z_i;\theta)\mathrm{p}(z_i;\theta)\, dz_i \\ &= \mathbb{E}_{p_{z_i}}\left(\mathrm{p}(y_i|z_i;\theta)\right). \end{aligned}$$

Thus, $\mathrm{p}(y_i;\theta)$ is now expressed as an expectation and can therefore be approximated by an empirical mean using Monte Carlo:

1. Draw M independent values $z_i^{(1)}, z_i^{(2)}, \ldots, z_i^{(M)}$ from the marginal distribution $p_{z_i}(\,\cdot\,;\theta)$.

2. Estimate $\mathrm{p}(y_i;\theta)$ with

$$\tilde{p}_{i,M} = \frac{1}{M}\sum_{m=1}^{M} \mathrm{p}(y_i|z_i^{(m)};\theta).$$

By construction, this estimator is unbiased:

$$\begin{aligned}\mathbb{E}\left(\tilde{p}_{i,M}\right) &= \mathbb{E}_{p_{z_i}}\left(\mathrm{p}(y_i|z_i^{(m)};\theta)\right)\\ &= \mathrm{p}(y_i;\theta).\end{aligned}$$

Furthermore, it is consistent since its variance decreases as $1/M$:

$$\mathrm{Var}\left(\tilde{p}_{i,M}\right) = \frac{1}{M}\mathrm{Var}_{p_{z_i}}\left(\mathrm{p}(y_i|z_i^{(m)};\theta)\right).$$

We could consider ourselves satisfied with this estimator since we "only" have to select M large enough to get an estimator with a small variance. Nevertheless, we will see now that it is possible to improve its statistical properties. For any distribution $\tilde{p}_{z_i}$ that is absolutely continuous with respect to the marginal distribution p_{z_i}, we can write

$$\begin{aligned}\mathrm{p}(y_i;\theta) &= \int \mathrm{p}(y_i, z_i;\theta)\, dz_i\\ &= \int \mathrm{p}(y_i|z_i;\theta)\frac{\mathrm{p}(z_i;\theta)}{\tilde{\mathrm{p}}(z_i;\theta)}\tilde{\mathrm{p}}(z_i;\theta)\, dz_i\\ &= \mathbb{E}_{\tilde{p}_{z_i}}\left(\mathrm{p}(y_i|z_i;\theta)\frac{\mathrm{p}(z_i;\theta)}{\tilde{\mathrm{p}}(z_i;\theta)}\right).\end{aligned}$$

We can now approximate $\mathrm{p}(y_i;\theta)$ using an *importance sampling* integration method with $\tilde{p}_{z_i}$ as the proposal distribution:

1. Draw M independent values $z_i^{(1)}, z_i^{(2)}, \ldots, z_i^{(M)}$ from proposal distribution $\tilde{p}_{z_i}(\,\cdot\,;\theta)$.

2. Estimate $\mathrm{p}(y_i;\theta)$ with

$$\hat{p}_{i,M} = \frac{1}{M}\sum_{m=1}^{M} \mathrm{p}(y_i|z_i^{(m)};\theta)\frac{\mathrm{p}(z_i^{(m)};\theta)}{\tilde{\mathrm{p}}(z_i^{(m)};\theta)}.$$

By construction, this new estimator is also unbiased and its variance decreases as $1/M$:

$$\mathrm{Var}\left(\hat{p}_{i,M}\right) = \frac{1}{M}\mathrm{Var}_{\tilde{p}_{z_i}}\left(\mathrm{p}(y_i|z_i^{(m)};\theta)\frac{\mathrm{p}(z_i^{(m)};\theta)}{\tilde{\mathrm{p}}(z_i^{(m)};\theta)}\right).$$

There exist an infinite number of possible proposal distributions $\tilde{\mathrm{p}}$ which all provide the same rate of convergence $1/M$. The trick is to reduce the variance of the estimator by selecting a proposal distribution so that the numerator is as small as possible. Imagine that we use the conditional distribution $p_{z_i|y_i}$ as the proposal. Then, for any $m = 1, 2, \ldots, M$,

$$\begin{aligned}
\mathrm{p}(y_i|z_i^{(m)};\theta)\frac{\mathrm{p}(z_i^{(m)};\theta)}{\tilde{\mathrm{p}}(z_i^{(m)};\theta)} &= \mathrm{p}(y_i|z_i^{(m)};\theta)\frac{\mathrm{p}(z_i^{(m)};\theta)}{\mathrm{p}(z_i^{(m)}|y_i;\theta)} \\
&= \mathrm{p}(y_i;\theta),
\end{aligned}$$

which means that $\hat{p}_{i,M} = \mathrm{p}(y_i;\theta)$. Such an estimator is optimal since its variance is zero and only one draw from $p_{z_i|y_i}$ is required to exactly compute $\mathrm{p}(y_i;\theta)$. The problem is that it is not possible to generate the $z_i^{(m)}$ with this conditional distribution since this would require computing a normalizing constant, which is in fact $\mathrm{p}(y_i;\theta)$ here.

Nevertheless, this conditional distribution can be estimated using the MH algorithm described in Section 9.3 and a practical proposal "close" to the optimal proposal $p_{z_i|y_i}$ can be obtained. We can then expect to get a very accurate estimate with a relatively small Monte Carlo size M.

In Monolix, the mean and variance of the conditional distribution $p_{z_i|y_i}$ are estimated by MH for each individual i. Then, the $z_i^{(m)}$ are drawn with a noncentral t distribution:

$$z_i^{(m)} = \mu_i + \sigma_i T_{i,m},$$

where μ_i and σ_i^2 are estimates of $\mathbb{E}\left(z_i|y_i;\theta\right)$ and $\mathrm{Var}\left(z_i|y_i;\theta\right)$, and $(T_{i,m})$ a sequence of i.i.d. random variables from a Student's t distribution with ν degrees of freedom (d.f.). Monolix uses the default value $\nu = 5$. It is also possible to automatically test different d.f. from the set $\{2, 5, 10, 20\}$ and select the one that provides the smallest empirical variance for $\widehat{\mathcal{LL}}_{\boldsymbol{y}}(\theta) = \sum_{i=1}^{N}\log(\hat{p}_{i,M})$.

Remark: Even if $\widehat{\mathcal{L}}_{\boldsymbol{y}}(\theta) = \prod_{i=1}^{N}\hat{p}_{i,M}$ is an unbiased estimator of $\mathcal{L}_{\boldsymbol{y}}(\theta)$, $\widehat{\mathcal{LL}}_{\boldsymbol{y}}(\theta)$ is a biased estimator of $\mathcal{LL}_{\boldsymbol{y}}(\theta)$. Indeed, by Jensen's inequality, we have that

$$\mathbb{E}\left(\log(\widehat{\mathcal{L}}_{\boldsymbol{y}}(\theta))\right) \leq \log\mathbb{E}\left(\widehat{\mathcal{L}}_{\boldsymbol{y}}(\theta)\right) = \log(\mathcal{L}_{\boldsymbol{y}}(\theta)).$$

However, the bias decreases as M increases and also if $\widehat{\mathcal{L}}_{\boldsymbol{y}}(\theta)$ is close to $\mathcal{L}_{\boldsymbol{y}}(\theta)$. It is therefore highly recommended to use a proposal as close as possible to the conditional distribution $p_{z_i|y_i}$, which means having to estimate this conditional distribution before estimating the log-likelihood.

EXAMPLE 9.11 A mixture model is used for this example. The goal here is not to provide details about the model and the formulas used for its implementation. We only want to highlight the importance of the choice of the proposal distribution for estimating the likelihood. Figure 9.11 shows several estimated deviances $(-2 \times \mathcal{LL}_{\boldsymbol{y}}(\hat{\theta}))$ as functions of the Monte Carlo size.

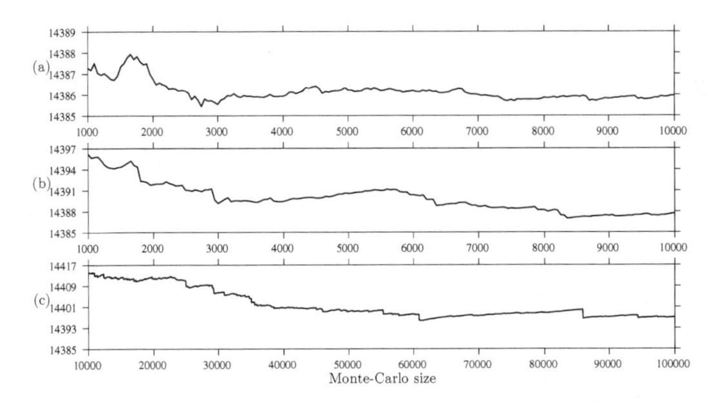

FIGURE 9.11: Estimation of the deviance as a function of the Monte Carlo size. The conditional distributions $\mathrm{p}(\psi_i|y_i;\widehat{\theta})$ are estimated using the MH algorithm in (a) and (b) and the last 30 SAEM iterations in (c); noncentral t distributions with 5 d.f. are used as proposal distributions in (a) and (c), normal distributions in (b).

In the first case, the conditional distributions of the individual parameters z_i are estimated using the MH algorithm (notice that only 100 MH iterations are required to correctly estimate the conditional mean and variance of the ψ_i). Then, noncentral t distributions with 5 d.f. are used as proposal distributions for estimating the deviance. We see in Figure 9.11(a) that there is no bias and an accurate estimate is obtained with a small Monte Carlo size (less than 3000). The estimated deviance is 14385.9 with a standard error (s.e.) of 0.7.

In the second case, normal distributions are used as proposals. The parameters of these distributions are the mean and variance of the conditional distributions of the z_i estimated using MH. Results are similar to those obtained with a t distribution (estimated deviance=14387.7, s.e. = 0.95) but Figure 9.11(b) shows that more simulations are required to eliminate the bias.

In the third case, only the last 30 SAEM iterations are used for estimating the conditional mean and variance of the z_i. Then, noncentral t distributions with 5 d.f. are used as proposal distributions. We see in Figure 9.11(c) that the bias decreases very slowly with the Monte Carlo size and is nonnegligible even after 10^5 simulations (estimated deviance=14397, s.e.=2.7).

9.5.2 Estimation using model linearization

For continuous data models, an alternative to the importance sampling approach is to use a linearization of the model like that proposed in Section 9.4.2 to approximate the observed Fisher information matrix. Indeed, the marginal distribution of a vector of continuous observations y_i can be approximated by the normal distribution with mean μ_i and variance Γ_i defined in (9.17). It is then straightforward to derive the associated likelihood. All of these calculations are described in Section 9.4.2.

This method can be much faster than importance sampling. It should be used by modelers for model selection purposes during the initial runs, when the goal is to identify significant differences between models. Importance sampling should be used when a more precise evaluation of the log-likelihood is required.

9.6 Examples of calculating the log-likelihood and its derivatives

For any $\theta \in \Theta$, let us define the following function of θ:

$$\mathcal{LL}_{\boldsymbol{y},\boldsymbol{z}}(\theta) = \ell(\boldsymbol{y}, \boldsymbol{z}; \theta) = \log \mathrm{p}(\boldsymbol{y}, \boldsymbol{z}; \theta).$$

As described Section 9.2, the kth iteration of SAEM requires maximization of $\mathcal{LL}_{\boldsymbol{y},\boldsymbol{z}^{(k)}}(\theta)$. Furthermore, computing the FIM requires the first and second derivatives of $\mathcal{LL}_{\boldsymbol{y},\boldsymbol{z}}(\theta)$. In the following, we will assume that θ can be split as (θ_y, θ_z) such that

$$\ell(\boldsymbol{y}, \boldsymbol{z}; \theta) = \ell(\boldsymbol{y}|\boldsymbol{z}; \theta_y) + \ell(\boldsymbol{z}; \theta_z).$$

We can then define the following functions of θ_y and θ_z:

$$\mathcal{LL}_{\boldsymbol{y}|\boldsymbol{z}}(\theta_y) = \ell(\boldsymbol{y}|\boldsymbol{z}; \theta_y)$$
$$\mathcal{LL}_{\boldsymbol{z}}(\theta_z) = \ell(\boldsymbol{z}; \theta_z).$$

Calculating the log-likelihood $\mathcal{LL}_{\boldsymbol{y},\boldsymbol{z}}(\theta)$ and its first and second derivatives therefore consists of calculating $\mathcal{LL}_{\boldsymbol{y}|\boldsymbol{z}}(\theta_y)$ and $\mathcal{LL}_{\boldsymbol{z}}(\theta_z)$ and their first and second derivatives:

$$\begin{aligned}
\mathcal{LL}_{\boldsymbol{y},\boldsymbol{z}}(\theta) &= \mathcal{LL}_{\boldsymbol{y}|\boldsymbol{z}}(\theta_y) + \mathcal{LL}_{\boldsymbol{z}}(\theta_z) \\
\partial_\theta \mathcal{LL}_{\boldsymbol{y},\boldsymbol{z}}(\theta) &= \begin{pmatrix} \partial_{\theta_y} \mathcal{LL}_{\boldsymbol{y}|\boldsymbol{z}}(\theta_y) \\ \partial_{\theta_z} \mathcal{LL}_{\boldsymbol{z}}(\theta_z) \end{pmatrix} \\
\partial^2_\theta \mathcal{LL}_{\boldsymbol{y},\boldsymbol{z}}(\theta) &= \begin{pmatrix} \partial^2_{\theta_y} \mathcal{LL}_{\boldsymbol{y}|\boldsymbol{z}}(\theta_y) & 0 \\ 0 & \partial^2_{\theta_z} \mathcal{LL}_{\boldsymbol{z}}(\theta_z) \end{pmatrix}.
\end{aligned}$$

We can therefore treat $\mathcal{LL}_{\boldsymbol{y}|\boldsymbol{z}}(\theta_y)$ and $\mathcal{LL}_{\boldsymbol{z}}(\theta_z)$ separately for both parameter estimation and calculating the block structure of the FIM.

To begin, let us suppose that the variance-covariance matrix Ω is diagonal. This helps greatly simplify the calculations because the components of the vector z_i are independent and the expression for $\mathcal{LL}_{\boldsymbol{z}}(\theta_z)$ can therefore be split into simple terms. The calculations require the first and second derivatives of real-valued functions and thus pose no particular technical difficulties.

Things get more complicated when we are looking at models with covariates and/or ones where the variance-covariance matrix Ω is not necessarily diagonal. In these cases, we will use the methodology proposed by Magnus and Neudecker (1999) for calculating the first and second derivatives of $\mathcal{LL}_{\boldsymbol{z}}(\theta_z)$.

9.6.1 Models with diagonal Ω

Consider first the model without covariates:

$$z_i \underset{\text{i.i.d.}}{\sim} \mathcal{N}(\beta, \Omega),$$

where $\beta = (\beta_1, \ldots, \beta_d)^t$ and $\Omega = \text{diag}(\omega_1^2, \omega_2^2, \ldots, \omega_d^2)$ is a diagonal matrix. The vector of population parameters $\theta = (\beta_1, \ldots, \beta_d, \omega_1^2, \ldots, \omega_d^2)^t$ is a $2d \times 1$ vector and here

$$\begin{aligned}
\mathcal{LL}_{\boldsymbol{z}}(\theta_z) &= \sum_{m=1}^{d} \sum_{i=1}^{N} \ell(z_{i,m}; \beta_m, \omega_m^2) \\
&= -\frac{Nd}{2}\log(2\pi) - \frac{N}{2}\sum_{m=1}^{d}\log(\omega_m^2) - \sum_{m=1}^{d}\frac{1}{2\omega_m^2}\sum_{i=1}^{N}(z_{i,m} - \beta_m)^2.
\end{aligned}$$

The gradient of $\mathcal{LL}_{\boldsymbol{z}}$ is therefore given by

$$\partial_{\beta_m} \mathcal{LL}_{\boldsymbol{z}}(\theta_z) = \frac{1}{\omega_m^2} \sum_{i=1}^{N} (z_{i,m} - \beta_m)$$

$$\partial_{\omega_m^2} \mathcal{LL}_{\boldsymbol{z}}(\theta_z) = -\frac{N}{2\omega_m^2} + \frac{1}{2\,\omega_m^4} \sum_{i=1}^{N} (z_{i,m} - \beta_m)^2.$$

Setting this gradient to 0, we deduce that for $m = 1, \ldots, d$, the ML estimate of (β_m, ω_m^2) is

$$\hat{\beta}_m = \frac{1}{N} \sum_{i=1}^{N} z_{i,m} \quad \text{and} \quad \hat{\omega}_m^2 = \frac{1}{N} \sum_{i=1}^{N} (z_{i,m} - \hat{\beta}_m)^2.$$

The Hessian of $\mathcal{LL}_{\boldsymbol{z}}$ is given by

$$\partial^2_{\beta_m \beta_j} \mathcal{LL}_{\boldsymbol{z}}(\theta_z) = \begin{cases} -N/\omega_m^2 & \text{if } m = j \\ 0 & \text{otherwise} \end{cases}$$

$$\partial^2_{\omega_m^2 \omega_j^2} \mathcal{LL}_{\boldsymbol{z}}(\theta_z) = \begin{cases} N/2\omega_m^4 - \sum_{i=1}^{N} (z_{i,m} - \beta_m)^2/\omega_m^6 & \text{if } m = j \\ 0 & \text{otherwise} \end{cases}$$

$$\partial^2_{\beta_m \omega_j^2} \mathcal{LL}_{\boldsymbol{z}}(\theta_z) = \begin{cases} -\sum_{i=1}^{N} (z_{i,m} - \beta_m)/\omega_m^4 & \text{if } m = j \\ 0 & \text{otherwise.} \end{cases}$$

Now suppose that there are covariates in the model but Ω is still diagonal. Then, for $m = 1, 2, \ldots, d$, there exists an $L_m \times 1$ vector β_m and a $1 \times L_m$ vector $c_{i,m}$ for $i = 1, \ldots, N$ such that

$$z_{i,m} \underset{\text{i.i.d.}}{\sim} \mathcal{N}(c_{i,m}\beta_m, \omega_m^2).$$

If we assume that the β_m are disjoint, then $\theta_z = (\beta_1^t, \ldots, \beta_d^t, \omega_1^2, \ldots, \omega_d^2)^t$. For $m = 1, 2, \ldots, d$, let Z_m be the $N \times 1$ vector and C_m the $N \times L_m$ matrix defined as

$$Z_m = \begin{pmatrix} z_{1,m} \\ \vdots \\ z_{N,m} \end{pmatrix} \quad \text{and} \quad C_m = \begin{pmatrix} c_{1,m} \\ \vdots \\ c_{N,m} \end{pmatrix}.$$

Assume also that the columns of C_m are linearly independent (i.e., the rank of C_m is L_m). Then,

$$\begin{aligned} \mathcal{LL}_{\boldsymbol{z}}(\theta_z) &= \sum_{m=1}^{d} \sum_{i=1}^{N} \ell(z_{i,m}; \beta_m, \omega_m^2) \\ &= -\frac{Nd}{2} \log(2\pi) - \frac{N}{2} \sum_{m=1}^{d} \log(\omega_m^2) - \sum_{m=1}^{d} \frac{1}{2\omega_m^2} \|Z_m - C_m\beta_m\|^2. \end{aligned}$$

We can then deduce the gradient of $\mathcal{LL}_{\boldsymbol{z}}$:

$$\partial_{\beta_m} \mathcal{LL}_{\boldsymbol{z}}(\theta_z) = \frac{1}{\omega_m^2} C_m^t (Z_m - C_m \beta_m)$$
$$\partial_{\omega_m^2} \mathcal{LL}_{\boldsymbol{z}}(\theta_z) = -\frac{N}{2\omega_m^2} + \frac{1}{2\,\omega_m^4} \|Z_m - C_m \beta_m\|^2,$$

and an expression for the ML estimate of θ_z: for $m = 1, \dots, d$,

$$\hat{\beta}_m = (C_m^t C_m)^{-1} C_m^t Z_m \quad \text{and} \quad \hat{\omega}_m^2 = \frac{1}{N} \|Z_m - C_m \hat{\beta}_m\|^2.$$

Here, the Hessian of $\mathcal{LL}_{\boldsymbol{z}}$ is given by

$$\partial^2_{\beta_m \beta_j} \mathcal{LL}_{\boldsymbol{z}}(\theta_z) = \begin{cases} -C_m^t C_m / \omega_m^2 & \text{if } m = j \\ 0 & \text{otherwise} \end{cases}$$
$$\partial^2_{\omega_m^2 \omega_j^2} \mathcal{LL}_{\boldsymbol{z}}(\theta_z) = \begin{cases} N/2\omega_m^4 - \|Z_m - C_m \beta_m\|^2 / \omega_m^6 & \text{if } m = j \\ 0 & \text{otherwise} \end{cases}$$
$$\partial^2_{\beta_m \omega_j^2} \mathcal{LL}_{\boldsymbol{z}}(\theta_z) = \begin{cases} -C_m^t (Z_m - C_m \beta_m) / \omega_m^4 & \text{if } m = j \\ 0 & \text{otherwise.} \end{cases}$$

9.6.2 Linear models with covariates and nondiagonal Ω

Assume now that

$$z_i \underset{\text{i.i.d.}}{\sim} \mathcal{N}(C_i \beta, \Omega),$$

where the variance-covariance matrix Ω is any positive-definite matrix. To continue, we need to provide some further notation. For any symmetric $d \times d$ matrix Ω:

- v_Ω is the $d^2 \times 1$ vector obtained by stacking the d columns of Ω one underneath the other.
- $\overline{v}_\Omega$ is the $\frac{1}{2}d(d+1) \times 1$ vector obtained from v_Ω by eliminating the above-diagonal elements of Ω.
- $\mathcal{D}_d$ is the $\frac{1}{2}d(d+1) \times d^2$ *elimination matrix* which transforms v_Ω into $\overline{v}_\Omega$.

For example, if $d = 2$,

$$\Omega = \begin{pmatrix} \omega_1^2 & \omega_{12} \\ \omega_{12} & \omega_2^2 \end{pmatrix}$$
$$v_\Omega = (\omega_1^2, \omega_{12}, \omega_{12}, \omega_2^2)^t$$
$$\overline{v}_\Omega = (\omega_1^2, \omega_{12}, \omega_2^2)^t$$
$$\mathcal{D}_2 = \begin{pmatrix} 1 & 0 & 0 & 0 \\ 0 & 1 & 0 & 0 \\ 0 & 0 & 0 & 1 \end{pmatrix}.$$

Let us first compute the log-likelihood $\mathcal{LL}_{\boldsymbol{z}}(\theta_z)$ where $\theta_z = (\beta, \Omega)$. We get

$$\begin{aligned}\mathcal{LL}_{\boldsymbol{z}}(\theta_z) &= \ell(\boldsymbol{z};\theta_z)\\ &= \sum_{i=1}^{N} \ell(z_i;\beta,\Omega)\\ &= -\frac{Nd}{2}\log(2\pi) - \frac{N}{2}\log(|\Omega|) - \frac{1}{2}\sum_{i=1}^{N}(z_i - C_i\beta)^t\Omega^{-1}(z_i - C_i\beta).\end{aligned}$$

We show in Appendix B.3 that $\hat{\beta}$ and $\hat{\Omega}$ are given by

$$\hat{\beta} = \left(\sum_{i=1}^{N} C_i^t\hat{\Omega}^{-1}C_i\right)^{-1}\sum_{i=1}^{N} C_i^t\hat{\Omega}^{-1}z_i$$

$$\hat{\Omega} = \frac{1}{N}\sum_{i=1}^{N}(z_i - C_i\hat{\beta})(z_i - C_i\hat{\beta})^t.$$

Let $S = \sum_{i=1}^{N}(z_i - C_i\beta)(z_i - C_i\beta)^t$. We can then show that the Hessian matrix of $\mathcal{LL}_{\boldsymbol{z}}$ is

$$\partial_\theta^2\mathcal{LL}_{\boldsymbol{z}}(\theta_z) = \begin{pmatrix} \frac{\partial^2\mathcal{LL}_{\boldsymbol{z}}(\theta_z)}{\partial\beta\,\partial\beta^t} & \frac{\partial^2\mathcal{LL}_{\boldsymbol{z}}(\theta_z)}{\partial\beta\,\partial\overline{v}_\Omega^t} \\ \frac{\partial^2\mathcal{LL}_{\boldsymbol{z}}(\theta_z)}{\partial\overline{v}_\Omega\,\partial\beta^t} & \frac{\partial^2\mathcal{LL}_{\boldsymbol{z}}(\theta_z)}{\partial\overline{v}_\Omega\,\partial\overline{v}_\Omega^t} \end{pmatrix},$$

where

$$\begin{aligned}\frac{\partial^2\mathcal{LL}_{\boldsymbol{z}}(\theta_z)}{\partial\beta\,\partial\beta^t} &= -\sum_{i=1}^{N} C_i^t\Omega^{-1}C_i\\ \frac{\partial^2\mathcal{LL}_{\boldsymbol{z}}(\theta_z)}{\partial\beta\,\partial\overline{v}_\Omega^t} &= \left(\frac{\partial^2\mathcal{LL}_{\boldsymbol{z}}(\theta_z)}{\partial\overline{v}_\Omega\,\partial\beta^t}\right)^t = -\left(\sum_{i=1}^{N}((z_i - C_i\beta)^t\Omega^{-1})\otimes(C_i^t\Omega^{-1})\right)\mathcal{D}_p\\ \frac{\partial^2\mathcal{LL}_{\boldsymbol{z}}(\theta_z)}{\partial\overline{v}_\Omega\,\partial\overline{v}_\Omega^t} &= -\mathcal{D}_p^t\left(\Omega^{-1}\otimes\left(\Omega^{-1}(S - \frac{N}{2}\Omega)\Omega^{-1}\right)\right)\mathcal{D}_p.\end{aligned}$$

9.7 Automatic construction of visual predictive checks

Figure 9.12 illustrates how a visual predictive check (VPC) is constructed in MONOLIX:

(a) Observations $(y_{ij}, 1 \leq i \leq N, 1 \leq j \leq n_i)$ measured at times (t_{ij}) are pooled.

(b) Data is grouped into adjacent time intervals (bins). Empirical quantiles are computed for the data in each bin. Here, the 10th, 50th and 90th quantiles are calculated.

(c) These quantiles summarize the distribution of the observations; they are used as test statistics.

(d) A large number of datasets are simulated under the model being evaluated using the design of the original dataset.

(e) The data from each simulated dataset are grouped into the same original bins and the same quantiles are computed in each bin for each of the simulated datasets.

(f) Prediction intervals (PI) for each quantile are estimated using these simulated quantiles and the observed quantiles are compared with them. Here, 90% PI are computed.

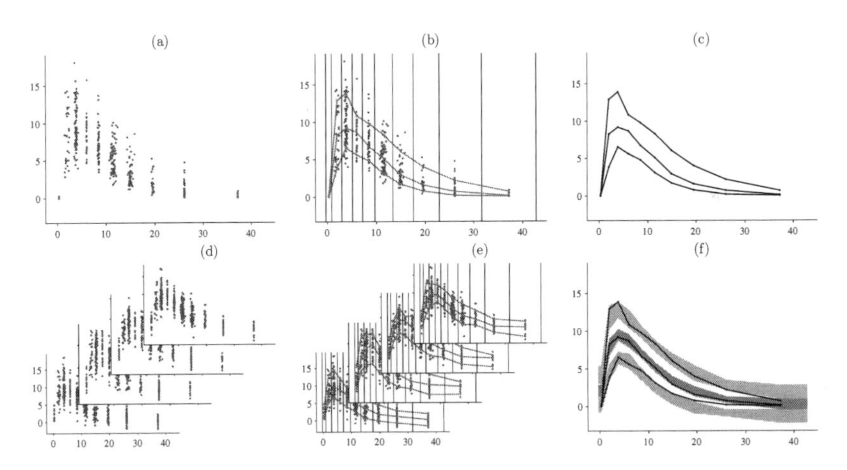

FIGURE 9.12: Visual predictive check construction.

The only technical difficulty in creating these graphs comes from the need to define the bins, i.e., the intervals into which the data are grouped. By data we usually mean observations, but the same approach can be used for any longitudinal sequence such as residuals or NPDEs.

In the population context, data from different individuals can be pooled so as to make one big set $(y_j; 1 \leq j \leq n)$ containing all measured data (at the set of times $(t_j, 1 \leq j \leq n)$). Here, n is the total number of data from the whole set of individuals and the index i referring to individuals can be omitted. The binning of this data then allows us to approximate its distribution by a piecewise-constant one (constant in each bin) and thus construct quantitative and graphical summaries such as VPCs (see Figure 7.10) and residuals (see Figure 7.9).

The choice of the set of bins is crucial as binning will always lead to a certain distortion between the original and approximated distributions. Defining K as the number of bins, the two simplest binning strategies are

- **equal-width binning**: The interval (t_{min}, t_{max}) is split into K bins of length $(t_{max}-t_{min})/K$, where t_{min} and t_{max} are such that $t_{min} \leq t_j \leq t_{max}$ for all j. This method is especially useful when the measurement times are uniformly spread across the interval (t_{min}, t_{max}). We see in Figure 9.13(a) that this is not at all the case when the times are spaced irregularly because some bins contain many points while others remain empty.

- **equal-size binning**: The n data points are distributed into K bins, each with n/K data points. If n is not a multiple of K, we make it so that each bin has either $\lfloor n/K \rfloor$ or $\lfloor n/K \rfloor + 1$ data points. This method is well-adapted to when individuals have similarly designed observation schedules, e.g., the same number of observations each, and at similar time points. Figure 9.13(b) shows that this method performs badly when the clusters of times/measurements have different numbers of points.

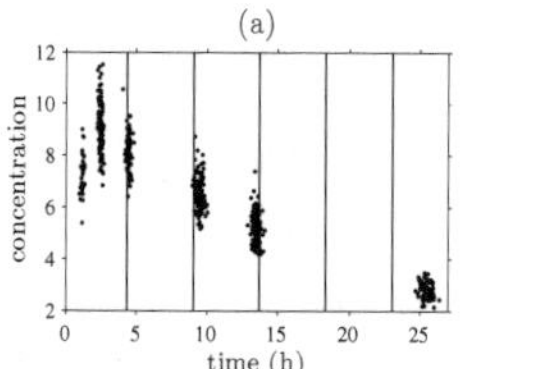

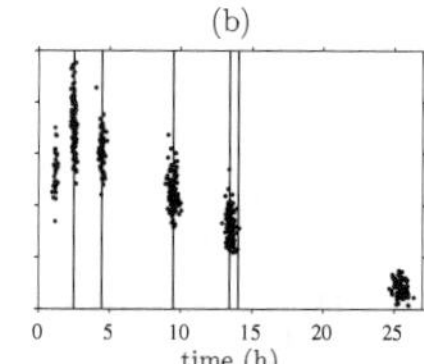

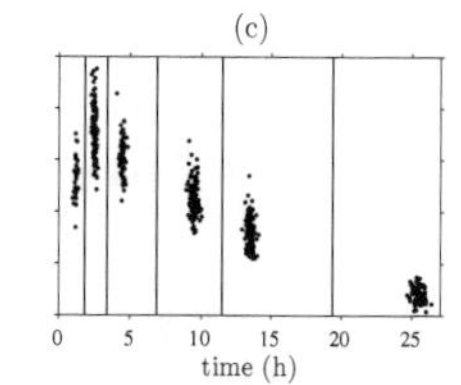

FIGURE 9.13: Three binnings of the same data using different strategies: (a) equal-width binning; (b) equal-size binning; (c) optimal binning $\widehat{I}_6$ obtained by minimizing J with $K = 6$.

In order to improve on these strategies, Lavielle and Bleakley (2011) have proposed a method for automatic segmentation of data into coherent subsets for both homogeneous and heterogenous data where the observation times and number of observations can vary between individuals. For a given number of bins, the locations of the bin edges are chosen so as to minimize heterogeneity of data in each bin.

Often, we have data which is "clustered" around certain time points (the scheduled observation times in a clinical trial, for example). One way to resolve the general binning problem is to interpret binning as *clustering* or 1*d-segmentation*, i.e., grouping the n time points $t_1 \leq t_2 \leq \ldots \leq t_n$ into K clusters or segments along the time axis. One possible way to do this is by 1d K-means clustering (Hartigan, 1975). Let us define

$$J(I) = \sum_{k=1}^{K} \sum_{j \in I_k} \left(t_j - \bar{t}_k\right)^2, \tag{9.18}$$

where $\bar{t}_k = \frac{1}{n_k} \sum_{j \in I_k} t_j$ is the empirical mean of the t_j in bin I_k, n_k being the number of points in the bin. Then, the K-means solution $\widehat{I}_K$ is found by minimizing J over all possible segmentations $I = (I_1, I_2, \ldots, I_K)$ of the data into K bins. In practice, this type of minimization can be done using dynamic programming (Kay, 1998). The binning obtained by minimizing J with $K = 6$ is shown in Figure 9.13(c) and would appear to be optimal.

The number of bins must also be carefully chosen, i.e., we require a good tradeoff between a large number of bins and a large number of observations in each bin. Indeed, the true distribution can be accurately approximated by a piecewise-constant distribution with a large number of bins, while a large number of observations in each bin is required to accurately estimate this true distribution.

The question therefore arises as to which number of segments K to choose. A small number of bins leads to a poor approximation (large bias) but a good estimation (small variance) of the data's distribution. On the other hand, a large number of bins will lead to a good approximation (small bias) but poor estimation (large variance) because of the small number of data per bin. In order to obtain a good compromise between these two, Lavielle and Bleakley (2011) propose to automatically select the number of bins using a model selection approach with the following penalized criterion:

$$U(I, \lambda) = \log\left(J(I)\right) + \lambda K(I),$$

where $K(I)$ is the number of bins in binning I. We choose the I (and thus the K) that minimizes $U(I, \lambda)$ for λ fixed. The larger the λ, the fewer the bins selected.

Let $J_K = J(\widehat{I}_K)$ be the minimum value of J over all segmentations with K bins. Then, the estimated number of bins $\hat{K}$ minimizes $U_K = \log(J_K) + \lambda K$ and the associated segmentation is therefore $\widehat{I}_{\hat{K}}$. Figure 9.14 displays the sequence of least-square criteria $(\log(J_K), 1 \leq K \leq 20)$ and the sequence of penalized criteria $(U_K, 1 \leq K \leq 20)$ with $\lambda = 0.3$.

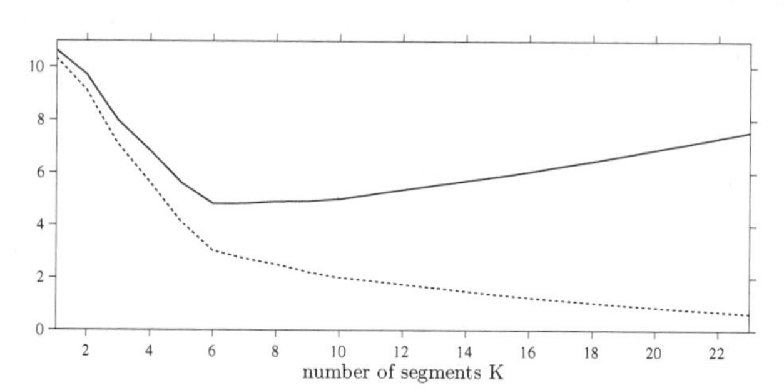

FIGURE 9.14: Criterion $\log(J_K)$ is displayed as a dotted line and penalized criterion U_K as a solid line.

The J defined in (9.18) is a least-squares criterion that supposes we are dealing with a homoscedastic model, i.e., the data spread (with respect to time) inside each cluster is similar. This is not always the case, as seen, for example, in Figure 9.15. Here the combined variability of the first two clusters is similar to that of each of the third, fourth and fifth, whereas the variability of the sixth cluster is significantly greater than all the others. In this case, the J criterion may not be optimal. Figure 9.15(a) shows that it groups the first two clusters together and splits the sixth cluster in two.

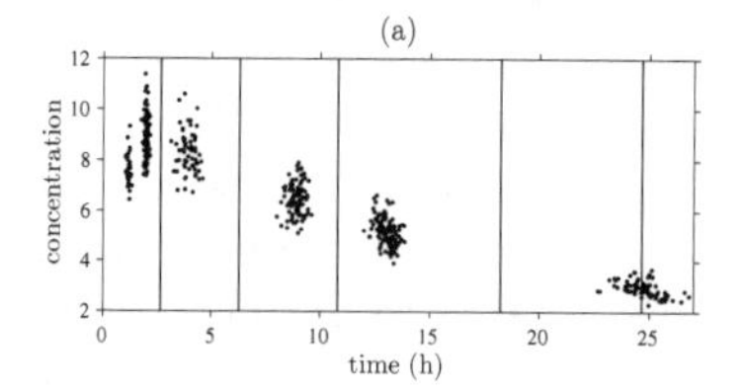

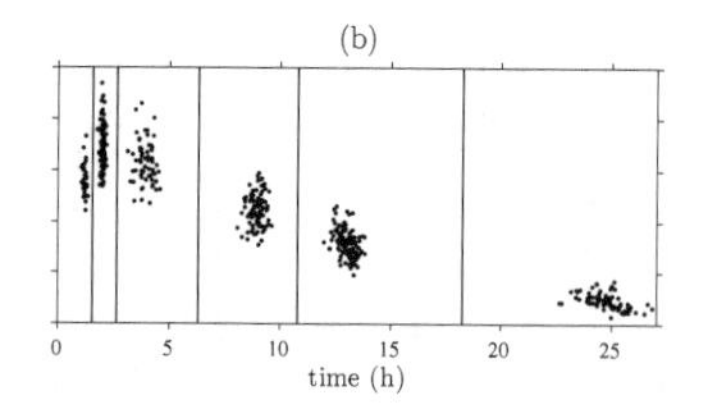

FIGURE 9.15: Two segmentations of the same data obtained by minimizing $U(I;\lambda,\beta)$ with $\lambda = 0.3$ and (a) $\beta = 1$; (b) $\beta = 0.4$.

Lavielle and Bleakley (2011) propose to better take into account heteroscedasticity by using the following criterion:

$$J(I;\beta) = \sum_{k=1}^{K} n_k (\sigma_k^2)^\beta,$$

where $\beta \in (0,1]$ and σ_k^2 is the empirical variance of the t_j in bin I_k:

$$\sigma_k^2 = \frac{1}{n_k} \sum_{j \in I_k} \left(t_j - \bar{t}_k\right)^2.$$

Then, the bins and their number can be simultaneously estimated by minimizing

$$U(I;\lambda,\beta) = \log\left(J(I;\beta)\right) + \lambda\beta K(I). \tag{9.19}$$

Figure 9.15(b) shows an intuitively optimal binning, obtained by minimizing $U(I;\lambda,\beta)$ when $\beta = 0.4$ and $\lambda = 0.3$. Note that in this example, the same binning is obtained for any value of β in $[0.03\,,\ 0.6]$.

Remarks:

1. The criterion J defined in (9.18) is the criterion $J(\cdot;\beta)$ with $\beta = 1$. Then, as β is set closer and closer to 0, more emphasis is made on selecting bins with different variability. $\beta = 0.4$ is the default value proposed in MONOLIX.

2. The β term is included in the penalty introduced in (9.19) as it can be shown that when the t_j are uniformly distributed, $\log\left(J_K(\beta)\right) = J(\widehat{I}_K;\beta)$ decreases as a linear function of β for any K.

Part IV

Appendices

A

The Individual Approach

Before looking at modeling a whole population at the same time, let us consider only one individual from that population. Much of the basic methodology for modeling one individual follows through to population modeling. We will see that when stepping up from one individual to a population, the difference is that some parameters shared by individuals are considered to be drawn from a probability distribution.

Let us begin with a simple example. An individual receives 100mg of a drug at time $t = 0$. The concentration of the drug in the bloodstream is measured at twelve time points and plotted as shown in Figure A.1.

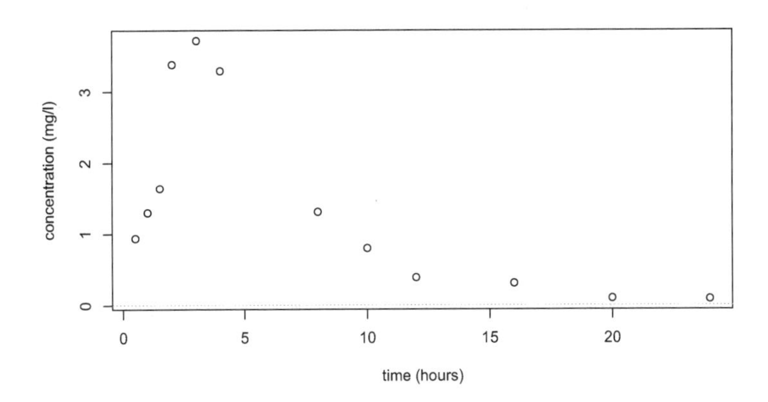

FIGURE A.1: Twelve measured concentration of a drug for a single subject.

We aim to find a mathematical model to describe what we see in the plot. A model for continuous data is presented in Section A.1, Section A.2 describes some standard methods for modeling such data, and Section A.3 shows how to implement them in R and use them. These methods essentially require the ability to manipulate conditional probability distributions.

This appendix is independent from the rest of the book. Several concepts, such as models and methods, presented here in the context of the individual approach are also presented in Part I and II for the population approach.

A.1 Models for the individual approach

In our example, the concentration is a *continuous* variable, so we will try to use continuous functions to model it. Different types of data (e.g., count data, categorical data, time-to-event data, etc.) require different types of models. All of these data types will be considered in due time, but for now let us concentrate on continuous data.

A model for continuous data can be represented mathematically as follows:

$$y_j = f(t_j; \phi) + e_j, \qquad 1 \le j \le n,$$

where

- f is called the *structural model.* It is a parametric function of time.
- $(t_1, t_2, \dots, t_n)$ is the vector of sampling times. Here, $t_1 = 0$ h and $t_n = t_{16} = 15$ h.
- $\phi = (\phi_1, \phi_2, \dots, \phi_d)$ is a vector of d structural parameters.
- $(e_1, e_2, \dots, e_n)$ are called the *residual errors.* It is common to assume that the residual errors are normally distributed but we can also use any centered probability distribution, i.e., such that $\mathbb{E}(e_j) = 0$.

We usually, however, state continuous data models in a slightly more flexible way:

$$y_j = f(t_j; \phi) + g(t_j; \phi, \xi)\varepsilon_j, \qquad 1 \le j \le n, \tag{A.1}$$

where now

- g is called the *residual error model.* It depends on some parameters ξ. It may also be a function of the time t_j and the parameters ϕ of the structural model.
- $(\varepsilon_1, \varepsilon_2, \dots, \varepsilon_n)$ are the *standardized* residual errors. For identifiability reasons, we suppose that these come from a probability distribution which is centered and has unit variance: $\mathbb{E}(\varepsilon_j) = 0$ and $\mathrm{Var}(\varepsilon_j) = 1$, such as the standard normal distribution $\mathcal{N}(0, 1)$.

The choice of a residual error model g is very flexible and allows us to account for many different hypotheses we may have on the error's distribution. Let $f_j = f(t_j; \phi)$. Here are some simple error models:

- *Constant error model*: $g = a$. That is, $y_j = f_j + a\varepsilon_j$ and $\xi = a$.
- *Proportional error model*: $g = bf$. That is, $y_j = f_j + bf_j\varepsilon_j$. This is for when we think the magnitude of the error is proportional to the value of the predicted value f. Here, $\xi = b$.
- *Combined error model*: $g = a+bf$. Here, $y_j = f_j+(a+bf_j)\varepsilon_j$ and $\xi = (a, b)$ (an alternative combined error model assumes $g^2 = a^2+b^2f^2$).
- *Exponential error model*: Here, the model is instead $\log(y_j) = \log(f_j) + a\varepsilon_j$, that is, $\xi = a$. It is exponential in the sense that if we exponentiate, we end up with $y_j = f_j e^{a\varepsilon_j}$. We remark that when a is small, the exponential error model is similar to the proportional error one since $e^{a\varepsilon_j} \approx 1 + a\varepsilon_j$.

A.2 Tasks and methods

To model a vector of observations $y = (y_j, 1 \leq j \leq n)$, we must perform several tasks:

- For a given model, *estimate* the model's parameters ψ and compute confidence intervals in order to evaluate the reliability of the estimate.
- *Evaluate* whether the assumptions of the proposed model are reasonable, i.e., if the observed data could have been generated by the model.
- Among candidate models, *select* the best one(s), i.e., select the best structural model(s) f and best residual error model(s) g.

Parameter estimation: Given the observed data and the choice of a parametric model to describe it, our goal becomes to find the "best" parameters for the model. A traditional framework to solve this kind of problem is called *maximum likelihood estimation* (MLE).

Let $\psi = (\phi, \xi)$ be the vector of parameters to be estimated. The likelihood $\mathcal{L}_y$ is a function defined as

$$\mathcal{L}_y(\psi) \stackrel{\text{def}}{=} \mathrm{p}(y_1, y_2, \ldots, y_n; \psi),$$

i.e., the conditional joint density function of (y_j) given the parameters ψ, but looked at as if the data are known and the parameters not. The $\hat{\psi}$ which maximizes $\mathcal{L}_y$ is known as the *maximum likelihood estimator* of ψ.

Suppose that we have chosen a structural model f and residual error model g. If we assume for instance that the ε_j are independent and identically distributed (i.i.d.) and that $\varepsilon_j \sim \mathcal{N}(0,1)$, then the y_j are mutually independent and (A.1) implies that:

$$y_j \sim \mathcal{N}\left(f(t_j;\phi), g(t_j;\phi,\xi)^2\right), \qquad 1 \leq j \leq n.$$

Due to this independence, the probability density function (pdf) of $y = (y_1, y_2, \ldots, y_n)$ is the product of the pdfs of each y_j:

$$\begin{aligned} \mathrm{p}(y_1, y_2, \ldots y_n; \psi) &= \prod_{j=1}^{n} \mathrm{p}(y_j; \phi, \xi) \\ &= \frac{(2\pi)^{-n/2}}{\prod_{j=1}^{n} g(t_j;\phi,\xi)} \exp\left\{-\frac{1}{2}\sum_{j=1}^{n}\left(\frac{y_j - f(t_j;\phi)}{g(t_j;\phi,\xi)}\right)^2\right\}. \end{aligned}$$

This is the same thing as the likelihood function $\mathcal{L}_y$ when seen as a function of ψ. Maximizing $\mathcal{L}_y$ is equivalent to minimizing the deviance, i.e., -2 $\times$ the log-likelihood:

$$\begin{aligned} \hat{\psi} &= \arg\min_{\psi} \left\{-2\,\mathcal{LL}_y(\psi)\right\} \\ &= \arg\min_{\psi} \left\{-2\,\log\left(\mathrm{p}(y_1, y_2, \ldots, y_n; \psi)\right)\right\}. \end{aligned}$$

Thus, $\hat{\psi} = (\hat{\phi}, \hat{\xi})$ is a solution of the following minimization problem:

$$(\hat{\phi}, \hat{\xi}) = \arg\min_{(\phi,\xi)} \left\{\sum_{j=1}^{n} \log\left(g(t_j;\phi,\xi)^2\right) + \sum_{j=1}^{n}\left(\frac{y_j - f(t_j;\phi)}{g(t_j;\phi,\xi)}\right)^2\right\}. \qquad \text{(A.2)}$$

This minimization problem does not usually have an analytical solution for nonlinear models, so an optimization procedure needs to be used. However, for a few specific models, analytic solutions do exist. For instance, suppose we have a constant error model: $y_j = f(t_j;\phi) + a\,\varepsilon_j$, $1 \leq j \leq n$, i.e., $g(t_j;\phi,\xi) = a$ and $\xi = a$. Then, (A.2) simplifies to

$$(\hat{\phi}, \hat{a}) \quad = \quad \arg\min_{(\phi,a)} \left\{ n\log(a^2) + \sum_{j=1}^{n}\left(\frac{y_j - f(t_j;\phi)}{a}\right)^2\right\}.$$

The solution is then

$$\begin{aligned}\hat{\phi} &= \arg\min_{\phi} \sum_{j=1}^{n} (y_j - f(t_j;\phi))^2 \\ \hat{a}^2 &= \frac{1}{n}\sum_{j=1}^{n}\left(y_j - f(t_j;\hat{\phi})\right)^2,\end{aligned}$$

where $\hat{a}^2$ is found by setting the partial derivative of $-2LL$ to zero. Whether this has an analytical solution or not depends on the form of f. For example, if $f(t_j;\phi)$ is a linear function of the components of the vector ϕ, we can represent it as a matrix F whose jth row gives the coefficients at time t_j. Therefore, we have the matrix equation $y = F\phi + a\varepsilon$. The solution for $\hat{\phi}$ is thus the least-squares one, and for $\hat{a}^2$ it is the same as previously:

$$\begin{aligned}\hat{\phi} &= (F'F)^{-1}F'y \\ \hat{a}^2 &= \frac{1}{n}\sum_{j=1}^{n}\left(y_j - F_j\hat{\phi}\right)^2.\end{aligned}$$

Computing the Fisher information matrix: The Fisher information matrix (FIM) is a way of measuring the amount of information that an observable random variable carries about an unknown parameter upon which its probability distribution depends.

Let $\psi^* = (\phi^*, \xi^*)$ be the true unknown value of ψ, and let $\hat{\psi}$ be its maximum likelihood estimator. Following Section B.2 of Appendix B, if the observed likelihood function is sufficiently smooth, asymptotic theory for maximum likelihood estimation holds and the distribution of $\hat{\psi}$ can be approximated by a normal one:

$$\hat{\psi} \approx \mathcal{N}(\psi^*\,,\, I_n(\hat{\psi})^{-1}), \tag{A.3}$$

where $I_n(\hat{\psi})$ is (minus) the Hessian of the log-likelihood:

$$I_n(\hat{\psi}) = -\frac{\partial^2}{\partial\psi\partial\psi'}\mathcal{LL}_y(\hat{\psi}).$$

$I_n(\hat{\psi})$ is known as the *observed Fisher information matrix*. Here, *observed* means that it is a function of observed variables $y_1, y_2, \ldots, y_n$. Thus, an estimate of the variance-covariance matrix of $\hat{\psi}$ is the inverse of the observed FIM:

$$C(\hat{\psi}) = I_n(\hat{\psi})^{-1}.$$

Deriving confidence intervals for parameters: Let ψ_k be the kth of d components of ψ. Imagine that we have estimated ψ_k with $\hat{\psi}_k$, the kth component of the MLE $\hat{\psi}$, that is, a random variable that converges to ψ_k^* when $n \to \infty$ under very general conditions. An estimate of its variance is the kth element of the diagonal of the covariance matrix $C(\hat{\psi})$:

$$\widehat{\mathrm{Var}}(\hat{\psi}_k) = C_{kk}(\hat{\psi}).$$

We can thus derive an estimate of its standard error:

$$\widehat{\mathrm{s.e.}}(\hat{\psi}_k) = \sqrt{C_{kk}(\hat{\psi})},$$

and a confidence interval of level $1-\alpha$ for ψ_k^*:

$$\mathrm{CI}(\psi_k^*) = \left[\hat{\psi}_k + \widehat{\mathrm{s.e.}}(\hat{\psi}_k)\, q_{\alpha/2},\ \hat{\psi}_k + \widehat{\mathrm{s.e.}}(\hat{\psi}_k)\, q_{1-\alpha/2}\right],$$

where q_α is the quantile of order α of a $\mathcal{N}(0,1)$ distribution.

Remark: Approximating $\hat{\psi}/\widehat{\mathrm{s.e}}(\hat{\psi}_k)$ by the normal distribution is a "good" approximation only when the number of observations n is large. A better approximation should be used for small n. In the model $y_j = f(t_j;\phi)+a\varepsilon_j$, the distribution of $\hat{a}^2$ can be approximated by a chi-squared distribution with $(n-d)$ degrees of freedom where d is the dimension of ϕ. The quantiles of the normal distribution can then be replaced by those of a Student's t-distribution with $(n-d)$ degrees of freedom.

Deriving confidence intervals for predictions: Once ϕ has been estimated, the structural model can be used for prediction at arbitrary values of t using $f(t;\hat{\phi})$. For any t, we can then derive a confidence interval for $f(t,\phi)$ using the estimated variance of $\hat{\phi}$. Indeed, as a first approximation we have

$$f(t;\hat{\phi}) \simeq f(t;\phi^*) + \partial_\phi f(t,\phi^*)(\hat{\phi}-\phi^*),$$

where $\partial_\phi f(t,\phi^*)$ is the gradient of f at ϕ^*, i.e., the vector of the first-order partial derivatives of f with respect to the components of ϕ, evaluated at ϕ^*. Of course, we do not actually know ϕ^*, but can estimate $\partial_\phi f(t,\phi^*)$ with $\partial_\phi f(t,\hat{\phi})$. The variance of $f(t;\hat{\phi})$ can then be estimated by

$$\widehat{\mathrm{Var}}\left(f(t;\hat{\phi})\right) \simeq \partial_\phi f(t,\hat{\phi})\widehat{\mathrm{Var}}(\hat{\phi})\left(\partial_\phi f(t,\hat{\phi})\right)'.$$

We can then derive an estimate of the standard error of $f(t,\hat{\phi})$ for any t:

$$\widehat{\mathrm{s.e.}}(f(t;\hat{\phi})) = \sqrt{\widehat{\mathrm{Var}}\left(f(t;\hat{\phi})\right)},$$

and a confidence interval (CI) of level $1-\alpha$ for $f(t;\phi^*)$:

$$\mathrm{CI}(f(t;\phi^*)) = \left[f(t;\hat{\phi}) + \widehat{\mathrm{s.e.}}(f(t;\hat{\phi}))\, q\left(\frac{\alpha}{2}\right),\ f(t;\hat{\phi}) + \widehat{\mathrm{s.e.}}(f(t;\hat{\phi}))\, q\left(1-\frac{\alpha}{2}\right)\right].$$

Estimating confidence intervals using Monte Carlo simulation: The use of Monte Carlo methods to estimate a distribution does not require any approximation of the model. We proceed in the following way. Suppose we have found the MLE $\hat{\psi} = (\hat{\phi}, \hat{\xi})$ of ψ. We then draw a data vector $y^{(1)}$ by first randomly generating the vector $\varepsilon^{(1)}$ and calculating for $1 \leq j \leq n$,

$$y_j^{(1)} = f(t_j;\hat{\phi}) + g(t_j;\hat{\phi},\hat{\xi})\varepsilon_j^{(1)}.$$

In a sense, this gives us "new" data from the "same" model. We can then compute a new MLE $\hat{\psi}^{(1)}$ of ψ using $y^{(1)}$. Repeating this process M times gives M estimates of ψ from which we can obtain an empirical estimation of the distribution of $\hat{\psi}$ or any quantile we like.

Any confidence interval for ψ_k (respectively, $f(t,\phi_k)$) can then be approximated by a prediction interval for $\hat{\psi}_k$ (respectively, $f(t,\hat{\phi}_k)$). For instance, a two-sided confidence interval of level $1-\alpha$ for ψ_k^* can be estimated by the prediction interval

$$[\hat{\psi}_{k,(\lfloor\frac{\alpha}{2}M\rfloor)}\ ,\ \hat{\psi}_{k,(\lfloor(1-\frac{\alpha}{2})M\rfloor)}],$$

where $\lfloor x \rfloor$ denotes the integer part of x and $(\psi_{k,(m)},\ 1 \leq m \leq M)$ the order statistic, i.e., the parameters $(\hat{\psi}_k^{(m)}, 1 \leq m \leq M)$ reordered so that $\hat{\psi}_{k,(1)} \leq \hat{\psi}_{k,(2)} \leq \ldots \leq \hat{\psi}_{k,(M)}$.

Model evaluation and model selection: We have seen how to estimate the parameters, confidence intervals and prediction intervals for a given model. These tasks essentially mean running well-adapted algorithms and using well-chosen mathematical formulas. Such procedures can easily be automated and do not require particular skills on the part of modelers who have access to good tools.

Things get more complicated when it comes to building a model. Indeed, modelers must be capable of assessing the quality and performance of a given model, improving it, then comparing it with several others. In the context we are interested in here, that of a single individual, this means being able to build the structural model f and residual error model g.

In the absence of biological (or other) information, we might suggest possible structural models just by looking at the graphs of time-evolution of the data. For example, if y_j is increasing with time, we might suggest a linear, quadratic or logarithmic model, depending on the approximate trend in the data. If y_j is instead decreasing, increasingly slowly, to zero, an exponential model might be appropriate.

This said, often we do have biological or physical (or other) information available to help us make our choice. In the context of pharmacokinetics modeling, for instance, if we have some knowledge about how a drug is absorbed, distributed and eliminated from the body, the pharmacokinetics process can usually be mathematically represented by a system of differential equations. The solution to these equations may provide the formula (i.e., structural model) we are seeking.

In the real world, it is often not enough to look at the data, choose one possible model and estimate the parameters. The chosen structural model may or may not be "good" at representing the data. It may be good but the chosen residual error model bad, meaning that the overall model is poor, and so on. That is why in practice we may want to try out several structural and residual error models. After performing parameter estimation for each model, we require graphical diagnostic tools in order to verify that the hypotheses made in the models are valid. These diagnostic plots can then be used for eliminating "poor candidates" and also for improving models. Statistical criteria (tests and information criteria) can then be used to compare the models that remain.

We are not going to review all of these criteria in this appendix. In the application we will present, we content ourselves with using the Bayesian information criterion (BIC) to compare models and select the best one. Once the estimate $\hat{\psi}$ has been calculated, the BIC is defined as a penalized likelihood criterion:

$$BIC = -2\,\mathcal{LL}_y(\hat{\psi}) + \log(n)\,d,$$

where n is the number of observations and d the number of model parameters, i.e., the length of the parameter vector ψ. The model we select is the one that minimizes the BIC.

A.3 A pharmacokinetics example

We will illustrate this modeling process using a pharmacokinetics (PK) example. The point of this example is to show how several of the tasks described earlier can be easily implemented using the statistical software R. Some knowledge of statistics and R is necessary for following the various modeling steps and implementing the methods.

The data: Let us consider a dose D = 50 mg of a drug administered orally to a patient at time $t = 0$. The concentration of the drug in the bloodstream $(y_j, 1 \leq j \leq 12)$ is then measured at times $(t_j, 1 \leq j \leq 12)$:

time (h)	0.5	1.0	1.5	2.0	3.0	4.0
concentration (mg/l)	0.94	1.30	1.64	3.38	3.72	3.29
time (h)	8.0	10.0	12.0	16.0	20.0	24.0
concentration (mg/l)	1.31	0.80	0.39	0.31	0.10	0.09

First, we import the data stored in the data file `individualFitting_data.txt` and plot it to have an initial look:

```
> pk1=read.table("individualFitting_data.txt",header=T)
> t=pk1$time
> y=pk1$concentration
> n=length(t)
> plot(t,y,xlab="time (hours)",ylab="concentration (mg/l)")
> abline(a=0,b=0,lty=3,col="grey")
```

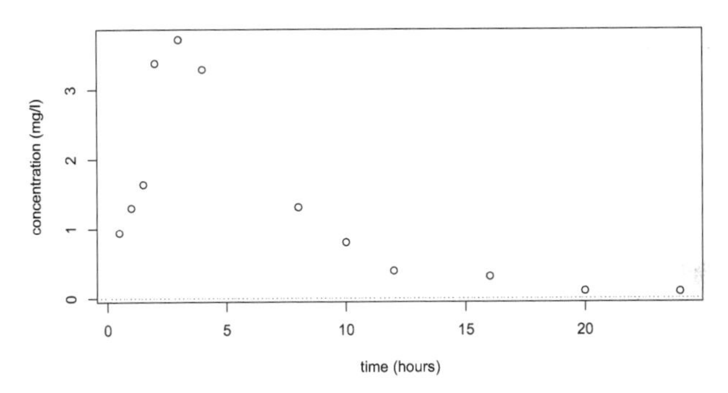

Fitting two PK models We are going to consider two possible structural models that may describe the observed time-course of the concentration:

1. A one-compartment model with first-order absorption and first-order elimination,

$$\begin{aligned} \phi_1 &= (ka, V, ke) \\ f_1(t;\phi_1) &= \frac{D\,ka}{V(ka - ke)}\left(e^{-ke\,t} - e^{-ka\,t}\right). \end{aligned}$$

2. A one-compartment model with zero-order absorption and first-order elimination,

$$\begin{aligned} \phi_2 &= (Tk0, V, ke) \\ f_2(t;\phi_2) &= \begin{cases} \frac{D}{V\,Tk0\,ke}\left(1 - e^{-ke\,t}\right) & \text{if } t \leq Tk0 \\ \frac{D}{V\,Tk0\,ke}\left(1 - e^{-ke\,Tk0}\right)e^{-ke\,(t-Tk0)} & \text{otherwise.} \end{cases} \end{aligned}$$

We define each of these functions in R:

```
> predc1=function(t,x){
+     f=50*x[1]/x[2]/(x[1]-x[3])*(exp(-x[3]*t)-exp(-x[1]*t)) }
>
> predc2=function(t,x){
+   f=50/x[1]/x[2]/x[3]*(1-exp(-x[3]*t))
+     f[t>x[1]]=50/x[1]/x[2]/x[3]*(1-exp(-x[3]*x[1]))*
+               exp(-x[3]*(t[t>x[1]]-x[1]))
+     return(f)}
```

We then define two models $\mathcal{M}_1$ and $\mathcal{M}_2$ that assume (for now) constant residual error models:

$$\begin{aligned} \mathcal{M}_1 : \quad y_j &= f_1(t_j;\phi_1) + a_1\varepsilon_j \\ \mathcal{M}_2 : \quad y_j &= f_2(t_j;\phi_2) + a_2\varepsilon_j. \end{aligned}$$

We can fit these two models to our data by computing the MLE $\hat{\psi}_1 = (\hat{\phi}_1, \hat{a}_1)$ and $\hat{\psi}_2 = (\hat{\phi}_2, \hat{a}_2)$ of ψ under each model. We can use the `nlm` R function for nonlinear minimization. This function requires an initial value $\psi_0 = (\phi_0, a_0)$:

```
> fmin1=function(x,y,t){
+     f=predc1(t,x)
+     g=x[4]
+     e=sum( ((y-f)/g)^2 + log(g^2))
+ return(e)}
>
> fmin2=function(x,y,t){
+     f=predc2(t,x)
+     g=x[4]
+     e=sum( ((y-f)/g)^2 + log(g^2))
+ return(e)}
> phi0=c(0.3,6,0.2)
> a0=1
> pk.nlm1=nlm(fmin1, c(phi0,a0), y, t, hessian="true")
> psi1=pk.nlm1$estimate
>
> phi0=c(3,10,0.2)
> a0=4
> pk.nlm2=nlm(fmin2, c(phi0,a0), y, t, hessian="true")
> psi2=pk.nlm2$estimate
```

Here are the parameter estimation results:

```
> cat(" psi1 =",psi1,"\n\n")
 psi1 = 0.3240916 6.001204 0.3239337 0.4366948

> cat(" psi2 =",psi2,"\n\n")
 psi2 = 3.203111 8.999746 0.229977 0.2555242
```

Evaluating and selecting PK models: The estimated parameters $\hat{\phi}_1$ and $\hat{\phi}_2$ can then be used for computing the predicted concentrations $\hat{f}_1(t)$ and $\hat{f}_2(t)$ under both models at any time t. These curves can be plotted over the original data and compared:

```
> tc=seq(from=0,to=25,by=0.1)
> phi1=psi1[c(1,2,3)]
```

```
> fc1=predc1(tc,phi1)
> phi2=psi2[c(1,2,3)]
> fc2=predc2(tc,phi2)
>
> par(mfrow= c(1,1))
> plot(t,y,ylim=c(0,4.1),xlab="time (hours)",ylab="concentration (mg/l)")
> lines(tc,fc1, type = "l", col = "black", lwd=1, lty=1)
> lines(tc,fc2, type = "l", col = "black", lwd=1, lty=4)
> abline(a=0,b=0,lty=3,col="grey")
> legend(13,4,
+     c("observations","first-order absorption","zero-order absorption"),
+     lty=c(-1,1,4), pch=c(1,-1,-1), lwd=1)
```

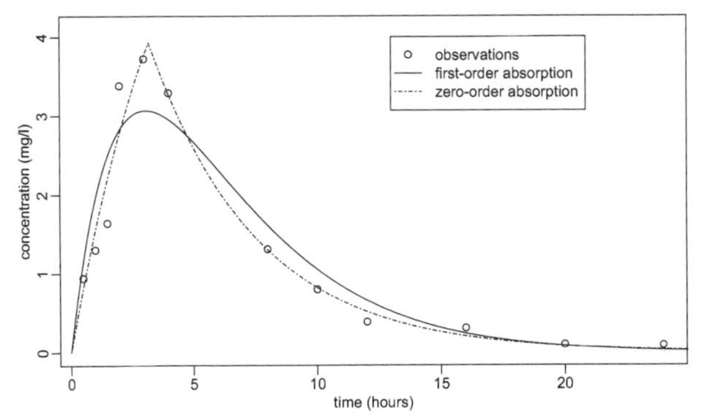

We clearly see that a much better fit is obtained with model $\mathcal{M}_2$, i.e., assuming a zero-order absorption process.

Another useful goodness-of-fit plot can be obtained by plotting the observations (y_j) versus the predictions $\hat{y}_j = f(t_j; \hat{\psi})$ given by the models:

```
> f1=predc1(t,phi1)
> f2=predc2(t,phi2)
>
> par(mfrow= c(1,2))
> plot(f1,y,xlim=c(0,4),ylim=c(0,4), main="model 1")
> abline(a=0,b=1,lty=1)
> plot(f2,y,xlim=c(0,4),ylim=c(0,4), main="model 2")
> abline(a=0,b=1,lty=1)
```

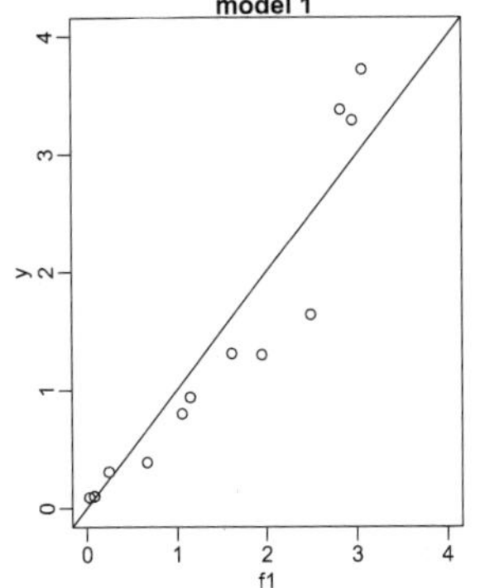

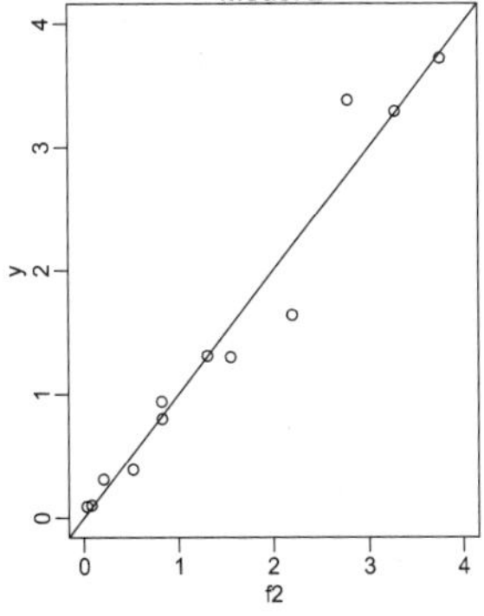

Model selection: According to the previous diagnostic plots, $\mathcal{M}_2$ would seem to have a slight edge. This can be tested more analytically using the BIC:

```
> deviance1=pk.nlm1$minimum + n*log(2*pi)
> bic1=deviance1+log(n)*length(psi1)
> deviance2=pk.nlm2$minimum + n*log(2*pi)
> bic2=deviance2+log(n)*length(psi2)
>
> cat(" bic1 =",bic1,"\n\n")
 bic1 = 24.10972

> cat(" bic2 =",bic2,"\n\n")
 bic2 = 11.24769
```

A smaller BIC is better. Therefore, this result also suggests that model $\mathcal{M}_2$ should be selected.

Fitting different error models: For the moment, we have considered only constant error models. However, the "observations vs predictions" plot hints that the amplitude of the residual errors may increase with the size of the predicted value. Let us therefore take a closer look at four different residual error models, each of which we will associate with the "best" structural model f_2:

$\mathcal{M}_2$	constant error model:	$y_j = f_2(t_j; \phi_2) + a_2\varepsilon_j$
$\mathcal{M}_3$	proportional error model:	$y_j = f_2(t_j; \phi_3) + b_3 f_2(t_j; \phi_3)\varepsilon_j$
$\mathcal{M}_4$	combined error model:	$y_j = f_2(t_j; \phi_4) + (a_4 + b_4 f_2(t_j; \phi_4))\varepsilon_j$
$\mathcal{M}_5$	exponential error model:	$\log(y_j) = \log(f_2(t_j; \phi_5)) + a_5\varepsilon_j.$

The three new models need to be entered into R:

```
> fmin3=function(x,y,t){
+     f=predc2(t,x)
+     g=x[4]*f
+     e=sum( ((y-f)/g)^2 + log(g^2))
+ return(e)}
>
> fmin4=function(x,y,t){
+     f=predc2(t,x)
+     g=abs(x[4])+abs(x[5])*f
+     e=sum( ((y-f)/g)^2 + log(g^2))
+ return(e)}
>
> fmin5=function(x,y,t){
+     f=predc2(t,x)
+     g=x[4]
+     e=sum( ((log(y)-log(f))/g)^2 + log(g^2))
+ return(e)}
```

We can now compute the MLEs $\hat{\psi}_3 = (\hat{\phi}_3, \hat{b}_3)$, $\hat{\psi}_4 = (\hat{\phi}_4, \hat{a}_4, \hat{b}_4)$ and $\hat{\psi}_5 = (\hat{\phi}_5, \hat{a}_5)$ of ψ under models $\mathcal{M}_3$, $\mathcal{M}_4$ and $\mathcal{M}_5$:

```
> pk.nlm3=nlm(fmin3, c(phi2,0.1), y, t, hessian="true")
> psi3=pk.nlm3$estimate
>
> pk.nlm4=nlm(fmin4, c(phi2,1,0.1), y, t, hessian="true")
> psi4=pk.nlm4$estimate
> psi4[c(4,5)]=abs(psi4[c(4,5)])
>
> pk.nlm5=nlm(fmin5, c(phi2,0.1), y, t, hessian="true")
> psi5=pk.nlm5$estimate
>
> cat(" psi3 =",psi3,"\n\n")
 psi3 = 2.642409 11.44113 0.1838779 0.2189221

> cat(" psi4 =",psi4,"\n\n")
 psi4 = 2.890066 10.16836 0.2068221 0.02741416 0.1456332

> cat(" psi5 =",psi5,"\n\n")
 psi5 = 2.710984 11.2744 0.188901 0.2310001
```

Selecting the error model: As previously, these curves can be plotted over the original data and compared:

```
> phi3=psi3[c(1,2,3)]
> fc3=predc2(tc,phi3)
> phi4=psi4[c(1,2,3)]
> fc4=predc2(tc,phi4)
> phi5=psi5[c(1,2,3)]
> fc5=predc2(tc,phi5)
>
> par(mfrow= c(1,1))
> plot(t,y,ylim=c(0,4.1),xlab="time (hours)",ylab="concentration (mg/l)")
> lines(tc,fc2, type = "l", lwd=1)
> lines(tc,fc3, type = "l", lwd=1, lty=3)
> lines(tc,fc4, type = "l", lwd=1, lty=4)
> lines(tc,fc5, type = "l", lwd=1, lty=2)
> abline(a=0,b=0,lty=3,col="grey")
> legend(13,4,c("observations","constant error model",
+    "proportional error model", "combined error model",
+    "exponential error model"), lty=c(-1,1,3,4,2), pch=c(1,-1,-1,-1,-1))
```

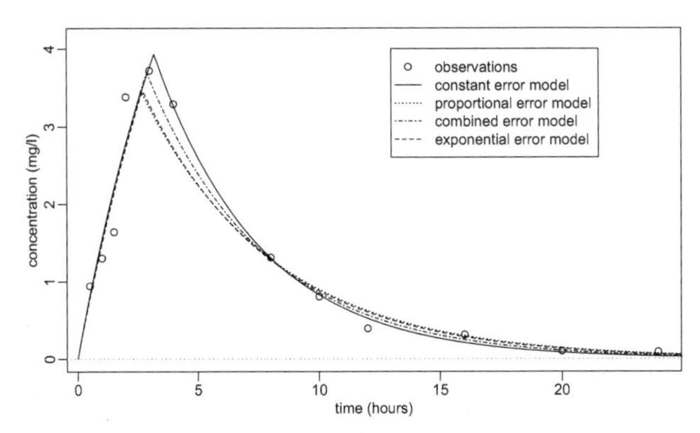

The predicted concentrations obtained with models $\mathcal{M}_3$, $\mathcal{M}_4$ and $\mathcal{M}_5$ are quite similar. We now calculate the BIC for each:

```
> deviance3=pk.nlm3$minimum + n*log(2*pi)
```

```
> bic3=deviance3 + log(n)*length(psi3)
> deviance4=pk.nlm4$minimum + n*log(2*pi)
> bic4=deviance4 + log(n)*length(psi4)
> deviance5=pk.nlm5$minimum + 2*sum(log(y)) + n*log(2*pi)
> bic5=deviance5 + log(n)*length(psi5)
>
> cat(" bic3 =",bic3,"\n\n")
 bic3 = 3.443607

> cat(" bic4 =",bic4,"\n\n")
 bic4 = 3.475841

> cat(" bic5 =",bic5,"\n\n")
 bic5 = 4.108521
```

All of these BICs are lower than the constant residual error one. There is not however a large difference between them, though the proportional and combined error models give the smallest and essentially identical BICs. We will use the combined error model $\mathcal{M}_4$ in the following (the same types of analyses could be done with the proportional error model).

A 90% confidence interval for ψ_4 can derived from the Hessian (i.e., the square matrix of second-order partial derivatives) of the objective function (i.e., -2 $\times$ LL):

```
> alpha=0.9
> df=n-length(phi4)
> I4=pk.nlm4$hessian/2
> H4=solve(I4)
> s4=sqrt(diag(H4)*n/df)
> delta4=s4*qt(0.5+alpha/2,df)
> ci4=matrix(c(psi4-delta4,psi4+delta4),ncol=2)
> print(ci4)
             [,1]        [,2]
[1,]  2.22576690  3.55436561
[2,]  7.93442421 12.40228967
[3,]  0.16628224  0.24736196
[4,] -0.02444571  0.07927403
[5,]  0.04119983  0.25006660
```

We can also calculate a 90% confidence interval for $f_4(t)$ using the central limit theorem (see (A.3)):

```
> nlpredci=function(phi,f,H){
+    dphi=length(phi)
+    nf=length(f)
+    H=H*n/(n-dphi)
+    S=H[seq(1,dphi),seq(1,dphi)]
+    G=matrix(nrow=nf,ncol=dphi)
+    for (k in seq(1,dphi)) {
+       dk=phi[k]*(1e-5)
+       phid=phi
+       phid[k]=phi[k] + dk
+       fd=predc2(tc,phid)
+       G[,k]=(f-fd)/dk
+    }
+    M=rowSums((G%*%S)*G)
+    deltaf=sqrt(M)*qt(0.5+alpha/2,df)
+ return(deltaf)}
>
> deltafc4=nlpredci(phi4,fc4,H4)
```

This can then be plotted:

```
> plot(t,y,ylim=c(0,4.5),xlab="time (hours)",ylab="concentration (mg/l)")
> lines(tc,fc4, type = "l", lwd=2)
> lines(tc,fc4-deltafc4, type = "l", lwd=1, lty=3)
> lines(tc,fc4+deltafc4, type = "l", lwd=1, lty=3)
> abline(a=0,b=0,lty=3,col="grey")
> legend(10.5,4.5,c("observed concentrations","predicted concentration",
+       "PI for predicted concentration"),lty=c(-1,1,3), pch=c(1,-1,-1),
        lwd=c(2,2,1))
```

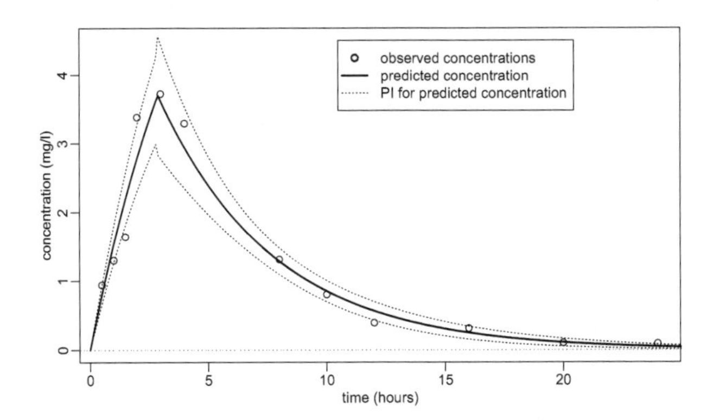

Alternatively, prediction intervals for $\hat{\psi}_4$, $\hat{f}_4(t;\hat{\psi}_4)$ and new observations at any time t can be estimated by Monte Carlo simulation:

```
> f=predc2(t,phi4)
> a4=psi4[4]
> b4=psi4[5]
> g=a4+b4*f
> dpsi=length(psi4)
> nc=length(tc)
> N=1000
> qalpha=c(0.5 - alpha/2,0.5 + alpha/2)
> PSI=matrix(nrow=N,ncol=dpsi)
> FC=matrix(nrow=N,ncol=nc)
> Y=matrix(nrow=N,ncol=nc)
> for (k in seq(1,N)) {
+    eps=rnorm(n)
+    ys=f+g*eps
+    pk.nlm=nlm(fmin4, psi4, ys, t)
+    psie=pk.nlm$estimate
+    psie[c(4,5)]=abs(psie[c(4,5)])
+    PSI[k,]=psie
+    fce=predc2(tc,psie[c(1,2,3)])
+    FC[k,]=fce
+    gce=a4+b4*fce
+    Y[k,]=fce + gce*rnorm(1)
+ }
> mean4s=apply(PSI,2,mean)
> median4s=apply(PSI,2,median)
> sd4s=apply(PSI,2,sd)
> matrix(c(mean4s,median4s,sd4s),nrow=dpsi)
> ci4s=matrix(nrow=dpsi,ncol=2)
> for (k in seq(1,dpsi)){
+    ci4s[k,]=quantile(PSI[,k],qalpha,names=FALSE)
+ }
> print(matrix(c(mean4s,median4s,sd4s),nrow=dpsi))
```

```
              [,1]        [,2]       [,3]
[1,]  2.90457137  2.88882014 0.33326934
[2,] 10.18906412 10.16458483 1.08848877
[3,]  0.20841538  0.20687597 0.01828873
[4,]  0.02755847  0.02194732 0.02828348
[5,]  0.11441976  0.11497724 0.05312626
> print(ci4s)
             [,1]        [,2]
[1,] 2.405311e+00  3.49257471
[2,] 8.430377e+00 12.11876046
[3,] 1.824481e-01  0.24093729
[4,] 8.307916e-09  0.08361688
[5,] 1.513002e-02  0.20225225
>
> cifc4s=matrix(nrow=nc,ncol=2)
> ciy4s=matrix(nrow=nc,ncol=2)
> for (k in seq(1,nc)){
+    cifc4s[k,]=quantile(FC[,k],qalpha,names=FALSE)
+    ciy4s[k,]=quantile(Y[,k],qalpha,names=FALSE)
+ }
>
> par(mfrow= c(1,1))
> plot(t,y,ylim=c(0,4.5),xlab="time (hours)",ylab="concentration (mg/l)")
> lines(tc,fc4, type = "l", lwd=2)
> lines(tc,cifc4s[,1], type = "l", lwd=1, lty=3)
> lines(tc,cifc4s[,2], type = "l", lwd=1, lty=3)
> lines(tc,ciy4s[,1], type = "l",  lwd=1, lty=2)
> lines(tc,ciy4s[,2], type = "l",  lwd=1, lty=2)
> abline(a=0,b=0,lty=3,col="grey")
> legend(10.5,4.5,c("observed concentrations","predicted concentration",
+     "PI for predicted concentration","PI for observed concentrations"),
+     lty=c(-1,1,3,2), pch=c(1,-1,-1,-1), lwd=c(2,2,1,1))
```

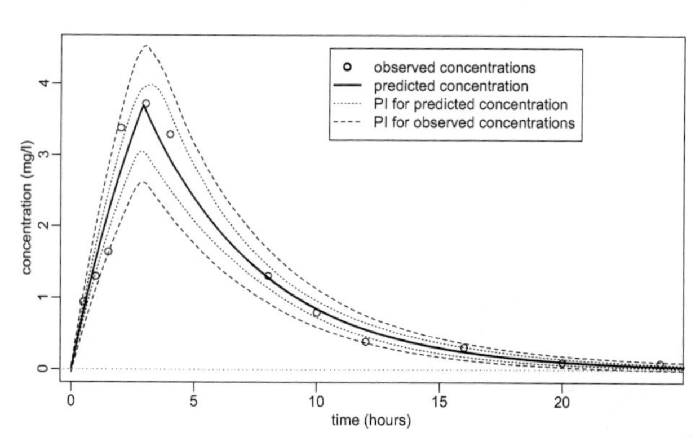

B

Some Useful Results

B.1 Continuous probability distributions

An (absolutely) continuous probability distribution is one that has a *probability density function* (pdf). Let p_x be a continuous nonnegative Lebesgue integrable function. A continuous random variable x that takes its values in $\mathbb{R}$ has density p_x if for any interval $(a, b) \subset \mathbb{R}$,

$$\mathbb{P}(a \leq x \leq b) = \int_a^b p_x(u)\, du.$$

The *cumulative distribution function* (cdf) F_x of x is such that, for any $a \in \mathbb{R}$,

$$\begin{aligned} F_x(a) &= \mathbb{P}(x \leq a) \\ &= \int_{-\infty}^{a} p_x(u)\, du, \end{aligned}$$

and

$$p_x(a) = F_x'(a).$$

Proposition 1. *Let h be a continuously differentiable and strictly increasing function. Let p_x be the pdf of a continuous random variable x and p_y the pdf of $y = h(x)$. Then, for any $a \in \mathbb{R}$,*

$$p_x(a) = h'(a)p_y(h(a)).$$

Proof. Since h is strictly increasing,

$$\mathbb{P}(x \leq a) = \mathbb{P}(h(x) \leq h(a)),$$

i.e.,

$$F_x(a) = F_y(h(a)).$$

Differentiating both terms with respect to a leads to the result $p_x(a) = h'(a)p_y(h(a))$. □

Proposition 2. *Let ψ_i be an individual parameter that takes its values in $\mathbb{R}$ and let h be a nonlinear, twice continuously differentiable and strictly increasing function such that*

$$h(\psi_i) \sim \mathcal{N}(h(\psi_{\text{pop}}), \omega^2).$$

Then, the reference parameter ψ_{pop} is the median of the distribution of ψ_i. In general, ψ_{pop} is neither the mean nor the mode of this distribution, including when h is strictly concave or convex, and more generally if $h''(\psi_{\text{pop}}) \neq 0$.

Proof. Since h is a strictly increasing function,

$$\begin{aligned}\mathbb{P}(\psi_i \leq \psi_{\text{pop}}) &= \mathbb{P}(h(\psi_i) \leq h(\psi_{\text{pop}})) \\ &= 0.5.\end{aligned}$$

In other words, ψ_{pop} is the median of the distribution of ψ.

If h is strictly concave or convex, then $h(\mathbb{E}(\psi_i)) \neq \mathbb{E}(h(\psi_i)) = h(\psi_{\text{pop}})$. Thus, $\mathbb{E}(\psi_i) \neq \psi_{\text{pop}}$. Let p be the pdf of ψ_i and p_h be the pdf of $h(\psi_i)$. By definition, for any $h(x) \in \mathbb{R}$,

$$p(x) = h'(x)p_h(h(x)).$$

Thus,

$$p'(x) = h''(x)p_h(h(x)) + h'^2(x)p'_h(h(x)).$$

By the definition of the mode, $p'_h(h(\psi_{\text{pop}})) = 0$. Thus, $p'(\psi_{\text{pop}}) \neq 0$ if $h''(\psi_{\text{pop}}) \neq 0$. □

B.2 Fisher information and maximum likelihood estimation

Let $y_1, y_2, \ldots, y_N$ be N *independent and identically distributed* (i.i.d.) random variables with parametric probability distribution $\mathrm{p}(\cdot\,, \theta^*)$ where $\theta^* \in \Theta$ is a $d \times 1$ vector of parameters. The joint distribution of $\boldsymbol{y} = (y_1, \ldots, y_N)$ is therefore

$$\mathrm{p}(y_1, \ldots y_N; \theta^*) = \prod_{i=1}^{N} \mathrm{p}(y_i; \theta^*).$$

For any $\theta \in \Theta$, the log-likelihood is defined as

$$\mathcal{LL}_{\boldsymbol{y}}(\theta) = \log \mathrm{p}(y_1, \ldots y_N; \theta) = \sum_{i=1}^{N} \log \mathrm{p}(y_i; \theta),$$

and the maximum likelihood estimator of θ^* as the function of $\boldsymbol{y}$ that maximizes the likelihood, i.e., maximizes the log-likelihood:

$$\widehat{\theta} = \arg\max_{\theta \in \Theta} \mathcal{LL}_{\boldsymbol{y}}(\theta).$$

The partial derivative of the log-likelihood with respect to θ is called the *score*. Under general regularity conditions, the expected value of the score is 0. Indeed, for any $i = 1, \ldots, N$, it is easy to show that

$$\mathbb{E}\left(\frac{\partial}{\partial \theta} \log \mathrm{p}(y_i; \theta^*)\right) = 0.$$

The variance of this individual score is called the *Fisher information matrix* (FIM):

$$I(\theta^*) = \mathbb{E}\left(\left(\frac{\partial}{\partial \theta} \log \mathrm{p}(y_i; \theta^*)\right)\left(\frac{\partial}{\partial \theta} \log \mathrm{p}(y; \theta^*)\right)'\right).$$

Furthermore, it can be shown that if $\mathcal{LL}_{\boldsymbol{y}}(\theta)$ is twice differentiable with respect to θ,

$$I(\theta^*) = -\mathbb{E}\left(\frac{\partial^2}{\partial \theta \partial \theta'} \log \mathrm{p}(y_i; \theta^*)\right).$$

In addition to this, the following central limit theorem (CLT) holds under certain regularity conditions (Lehmann and Casella, 1998):

$$\sqrt{N}(\widehat{\theta} - \theta^*) \underset{N \to \infty}{\longrightarrow} \mathcal{N}(0, I(\theta^*)^{-1}). \tag{B.1}$$

This theorem shows that under relevant hypotheses, the estimator $\widehat{\theta}$ is consistent and converges to θ^* at rate $\sqrt{N}$, i.e., to decrease on average the estimation error by a factor of k, we have to increase the sample size by a factor of k^2. The limiting variance $I(\theta^*)^{-1}$ is unknown because it depends on the unknown parameter θ^*. We can use instead the *observed Fisher information*:

$$\begin{aligned} I_{\boldsymbol{y}}(\widehat{\theta}) &= -\frac{\partial^2}{\partial \theta^2} \mathcal{LL}_{\boldsymbol{y}}(\widehat{\theta})) \\ &= \sum_{i=1}^{N} \frac{\partial^2}{\partial \theta^2} \log \mathrm{p}(y_i; \widehat{\theta}). \end{aligned} \tag{B.2}$$

Using the fact that $I_{\boldsymbol{y}}(\widehat{\theta})/N \to I(\theta^*)$, we can approximate the distribution of $\widehat{\theta}$ by a normal distribution with mean θ^* and variance-covariance matrix $I_{\boldsymbol{y}}(\widehat{\theta})^{-1}$:

$$\widehat{\theta} \approx \mathcal{N}(\theta^*, I_{\boldsymbol{y}}(\widehat{\theta})^{-1}). \tag{B.3}$$

The square roots of the diagonal elements of $I_{\boldsymbol{y}}(\widehat{\theta})^{-1}$ are called the *standard errors* (s.e.) of the elements of $\widehat{\theta}$.

It is unrealistic to suppose that observations $y_i = (y_{ij}, 1 \leq j \leq n_i)$ are identically distributed in most of the situations that interest us. In effect, the design (observation and administration times) often differs between patients, and in any case observations y_i are not identically distributed whenever the model depends on individual covariates. In this context, CLT (B.1) is meaningless because the very definition of asymptotics is not clearly defined. Nevertheless, we can still define the *observed Fisher information* $I_{\boldsymbol{y}}(\widehat{\theta})$ as in (B.2) and use the Gaussian approximation in (B.3).

Notice also that the Fisher information depends on the problem's parametrization. Suppose that there exists another parametrization based on another $d \times 1$ parameter vector $\zeta(\theta)$ where ζ is a continuously differentiable function of θ. Then, the Fisher information $\tilde{I}(\zeta(\theta))$ obtained using this new parametrization satisfies

$$I(\theta) = J^t \tilde{I}(\zeta(\theta))J,$$

where J is the Jacobian matrix $(\partial\zeta_i(\theta)/\partial\theta_j\,,\, 1 \leq i,j \leq d)$.

The use of the CLT with limiting variance $\tilde{I}(\zeta(\theta))^{-1} = J^t I(\theta)^{-1} J$ for approximating the distribution of $\hat{\zeta} = \zeta(\widehat{\theta})$ is equivalent to using the *delta method* (Casella and Berger, 1990):

$$\zeta(\widehat{\theta}) \approx \mathcal{N}(\zeta(\theta^*), J^t I_{\boldsymbol{y}}(\widehat{\theta})^{-1} J).$$

B.3 Computing the Hessian of the log-likelihood

The log-likelihood $\mathcal{LL}_{\boldsymbol{z}}(\theta_z)$ defined in Section 9.6.2, where $\theta_z = (\beta, \Omega)$, is

$$\mathcal{LL}_{\boldsymbol{z}}(\theta_z) = -\frac{Nd}{2}\log(2\pi) - \frac{N}{2}\log(|\Omega|) - \frac{1}{2}\sum_{i=1}^{N}(z_i - C_i\beta)^t\Omega^{-1}(z_i - C_i\beta).$$

Let

$$S = \sum_{i=1}^{N}(z_i - C_i\beta)(z_i - C_i\beta)^t.$$

Using the fact that for any vectors u and v of the same size, $u^t v = \mathrm{tr}\{u^t v\} = \mathrm{tr}\{vu^t\}$, we get

$$\mathcal{LL}_{\boldsymbol{z}}(\theta_z) = -\frac{Nd}{2}\log(2\pi) - \frac{N}{2}\log(|\Omega|) - \frac{1}{2}\mathrm{tr}\{\Omega^{-1}S\}. \tag{B.4}$$

Differentiating (B.4) yields

$$
\begin{aligned}
&\mathsf{d}\,\mathcal{LL}_{\boldsymbol{z}}(\theta_z;\mathsf{d}\,\beta,\mathsf{d}\,\Omega)\\
&= -\frac{N}{2}\mathsf{d}\,\log(|\Omega|) - \frac{1}{2}\mathsf{d}\,\mathrm{tr}\{\Omega^{-1}S\}\\
&= -\frac{N}{2}\mathrm{tr}\{\Omega^{-1}\mathsf{d}\,\Omega\} - \frac{1}{2}\mathrm{tr}\{(\mathsf{d}\,\Omega^{-1})S\} - \frac{1}{2}\mathrm{tr}\{\Omega^{-1}\mathsf{d}\,S\}\\
&= -\frac{N}{2}\mathrm{tr}\{\Omega^{-1}\mathsf{d}\,\Omega\} + \frac{1}{2}\mathrm{tr}\{\Omega^{-1}(\mathsf{d}\,\Omega)\Omega^{-1}S\}\\
&\quad + \frac{1}{2}\mathrm{tr}\{\Omega^{-1}\sum_{i=1}^{N}\left((z_i - C_i\beta)(\mathsf{d}\,\beta)^t C_i^t + C_i(\mathsf{d}\,\beta)(z_i - C_i\beta)^t\right)\}\\
&= \frac{1}{2}\mathrm{tr}\{(\mathsf{d}\,\Omega)\Omega^{-1}(S - N\Omega)\Omega^{-1}\} + \mathrm{tr}\{(\mathsf{d}\,\beta)^t\sum_{i=1}^{N}C_i^t\Omega^{-1}(z_i - C_i\beta)\}.
\end{aligned}
$$

This derivative is zero for any $(\mathsf{d}\,\beta,\mathsf{d}\,\Omega)$ at $(\hat{\beta},\hat{\Omega})$, the maximum likelihood estimate of (β,Ω). Thus,

$$
\begin{aligned}
\hat{\Omega}^{-1}(S - N\hat{\Omega})\hat{\Omega}^{-1} &= 0\\
\sum_{i=1}^{N}C_i^t\hat{\Omega}^{-1}(z_i - C_i\hat{\beta}) &= 0.
\end{aligned}
$$

$\hat{\beta}$ and $\hat{\Omega}$ are therefore given by

$$
\begin{aligned}
\hat{\beta} &= \left(\sum_{i=1}^{N}C_i^t\hat{\Omega}^{-1}C_i\right)^{-1}\sum_{i=1}^{N}C_i^t\hat{\Omega}^{-1}z_i\\
\hat{\Omega} &= \frac{1}{N}\sum_{i=1}^{N}(z_i - C_i\hat{\beta})(z_i - C_i\hat{\beta})^t.
\end{aligned}
$$

For any $d \times d$ matrix M, let v_M be the $d^2 \times 1$ vector obtained by stacking the d columns of M one underneath the other. Using the fact that $\mathrm{tr}\{ABCD\} = (v_{A^t})^t(D^t \otimes B)v_C$, we can now write the derivative of $\mathcal{LL}_{\boldsymbol{z}}$ as follows:

$$
\begin{aligned}
&\mathsf{d}\,\mathcal{LL}_{\boldsymbol{z}}(\theta_z;\mathsf{d}\,\beta,\mathsf{d}\,v_\Omega)\\
&= (\mathsf{d}\,\beta)^t\sum_{i=1}^{N}C_i^t\Omega^{-1}(z_i - C_i\beta) + \frac{1}{2}(v_{\mathsf{d}\,\Omega})^t(\Omega^{-1}\otimes\Omega^{-1})v_{(S-N\Omega)}.
\end{aligned}
$$

Next we use the fact that Ω is symmetric. The parameters defining Ω are therefore $\overline{v}_\Omega$ (see Section 9.6.2) and we thus have to calculate the derivative of $\mathcal{LL}_{\boldsymbol{z}}$ as a function of $\mathsf{d}\,\overline{v}_\Omega$ rather than $\mathsf{d}\,v_\Omega$:

$$\begin{aligned}
&\mathsf{d}\,\mathcal{LL}_{\boldsymbol{z}}(\theta_z;\mathsf{d}\,\beta,\mathsf{d}\,\overline{v}_\Omega)\\
&= (\mathsf{d}\,\beta)^t \sum_{i=1}^{N} C_i^t\Omega^{-1}(z_i - C_i\beta) + \frac{1}{2}(\mathsf{d}\,\overline{v}_\Omega)^t\mathcal{D}_d^t(\Omega^{-1}\otimes\Omega^{-1})v_{(S-N\Omega)}.
\end{aligned} \tag{B.5}$$

where $\mathcal{D}_d$ is the *elimination matrix* defined Section 9.6.2. We can then obtain from (B.5) the gradient of the log-likelihood, i.e., the partial derivatives of $\mathcal{LL}_{\boldsymbol{z}}$ with respect to the components of β and $\overline{v}_\Omega$. Indeed, by definition, $\mathsf{d}\,f(\theta;\mathsf{d}\,\theta) = (\mathsf{d}\,\theta)^t\partial_\theta f(\theta)$. Thus,

$$\begin{aligned}
\partial_\beta\mathcal{LL}_{\boldsymbol{z}}(\theta) &= \sum_{i=1}^{N} C_i^t\Omega^{-1}(z_i - C_i\beta)\\
\partial_{\overline{v}_\Omega}\mathcal{LL}_{\boldsymbol{z}}(\theta) &= \frac{1}{2}\mathcal{D}_d^t(\Omega^{-1}\otimes\Omega^{-1})v_{(S-N\Omega)}.
\end{aligned}$$

Let us now obtain the second-order derivative of $\mathcal{LL}_{\boldsymbol{z}}$ from (B.5). We have

$$\begin{aligned}
&\mathsf{d}^2\,\mathcal{LL}_{\boldsymbol{z}}(\theta_z;\mathsf{d}\,\beta,\mathsf{d}\,v_\Omega)\\
&= -(\mathsf{d}\,\beta)^t\left(\sum_{i=1}^{N} C_i^t\Omega^{-1}C_i\right)\mathsf{d}\,\beta + (\mathsf{d}\,\beta)^t\left(\sum_{i=1}^{N} C_i^t(\mathsf{d}\,\Omega^{-1})(z_i - C_i\beta)\right)\\
&\quad + \frac{1}{2}\mathrm{tr}\{(\mathsf{d}\,\Omega)(\mathsf{d}\,\Omega^{-1})(S - N\Omega)\Omega^{-1}\} + \frac{1}{2}\mathrm{tr}\{(\mathsf{d}\,\Omega)\Omega^{-1}(S - N\Omega)(\mathsf{d}\,\Omega^{-1})\}\\
&\quad + \frac{1}{2}\mathrm{tr}\{(\mathsf{d}\,\Omega)\Omega^{-1}(\mathsf{d}\,S - N\mathsf{d}\,\Omega)\Omega^{-1}\}\\
&= -(\mathsf{d}\,\beta)^t\left(\sum_{i=1}^{N} C_i^t\Omega^{-1}C_i\right)\mathsf{d}\,\beta - \mathrm{tr}\{(\mathsf{d}\,\Omega)\Omega^{-1}S\Omega^{-1}(\mathsf{d}\,\Omega)\Omega^{-1}\}\\
&\quad + \frac{N}{2}\mathrm{tr}\{(\mathsf{d}\,\Omega)\Omega^{-1}(\mathsf{d}\,\Omega)\Omega^{-1}\} - 2\mathrm{tr}\{(\mathsf{d}\,\beta)^t\sum_{i=1}^{N} C_i^t\Omega^{-1}(\mathsf{d}\,\Omega)\Omega^{-1}(z_i - C_i\beta)\}\\
&= -(\mathsf{d}\,\beta)^t\left(\sum_{i=1}^{N} C_i^t\Omega^{-1}C_i\right)\mathsf{d}\,\beta - \mathrm{tr}\{(\mathsf{d}\,\Omega)\Omega^{-1}(S - \frac{N}{2}\Omega)\Omega^{-1}(\mathsf{d}\,\Omega)\Omega^{-1}\}\\
&\quad - 2\sum_{i=1}^{N}\mathrm{tr}\{(\mathsf{d}\,\beta)^tC_i^t\Omega^{-1}(\mathsf{d}\,\Omega)\Omega^{-1}(z_i - C_i\beta)\}
\end{aligned}$$

$$= -(\mathrm{d}\,\beta)^t \left(\sum_{i=1}^{N} C_i^t \Omega^{-1} C_i\right) \mathrm{d}\,\beta$$
$$- (\mathrm{d}\,v_\Omega)^t \left(\Omega^{-1} \otimes \left(\Omega^{-1}(S - \frac{N}{2}\Omega)\Omega^{-1}\right)\right) \mathrm{d}\,v_\Omega$$
$$- 2(\mathrm{d}\,\beta)^t \left(\sum_{i=1}^{N} \left((z_i - C_i\beta)^t\Omega^{-1}\right) \otimes \left(C_i^t\Omega^{-1}\right)\right) \mathrm{d}\,v_\Omega.$$

Then,

$$\mathrm{d}^2\, \mathcal{LL}_{\boldsymbol{z}}(\theta_z; \mathrm{d}\,\beta, \mathrm{d}\,\overline{v}_\Omega) = -(\mathrm{d}\,\beta)^t \left(\sum_{i=1}^{N} C_i^t \Omega^{-1} C_i\right) \mathrm{d}\,\beta$$
$$- (\mathrm{d}\,\overline{v}_\Omega)^t \mathcal{D}_p^t \left(\Omega^{-1} \otimes \left(\Omega^{-1}(S - \frac{N}{2}\Omega)\Omega^{-1}\right)\right) \mathcal{D}_p \mathrm{d}\,\overline{v}_\Omega$$
$$- 2(\mathrm{d}\,\beta)^t \left(\sum_{i=1}^{N} \left((z_i - C_i\beta)^t\Omega^{-1}\right) \otimes \left(C_i^t\Omega^{-1}\right)\right) \mathcal{D}_p \mathrm{d}\,\overline{v}_\Omega.$$

By definition, if $\mathrm{d}^2\, f(\theta; \mathrm{d}\,\theta) = (\mathrm{d}\,\theta)^t B(\theta) \mathrm{d}\,\theta$, where $B(\theta)$ is a symmetric matrix, then the Hessian of f at θ is $\partial_\theta^2 f(\theta) = B(\theta)$. Here, $\theta = (\beta, \overline{v}_\Omega)$. The Hessian of $\mathcal{LL}_{\boldsymbol{z}}$ is therefore

$$\partial_\theta^2 \mathcal{LL}_{\boldsymbol{z}}(\theta_z) = \begin{pmatrix} \frac{\partial^2 \mathcal{LL}_{\boldsymbol{z}}(\theta_z)}{\partial\beta\, \partial\beta^t} & \frac{\partial^2 \mathcal{LL}_{\boldsymbol{z}}(\theta_z)}{\partial\beta\, \partial(\overline{v}_\Omega)^t} \\ \frac{\partial^2 \mathcal{LL}_{\boldsymbol{z}}(\theta_z)}{\partial\overline{v}_\Omega\, \partial\beta^t} & \frac{\partial^2 \mathcal{LL}_{\boldsymbol{z}}(\theta_z)}{\partial\overline{v}_\Omega\, \partial(\overline{v}_\Omega)^t} \end{pmatrix},$$

where

$$\frac{\partial^2 \mathcal{LL}_{\boldsymbol{z}}(\theta_z)}{\partial\beta\, \partial\beta^t} = -\sum_{i=1}^{N} C_i^t \Omega^{-1} C_i$$
$$\frac{\partial^2 \mathcal{LL}_{\boldsymbol{z}}(\theta_z)}{\partial\beta\, \partial(\overline{v}_\Omega)^t} = \left(\frac{\partial^2 \mathcal{LL}_{\boldsymbol{z}}(\theta_z)}{\partial\overline{v}_\Omega\, \partial\beta^t}\right)^t = -\left(\sum_{i=1}^{N} \left((z_i - C_i\beta)^t\Omega^{-1}\right) \otimes \left(C_i^t\Omega^{-1}\right)\right) \mathcal{D}_p$$
$$\frac{\partial^2 \mathcal{LL}_{\boldsymbol{z}}(\theta_z)}{\partial\overline{v}_\Omega\, \partial(\overline{v}_\Omega)^t} = -\mathcal{D}_p^t \left(\Omega^{-1} \otimes \left(\Omega^{-1}(S - \frac{N}{2}\Omega)\Omega^{-1}\right)\right) \mathcal{D}_p.$$

C

Introduction to Pharmacokinetics Modeling

C.1 Introduction

A drug can be given to a patient in several ways: intravenously, orally, subcutaneously, or in less common ways such as intramuscularly, by skin patch or inhalation. Once a drug is administered, we usually describe subsequent processes within the organism by the pharmacokinetics (PK) process known as *ADME*: absorption, distribution, metabolism, excretion.

- *Absorption* is the movement of the drug into the bloodstream from an extravascular site. The extent of absorption of a drug into the systemic circulation is known as the *bioavailability*.
- After absorption, most drugs are distributed via the blood to body tissue. *Distribution* describes the reversible transfer of a drug between blood, tissue and organs.
- *Metabolism* refers to the biotransformation within the body of a drug into other molecules, called metabolites. Metabolites are often pharmacologically inactive, but can also be active or toxic. Some drugs, called pro-drugs, are inactive until they are metabolized.
- *Excretion* is the removal of a drug from the body. The kidneys, which excrete water soluble substances with urine, are the principal organ for this process. Bile flow from the liver is also an important route for elimination in feces. A drug may also leave the body by other natural routes: breath, tears, sweat, saliva, etc. Metabolism and excretion processes are often merged under the name *elimination process*.

Drug PK are very complex biological processes that are difficult to describe quantitatively. Pharmacometricians therefore simplify physiological processes by creating a compartmental model: the human body is described by a series of compartments in which the drug is distributed.

The depot compartment is the site at which a drug is deposited: the gut for oral administration, skin for the application of dermal patches, the bloodstream for intravenous administration, etc. The central compartment consists of blood and highly perfused organs (liver, kidney, lungs) and peripheral compartments of less perfused tissue (fat, skin, muscle).

This simplified framework can be turned into a mathematical model that is intended to give a good descriptive approximation of PK processes and is able to compute the concentration of a drug at any time in all parts of the body.

PK compartment models assume that drug concentration is perfectly homogeneous in each compartment of the body at all times. This strong assumption has the advantage of allowing a quantitative description of a PK model. Indeed, describing quantitatively a PK model turns into describing how the drug amount varies in each compartment. This means we typically need to describe three components:

- The *rate in* describes how the drug moves from the depot compartment to the central compartment.
- The *rate of distribution* describes exchanges of the drug between the central and peripheral compartments.
- The *rate out* describes how the drug is eliminated from the central compartment.

The final model will then bring together these three components into one model.

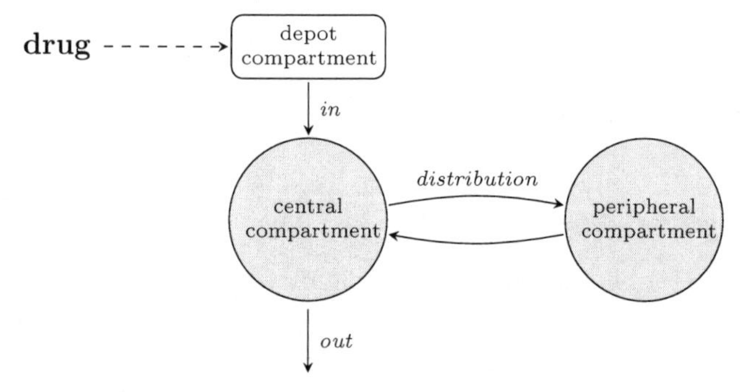

C.2 Dynamical systems for characterizing the ADME process

A PK model is a dynamical system mathematically represented by a system of ordinary differential equations (ODEs) which describe transfers between compartments and elimination from the central compartment. Let us look as several examples of dynamical systems for different types of administration.

Intravenous administration. Consider first a system for iv administration with only one central compartment. The only process that needs to be described is elimination.

There exist several several different mathematical models to describe the elimination process. For instance, *linear elimination* (or first-order elimination) means that the rate of elimination is directly proportional to the amount:

$$\dot{A}_c(t) = -ke \times A_c(t), \tag{C.1}$$

where $A_c(t)$ and $\dot{A}_c(t)$ are, respectively, the drug amount in the central compartment and its derivative at time t. The proportionality constant ke is the *elimination rate constant*. It is directly related to a corresponding *half-life*, i.e., the time required for half of the drug amount to leave the compartment:

$$t_{1/2} = \log(2)/ke.$$

Let V be the volume of distribution of the central compartment. Then, the *clearance*, defined as $Cl = ke/V$, relates the rate of elimination to the concentration $C = A_c/V$:

$$\dot{A}_c(t) = -Cl \times C(t).$$

Clearance is expressed in volume per unit of time. For drugs which are metabolized, the rate of elimination does not increase proportionately to drug concentration. *Saturable elimination* means that above a certain drug concentration, the elimination rate tends to reach a maximal value. Such capacity-limited elimination is best explained by the Michaelis-Menten equations:

$$\begin{aligned} \dot{A}_c(t) &= -\frac{V_m}{V\,K_m + A_c(t)}\,A_c(t) \qquad \text{(C.2)} \\ &= -\frac{V_m}{K_m + C(t)}\,C(t). \end{aligned}$$

Here, V_m is the maximum elimination capacity, i.e., the total drug amount that can be eliminated per unit time at saturation, and K_m the drug concentration eliminated at half maximum capacity. When the drug concentration is quite small with respect to K_m, the mixed-order process becomes similar to a first-order one and elimination is directly proportional to concentration. When the drug concentration is large in relation to K_m, the elimination rate approaches the constant value V_m.

Let us next introduce a peripheral compartment to the model and assume linear transfer between the central compartment and it. Assuming linear elimination from the central compartment, the mathematical representation of this model now consists of a system of two ODEs:

$$\begin{aligned}\dot{A}_c(t) &= k_{21}A_p(t) - k_{12}A_c(t) - k_e A_c(t) \\ \dot{A}_p(t) &= -k_{21}A_p(t) + k_{12}A_c(t),\end{aligned} \tag{C.3}$$

where A_p is the amount in the peripheral compartment and k_{12} and k_{21} the distribution rate constants.

Linear elimination can be replaced by other elimination processes such as the Michaelis-Menten one presented in (C.2). It is also straightforward to extend this model to more than one peripheral compartment. For example, a three-compartment model is characterized by three ODEs:

$$\begin{aligned}\dot{A}_c(t) &= k_{21}A_p(t) + k_{31}A_q(t) - (k_{12} + k_{13} + k_e)A_c(t) \\ \dot{A}_p(t) &= -k_{21}A_p(t) + k_{12}A_c(t) \\ \dot{A}_q(t) &= -k_{31}A_q(t) + k_{13}A_c(t).\end{aligned}$$

Oral administration. Once swallowed, a drug reaches the gastrointestinal tract and is absorbed into the bloodstream. Only a fraction F of an orally administered dose may reach systemic circulation due to factors such as breakdown in the intestine, poor absorption and presystemic extraction. F is known as the *bioavailability.*

A *zero-order absorption process* assumes that a drug is transferred from the depot compartment with constant rate R_0:

$$\dot{A}_d(t) = -R_0 \times \mathbb{1}_{A_d(t)>0}. \tag{C.4}$$

A *first-order absorption process* assumes that the absorption rate is proportional to the drug amount in the depot compartment:

$$\dot{A}_d(t) = -k_a \times A_d(t). \tag{C.5}$$

The absorption rate constant k_a is directly related to a corresponding absorption half-life:

$$t_{\text{abs},1/2} = \log(2)/k_a.$$

Remark: A zero-order absorption process can therefore be defined as the limit of the α-absorption process:

$$\dot{A}_d(t) = -R_\alpha \times A_d^\alpha(t),$$

as α tends to 0.

PK models for oral administration consist of a model each for absorption, distribution and elimination. For example, a one-compartment model with a first-order absorption process and linear elimination combines (C.5) and (C.1):

$$\begin{aligned}\dot{A}_d(t) &= -k_a\, A_d(t)\\ \dot{A}_c(t) &= k_a\, A_d(t) - k_e\, A_c(t).\end{aligned}$$

A two-compartment model with a zero-order absorption process and nonlinear elimination combines (C.4), (C.3) and (C.2):

$$\begin{aligned}\dot{A}_d(t) &= -R_0 \mathbb{1}_{A_d(t)>0}\\ \dot{A}_c(t) &= R_0 \mathbb{1}_{A_d(t)>0} + k_{21} A_p(t) - k_{12} A_c(t) - \frac{V_m}{V\,K_m + A_c(t)} A_c(t)\\ \dot{A}_p(t) &= -k_{21} A_p(t) + k_{12} A_c(t).\end{aligned}$$

C.3 Putting doses into a system

PK models do not describe how a drug is administered. Administered doses are *source terms*, i.e., *inputs* that dynamically modify the state of a system. This is important to note because it means that the same PK model can be used for different dose regimens.

The plasmatic concentration predicted by a model is the solution of a system of ODEs for a given series of inputs and initial conditions (we suppose in general that all compartments are empty before the first dose). When the system of ODEs is linear, an analytical solution can be calculated. Otherwise, numerical methods for ODEs are required for approximating the solution.

In the case of iv bolus, a drug is administered intravenously over a negligible period of time and achieves instantaneous distribution throughout the central compartment. Let D be the drug amount administered at time τ. Then,

$$A_c(\tau^+) = A_c(\tau^-) + D,$$

where τ^- and τ^+ are the times just before and after drug administration. If the compartment is empty before τ, the solution is

$$C(t) = \frac{D}{V}\, e^{-k_e\,(t-\tau)}\, \mathbb{1}_{t>\tau}.$$

If K doses $D_1, D_2, \ldots, D_K$ are administered at times $\tau_1, \tau_2, \ldots, \tau_K$, a superposition principle applies since the system is linear:

$$C(t) = \frac{1}{V} \sum_{k=1}^{K} D_k e^{-k_e\,(t-\tau_k)}\, \mathbb{I}_{t>\tau_k}.$$

In the case of iv infusion, a dose is administered with a constant rate R_{inf} during a certain infusion time period of length $T_{\text{inf}} = D/R_{\text{inf}}$. Assuming a unique dose is administered at time τ, the solution is

$$C(t) = \begin{cases} 0 & \text{if } t < \tau \\ R/(V\,k_e)(1 - e^{-k_e\,(t-\tau)}) & \text{if } \tau \leq t < \tau + T_{\text{inf}} \\ R/(V\,k_e)(1 - e^{-k_e\,T_{\text{inf}}})e^{-k_e\,(t-\tau-T_{\text{inf}})} & \text{if } t \geq \tau + T_{\text{inf}} \end{cases}$$

Note again that the same model was used for all these different examples; it is the changing inputs – here doses – which generate different solutions.

Consider now oral administration and let A_d be the drug amount in the depot compartment. If an amount D is instantaneously deposited at time τ (imagine, for instance, that the dose is swallowed all at once), then, denoting F the bioavailability, state variable A_d is modified at time τ:

$$A_d(\tau^+) = A_d(\tau^-) + F\,D.$$

If the central and depot compartments are empty before τ, the solution is

$$C(t) = \frac{F\,D\,k_a}{V(k_a - k_e)} \left(e^{-k_e\,(t-\tau)} - e^{-k_a\,(t-\tau)}\right) \mathbb{I}_{t>\tau}.$$

Similar types of solution can be obtained when there is zero-order absorption and/or two or three compartments; the solutions are linear combinations of decaying exponentials.

C.4 Implementing PK models with MLXTRAN

There are three main ways to implement PK models using MLXTRAN: first, the `pkmodel` function for defining standard PK models; second, PK macros for complex administrations and/or complex PK models; and third, equations for implementing any dynamical system. These options offer a lot of flexibility. Furthermore, the same implementation can be used for performing several tasks such as modeling and simulation.

1. Using the PKmodel function: PKmodel should be used when there is only one type of administration. It plays the role of PK model library; a model is selected by the choice of function arguments.

Model 1: One-compartment model for oral administration with lag-time, zero-order absorption and linear elimination. The model parameters are bioavailability F, lag-time $Tlag$, duration of absorption $Tk0$, volume of distribution V and clearance Cl.

```
[LONGITUDINAL]
input = {F, Tlag, Tk0, V, Cl}

EQUATION:
Cc = pkmodel(p=F, Tlag, Tk0, V, Cl)
```

Each of p, $Tlag$, $Tk0$, V and Cl is a reserved keyword automatically recognized by `pkmodel`; p is the fraction of the dose which is absorbed.

Model 2: Two-compartment model for iv administration, nonlinear elimination, including an effect compartment. The model parameters are distribution rate constants k_{12} and k_{21}, volume of distribution V, Michaelis-Menten parameters V_m and K_m, and transfer rate constant k_{e0}.

```
[LONGITUDINAL]
input = {k12, k21, V, Vm, Km, ke0}

EQUATION:
{Cc, Ce} = pkmodel(k12, k21, V, Vm, Km, ke0)
```

2. Using PK macros: PK macros can be used to define the components of a compartmental model (compartments, absorption, distribution, elimination, etc.).

Model 3: Sequential zero-order/first-order absorption process. A fraction F_0 of the dose is first absorbed with a zero-order absorption process, then the remaining $1 - F_0$ is absorbed with a first-order absorption process. The drug is eliminated from the central compartment by a linear process.

```
[LONGITUDINAL]
input = {F0, Tk0, ka, V, Cl)

PK:
compartment(cmt=1, amount=Ac)
oral(cmt=1, Tk0, p=F0)
oral(cmt=1, ka, Tlag=Tk0, p=1-F0)
elimination(cmt=1, k=Cl/V)
Cc = Ac/V
```

Model 4: Multiple administrations and multiple absorption processes. In this example, one type of dose is administered orally (`adm=1`) and absorbed into a latent compartment following a first-order absorption process, a second type is administered orally (`adm=2`) and absorbed into the central compartment following a zero-order absorption process, and a third type is directly administered intravenously to the central compartment (`adm=3`). There is linear transfer from the latent to the central compartment. A peripheral compartment is linked to the central compartment. The drug is eliminated by a linear process from the latent compartment and a nonlinear process from the central one. Here, A_l and A_c are the drug amounts in the latent and central compartments.

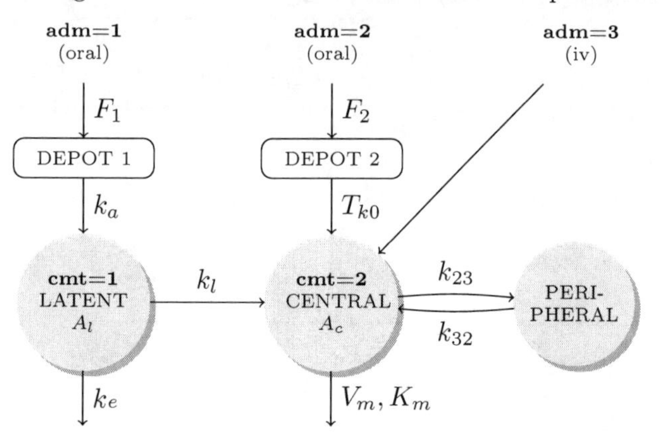


```
[LONGITUDINAL]
input = {F1, F2, ka, Tk0, kl, k23, k32, V, k, Vm, Km}

PK:
compartment(cmt=1, amount=Al)
compartment(cmt=2, amount=Ac)
peripheral(k23,k32)
oral(adm=1, cmt=1, ka,  p=F1)
oral(adm=2, cmt=2, Tk0, p=F2)
iv(adm=3, cmt=2)
transfer(from=1, to=2, kt=kl)
elimination(cmt=1, k)
elimination(cmt=2, Km, Vm)
Cc = Ac/V
```

3. Using equations: Equations can be used if we wish to represent a dynamical system by a system of ODEs and "deposit" the drug in any compartment, i.e., define administrations as source terms for any component of the system of ODEs.

Model 5: Combination of oral and iv administrations. Only a fraction F of the oral dose is absorbed with lag-time $Tlag$. Inputs of type 1 (adm=1) are oral administrations and inputs of type 2 (adm=2) are iv administrations.

```
[LONGITUDINAL]
input = {F, Tlag, ka, V, k}

PK:
depot(adm=1, target=Ad, p=F, Tlag)
depot(adm=2, target=Ac)

EQUATION:
ddt_Ad = -ka*Ad
ddt_Ac = ka*Ad - k*Ac
Cc = Ac/V
```

The model is now "ready" to receive any combination of oral and iv doses.

C.5 Using the same PK model for different tasks

In order to evaluate these types of models, in either the modeling or simulation situation, we need inputs, i.e., a dose regimen. For each dose being administered, we need specific information:

- the administration time,
- the drug amount administered,
- the rate (or duration) of infusion if this is the type of administration and
- the administration types if there are several of them.

Amounts and times must always be provided while rates and types are needed only in certain cases.

Suppose first that we want to visually explore the PK model in Example 5, stored in the text file pk_model.txt. The dose regimen now needs to be defined in an MLXPLORE script. Each administration type must be defined in the [ADMINISTRATION] section and the treatment in the [TREATMENT] section, here a combination of two administration types.

```
pk_mlxplore.txt
<MODEL>
file = 'pk_model.txt'

<DESIGN>
[ADMINISTRATION]
adm1={amount=40,time={0,24,48,72},type=1}
adm2={amount={50,75,50},time={12,36,60},
      type=2}
[TREATMENT]
trt = {adm1, adm2}

<PARAMETER>
F=0.8, Tlag=1.5, ka=0.7, V=10, k=0.1

<OUTPUT>
list=Cc
grid=0:0.1:100
```

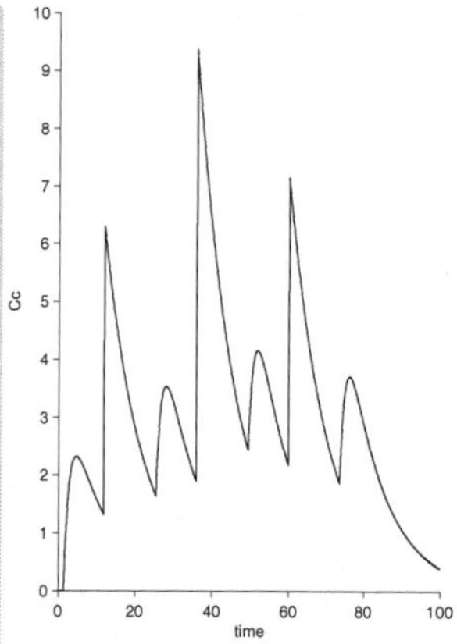

The same dose regimen can also be used for simulation with R function Simulx. In this case, each type of administration is defined as a list, and a treatment is a list of administrations. In this example we use Simulx for computing the predicted concentration C for a given set of PK parameters.

```
pk_simulx.R

adm1 <- list(amount=40,time=c(0,24,48,72), type=1)
adm2 <- list(amount=c(50,75,50),time=c(12,36,60), type=2)
trt  <- list(adm1, adm2)

psi  <- list(name=c('F','Tlag','ka','V','k'),
             value=c(0.8,1.5,0.7,10,0.1))
cc   <- list(name='Cc',time=seq(from=0, to=100, by=0.1))

res  <- simulx(model='pk_model.txt',treatment=trt,
               parameter=psi,output=cc)
```

We can do the same with the MATLAB version of Simulx. Here, administration types are structures and a treatment is a cell array with an administration in each cell.

```
pk_simulx.m

adm1 = struct('amount',40,'time',[0,24,48,72],'type',1);
adm2 = struct('amount',[50,75,50],'time',[12,36,60],'type',2);
trt  = {adm1,adm2};

psi  = struct('name',{{'F','Tlag','ka','V','k'}},...
              'value',[0.8,1.5,0.7,10,0.1]);
cc   = struct('name','Cc','time',0:0.1:100);

res=simulx('model','pk_model.txt','treatment',trt,...
           'parameter',psi,'output',cc);
```

If the dose regimen is defined in a data file, it should contain columns such as `time`, `amt`, `rate` and `adm`. Each row contains the complete set of information for a certain dose. Suppose for example that several patients receive several oral or intravenous doses at different times. If we want to use the same PK model again, a column with the administration type (oral=1 or iv=2) is required:

```
id   time   amt   adm
1    0      80    1
1    24     100   2
1    36     80    1
2    0      40    1
2    12     50    2
:    :      :     :
:    :      :     :
```

This design can then be used with either MONOLIX for modeling, MLXPLORE for exploration or Simulx for simulation.

D

Tools

The tools presented in this appendix all share the MLXTRAN language developed by Lixoft and Inria to implement mixed effects models.

MONOLIX, MLXPLORE and DATXPLORE are currently developed by Lixoft and are available at http://lixoft.com

Simulx was developed by Inria[1] and is available at https://team.inria.fr/popix/mlxtoolbox

The projects, models and data files used in this chapter are available at http://www.math.u-psud.fr/~lavielle/book

D.1 MLXPLORE for model exploration

MLXPLORE allows us to visualize not only the structural model but also the statistical model, which is of fundamental importance in the population approach. We can thus visualize the impact of covariates and inter-individual variability of model parameters on predictions. In the modeling context, we may also want to visually calibrate parameters in order to obtain predictions as close as possible to the observations.

The combination of MLXPLORE and MLXTRAN will allow us to explore pharmacokinetic models with complex administration schedules, include inter-individual variability in parameters, define a statistical model for covariates, etc.

To illustrate features of MLXPLORE, we are going to work with the tumor growth inhibition model proposed in Ribba et al. (2012). This model describes tumor size evolution in patients treated with chemotherapy:

[1]The R version of Simulx was developed by Inria for the DDMoRe project, http://www.ddmore.eu

$$\dot{C}(t) = -k_1 C(t)$$
$$\dot{A}(t) = \lambda A(t)(1 - P^\star(t)/S) - k_2 A(t) + k_3 D(t) - \gamma k_1 A(t) C(t)$$
$$\dot{Q}(t) = k_2 A(t) - \gamma k_1 Q(t) C(t)$$
$$\dot{D}(t) = \gamma k_1 Q(t) C(t) - k_3 D(t) - \delta D(t)$$

A tumor is considered to be composed of proliferative (A) cells and nonproliferative quiescent cells (Q). Treatment directly eliminates proliferative cells. Quiescent cells can also be affected by treatment and become damaged quiescent cells (D). The chemotherapy pharmacokinetics are modeled using a kinetic-pharmacodynamic approach. C represents the concentration of a virtual drug encompassing the various chemotherapeutic components of the treatment.

We are interested in the size of the tumor $P^\star = A + Q + D$, so let us begin by implementing this model for predicting $P^\star$ in MLXTRAN.

```
                                              tumor1_model.txt
[LONGITUDINAL]
input={k1, k2, k3, lambda, gamma, delta}

EQUATION:
S = 100
t0=0
A_0=5
Q_0 = 40
Pstar = A+Q+D
ddt_C = -k1*C
ddt_A = lambda*A*(1-Pstar/S) + k3*D - k2*A - gamma*k1*A*C
ddt_Q = k2*A - gamma*k1*Q*C
ddt_D = gamma*k1*Q*C - k3*D - delta*D
```

Initially, we would like to visualize how the tumor grows without treatment for a given set of parameters. To do so, we create an MLXPLORE script with all the necessary information: the model, parameter values k_1, k_2, k_3, λ, γ and δ, and the output we want to display.

```
                                           tumor1a_mlxplore.txt
<MODEL>
file = 'tumor1_model.txt'

<PARAMETER>
k1=0.3
k2=0.025
k3=0.004
lambda=0.12
gamma=1
delta=0.01
<OUTPUT>
list = {Pstar={xlabel='time (month)', ylabel='tumor size (mm)'}}
grid=0:1:100
```

If we now run this script, $P^{\star}$ is plotted, and then the MLXPLORE graphical interface allows us to interactively modify parameter values using sliders.

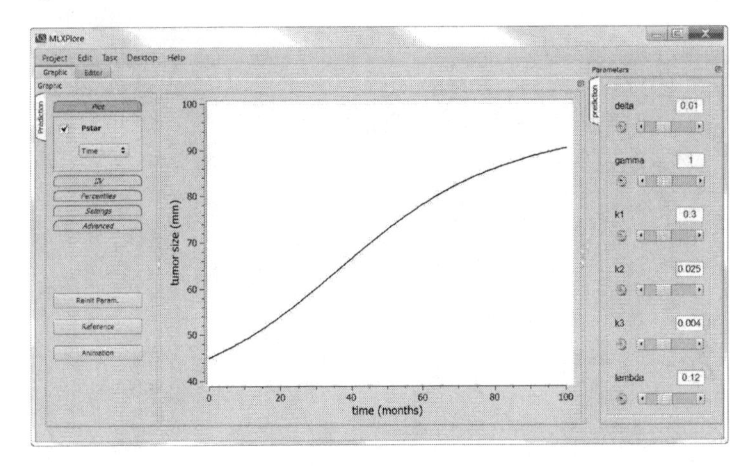

Next we may be interested in visualizing the impact of treatment on tumor growth. We may wish to compare two treatments, one consisting of administering one unit of the drug every twelve months, the other one quarter of a unit every three months. These schedules can be defined in the <DESIGN> section of the MLXPLORE script.

```
                                                   tumor1b_mlxplore.txt
<MODEL>
file = 'tumor1_model.txt'

<DESIGN>
[ADMINISTRATION]
adm1={time=12:12:48, amount=1,    target=C}
adm2={time=12:3:57,  amount=0.25, target=C}

<PARAMETER>
k1=0.3
k2=0.025
k3=0.004
lambda=0.12
gamma=1
delta=0.01

<OUTPUT>
list = {Pstar={xlabel='time (month)', ylabel='tumor size (mm)'}}
grid=0:1:100
```

Then, the two predicted tumor sizes can be displayed in the same plot.

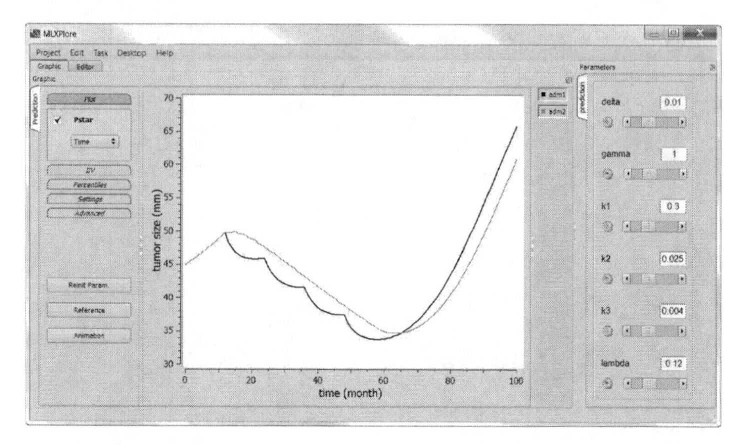

One of most useful features of MLXPLORE is its ability to graphically display the predicted distribution of the tumor size $P^{\star}$ when certain model parameters are assumed to be random variables. Suppose, for instance, that λ and γ are log-normally distributed. To take this into account, we simply insert an `[INDIVIDUAL]` section into the model file. The structural model defined in the `[LONGITUDINAL]` section remains unchanged.

```
                                                    tumor2_model.txt
[LONGITUDINAL]
input={k1, k2, k3, lambda, gamma, delta}

EQUATION:
t0=0
A_0=5
Q_0 = 40
Pstar = A+Q+D
ddt_C = -k1*C
ddt_A = lambda*A*(1-Pstar/100) + k3*D - k2*A - gamma*k1*A*C
ddt_Q = k2*A - gamma*k1*Q*C
ddt_D = gamma*k1*Q*C - k3*D - delta*D

;-----------------------------------------------------
[INDIVIDUAL]
input={lambda_pop,omega_lambda,gamma_pop,omega_gamma}

DEFINITION:
lambda={distribution=lognormal,reference=lambda_pop,sd=omega_lambda}
gamma={distribution=lognormal,reference=gamma_pop,sd=omega_gamma}
```

The model's parameters are now those of the population distributions for λ and γ, as well as k_1, k_2, k_3 and δ, considered constants in this example.

```
tumor2_mlxplore.txt
<MODEL>
file = 'tumor2_model.txt'

<DESIGN>
[ADMINISTRATION]
adm={time=12:12:48, amount=1, target=C}

<PARAMETER>
lambda_pop=0.12
gamma_pop=1
omega_lambda=0.3
omega_gamma=0.3

k1=0.3
k2=0.025
k3=0.004
delta=0.01

<OUTPUT>
list = {Pstar={xlabel='time (month)',ylabel='tumor size (mm)'}}
grid=0:1:95
```

As it is a function of two random variables, $P^{\star}$ is now itself random. MLXPLORE is able to display the order 10%, 20%, ..., 90% quantiles of its probability distribution.

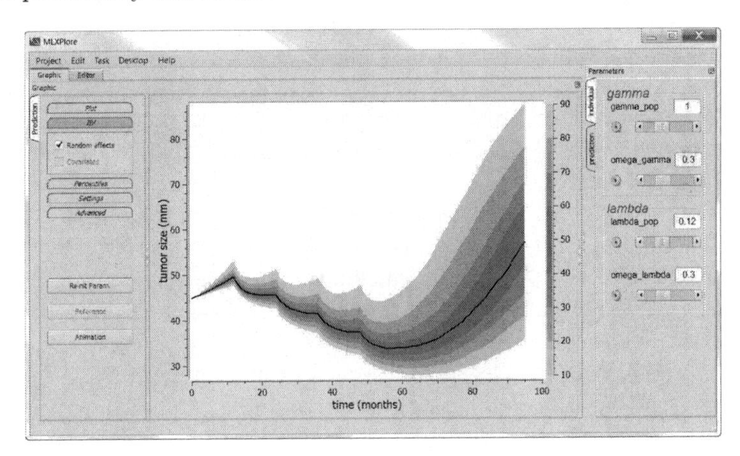

D.2 Simulx for data simulation

In Chapter 3 we proposed considering models as joint probability distributions of random variables. Then, the hierarchical structure of such models allowed us to decompose the joint distributions into products of conditional and marginal distributions. If a model includes observations $\boldsymbol{y}$, individual parameters $\boldsymbol{\psi}$, individual covariates $\boldsymbol{c}$ and population parameters θ, the joint distribution of these random variables can be written as

$$\mathrm{p}(\boldsymbol{y}, \boldsymbol{\psi}, \theta, \boldsymbol{c}; \boldsymbol{u}, \underline{\boldsymbol{t}}) = \mathrm{p}(\boldsymbol{y}|\boldsymbol{\psi}, \boldsymbol{u}, \underline{\boldsymbol{t}})\, \mathrm{p}(\boldsymbol{\psi}|\theta, \boldsymbol{c})\, \mathrm{p}(\boldsymbol{c}|\theta)\, \mathrm{p}(\theta), \tag{D.1}$$

where $\underline{\boldsymbol{t}}$ and $\boldsymbol{u}$ are observation times and source terms (e.g., doses). Simulating this model means successively drawing the model's variables under a given design $(\boldsymbol{u}, \underline{\boldsymbol{t}})$ and their associated submodels:

1. Draw population parameters θ from the distribution p_θ.
2. Then draw individual covariates $\boldsymbol{c}$ from the distribution p_c.
3. Next, draw individual parameters $\boldsymbol{\psi}$ from the distribution $p_{\psi|\theta,c}$ using the values of θ and $\boldsymbol{c}$ obtained in steps 1 and 2.
4. Lastly, draw observations $\boldsymbol{y}$ from the distribution $p_{y|\psi,u,t}$ using the design $(\boldsymbol{u}, \underline{\boldsymbol{t}})$ and the value of $\boldsymbol{\psi}$ obtained in step 3.

Clearly, if certain variables are present but not considered random, the associated simulation step is not performed.

If we now want to perform simulations, we can work with Simulx – both an R and MATLAB function – that lets us use MLXTRAN models in these environments. This combines the flexibility of the R and MATLAB environments with the ability of MLXTRAN to easily encode complex hierarchical models[2].

Let us consider again the tumor growth example used to illustrate MLXPLORE in Section D.1, and use it to present several features of Simulx. First, we would like to calculate the tumor size every 0.1 months from $t = 0$ to $t = 100$ months in the absence of treatment. We will use the following parameter values: $k_1 = 0.3$, $k_2 = 0.025$, $k_3 = 0.004$, $\lambda = 0.12$, $\gamma = 1$ and $\delta = 0.01$. The arguments of the Simulx function are the model name, model parameters and outputs required.

In R, the output of Simulx, i.e., the predicted values of $P^\star$, is stored in a list called `res` in this example:

```
tumor1a_simulx.R

psi <- list(name  = c('k1','k2','k3','lambda','gamma','delta'),
            value = c(0.3, 0.025, 0.004, 0.12, 1, 0.01))
f   <- list(name  = 'Pstar',time=seq(from=0, to=100, by=0.1));
res <- simulx(model='tumor1_model.txt',parameter=psi,output=f);
```

[2]Simulx also accepts models encoded with PharmML, the pharmacometrics markup language developed for the DDMoRe project, `http://pharmml.org`

In MATLAB, the output of Simulx is a cell array, also called `res` in this example:

```
                                             tumor1a_simulx.m

psi = struct('name',{{'k1','k2','k3','lambda','gamma','delta'}},...
             'value',[0.3, 0.025, 0.004, 0.12, 1, 0.01]);
f   = struct('name','Pstar','time',0:0.1:100);
res = simulx('model','tumor1_model.txt','parameter',psi,'output',f);
```

If we now want to compare two treatments, we can create two groups (by default each with one subject only) and apply one treatment to each group. In the same way, we can also use different parameter values and/or observation times for each group.

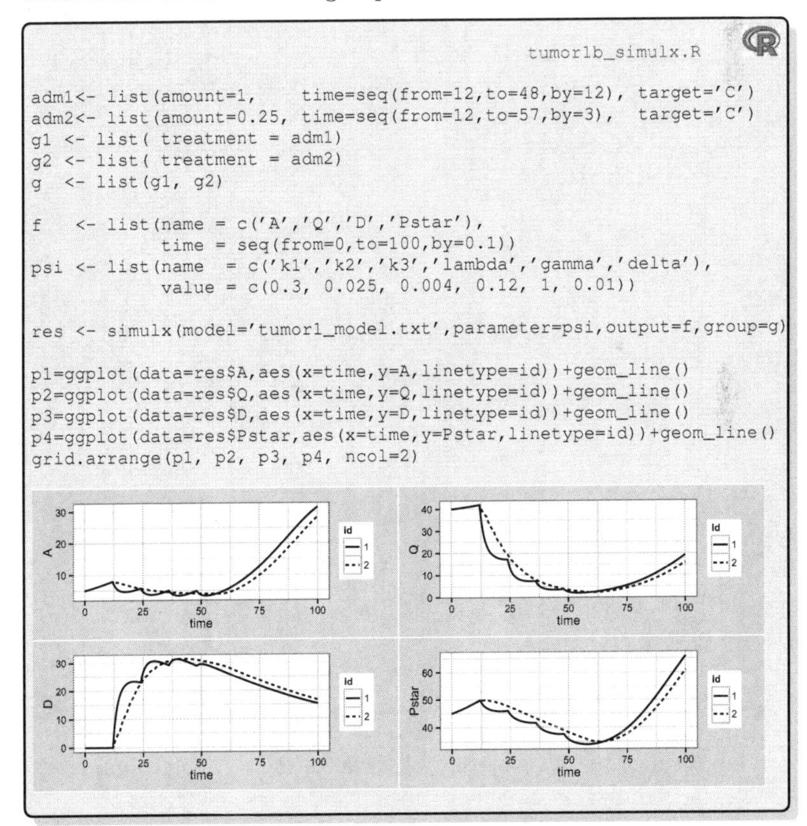

```
                                             tumor1b_simulx.R

adm1<- list(amount=1,    time=seq(from=12,to=48,by=12), target='C')
adm2<- list(amount=0.25, time=seq(from=12,to=57,by=3),  target='C')
g1 <- list( treatment = adm1)
g2 <- list( treatment = adm2)
g  <- list(g1, g2)

f   <- list(name = c('A','Q','D','Pstar'),
            time = seq(from=0,to=100,by=0.1))
psi <- list(name  = c('k1','k2','k3','lambda','gamma','delta'),
            value = c(0.3, 0.025, 0.004, 0.12, 1, 0.01))

res <- simulx(model='tumor1_model.txt',parameter=psi,output=f,group=g)

p1=ggplot(data=res$A,aes(x=time,y=A,linetype=id))+geom_line()
p2=ggplot(data=res$Q,aes(x=time,y=Q,linetype=id))+geom_line()
p3=ggplot(data=res$D,aes(x=time,y=D,linetype=id))+geom_line()
p4=ggplot(data=res$Pstar,aes(x=time,y=Pstar,linetype=id))+geom_line()
grid.arrange(p1, p2, p3, p4, ncol=2)
```


So far, we have used Simulx for making predictions defined as solutions of systems of ODEs. We can however also use it for simulating random variables, e.g., for the model in `tumor2_model.txt`. In the following example, three individuals from group 1 and three from group

2 are given different individual parameters drawn from the same population distribution.

```
tumor2_simulx.R

adm1 <- list(amount=1,time=seq(from=12,to=48,by=12),target='C')
adm2 <- list(amount=0.25,time=seq(from=12,to=57,by=3),target='C')
g1   <- list(size=3, treatment=adm1, level='individual')
g2   <- list(size=3,  treatment=adm2, level='individual')
g    <- list(g1, g2)

psi  <- list(name=c('lambda_pop','gamma_pop','omega_lambda',
                 'omega_gamma','k1','k2','k3','delta'),
            value= c(0.12, 1, 0.1, 0.1, 0.3, 0.025, 0.004, 0.01))
f    <- list(name='Pstar',time=seq(from=0,to=100,by=0.1))

res <-simulx(model='tumor2_model.txt',parameter=psi,output=f,group=g)
```

We can also define the distribution of the longitudinal observations (observed tumor size) by adding a `DEFINITION` block to the `[LONGITUDINAL]` section.

```
tumor3_model.txt

[LONGITUDINAL]
input={k1, k2, k3, lambda, gamma, delta, a}

EQUATION:
t0=0
A_0=5
Q_0 = 40
Pstar = A+Q+D
ddt_C = -k1*C
ddt_A = lambda*A*(1-Pstar/100) + k3*D - k2*A - gamma*k1*A*C
ddt_Q = k2*A - gamma*k1*Q*C
ddt_D = gamma*k1*Q*C - k3*D - delta*D

DEFINITION:
y = {distribution=normal, prediction=Pstar, sd=a}

;---------------------------------------------
[INDIVIDUAL]
input={lpop,omegal,gpop,omegag}

DEFINITION:
lambda={distribution=lognormal,reference=lpop,sd=omegal}
gamma={distribution=lognormal,reference=gpop,sd=omegag}
```

Simulx then lets us generate observations, every ten months, for example, by defining `y` as a new output via `f{2}`. Now, `res` is a list of data frames that contain the observed and predicted tumor sizes for the six simulated individuals.

tumor3_simulx.R

```
adm1 <- list(amount=1,time=seq(from=12,to=48,by=12),target='C')
adm2 <- list(amount=0.25,time=seq(from=12,to=57,by=3),target='C')
g1   <- list(size=3, treatment=adm1, level='individual')
g2   <- list(size=3, treatment=adm2, level='individual')
g    <- list(g1, g2)

psi  <- list(name=c('lambda_pop','gamma_pop','omega_lambda',
                    'omega_gamma','k1','k2','k3','delta','a'),
             value=c(0.12,1,0.1,0.1,0.3,0.025,0.004,0.01,1))
out1 <- list(name=c('Pstar'),time=seq(from=0,to=100,by=0.1))
out2 <- list(name=c('y'),time=seq(from=0,to=100,by=10))
o    <- list(out1, out2)

res <-simulx(model='tumor3_model.txt',parameter=psi,output=o,group=g)

p=ggplot() + geom_line(data=res$Pstar, aes(x=time, y=Pstar)) +
  geom_point(data=res$y, aes(x=time, y=y)) + facet_wrap( ~ id) +
   xlab("time (month)") + ylab("tumor size")
print(p)
```

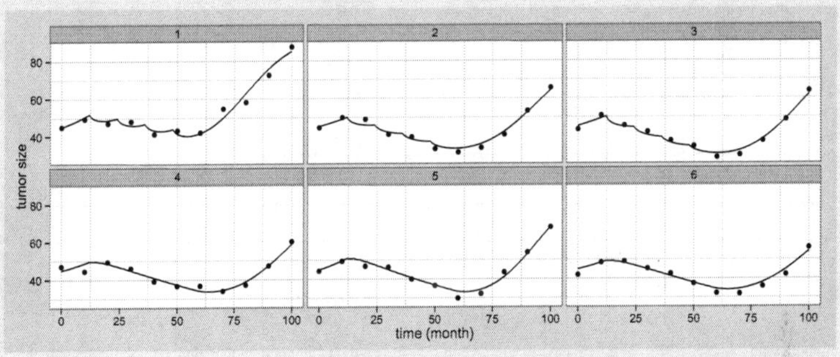

Simulx offers numerous other possibilities such as simulation of population parameters in order to simulate inter-population variability. It is also possible to use different parameters and designs for each individual. This type of information can be read from a data file.

D.3 DATXPLORE for data visualization

Before deciding to model data, it is often important to first be able to visualize it. This is especially the case for longitudinal data when we want to see how an outcome varies with time or as a function of another outcome. We may also want to visualize how the individual covariates are distributed, visually detect if there are relationships between variables, visually compare data from different groups, etc.

DATXPLORE creates graphical displays of continuous data using spaghetti plots. In the plot shown here, warfarin PK data are displayed as a function of time. Continuous and categorical covariates can be used in DATXPLORE to stratify data and split plots. In this example, data have been stratified by weight: patients with weights between 40 and 65 kg are displayed on the left and between 65 and 103 kg on the right.

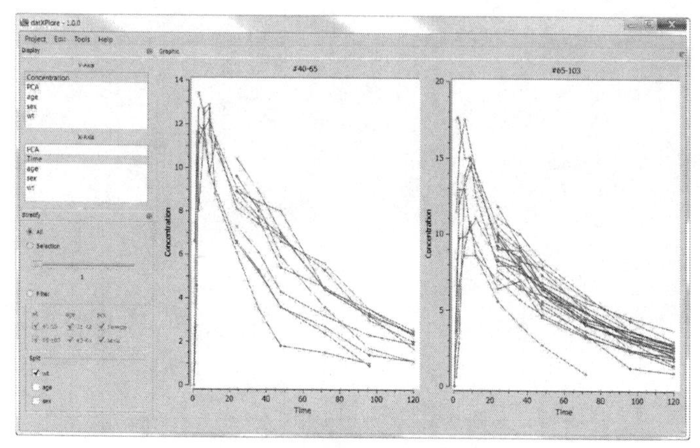

With DATXPLORE, it is also possible to plot PD data (PCA) on the y-axis and PK data (concentration) on the x-axis as we saw earlier in Figure 8.8, which allowed us in that example to detect a hysteresis phenomenon related to a delay in response after exposure. This type of plot is therefore extremely useful for helping modelers build PKPD models.

Furthermore, again using the warfarin data as an example, we have the possibility of showing the distribution of a covariate as a function of another one (for example, weight as a function of sex).

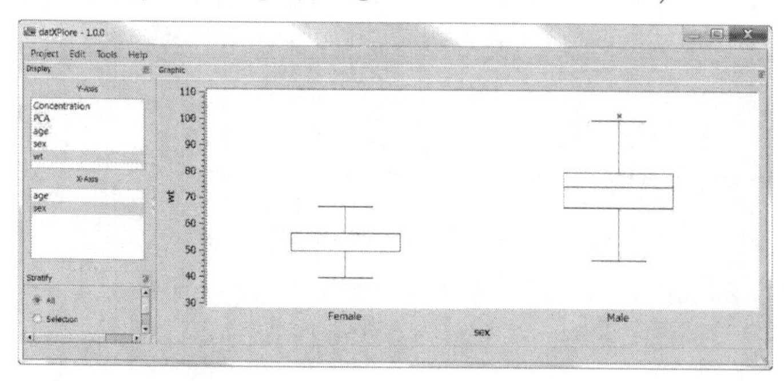

Lastly, we can represent time-to-event data using Kaplan-Meier plots, i.e., estimates of the survival function for the first event. In the case of repeated events, we can also represent the average cumulative number of events per individual. Covariates can be used to filter the data. Here, only arms A and C are displayed (and not B and D).

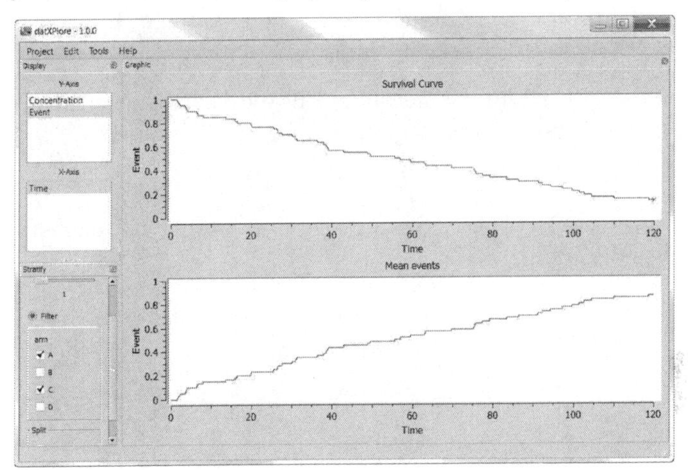

D.4 MONOLIX for data modeling

MONOLIX (MOdèles NOn LInéaires à effets miXtes) is a modeling platform for nonlinear mixed effects models that allows us to perform various tasks:

- Estimation of population parameters (using the SAEM algorithm, see Section 9.2).
- Estimation of the Fisher information matrix (using model linearization and/or stochastic approximation, see Section 9.4).
- Estimation of the individual parameters (using the conditional mean and/or median, see Section 9.3).
- Estimation of the observed log-likelihood (using model linearization and/or importance sampling Monte Carlo, see Section 9.5).
- Model evaluation using diagnostic plots and selection criteria (see Section 7.3).
- Simulation of new data.

MONOLIX offers a graphical user interface (GUI) for creating projects. A MONOLIX project contains information on the data, model and tasks to perform. All this information is stored in a project text file that can be edited. Such project files can be either loaded by the GUI or executed in batch mode.

Let us illustrate some basic features of MONOLIX[3] by modeling the warfarin PK data described in Section 7.1.

Loading data: Data are the measured PK and PD data, the dose regimen and several covariates (weight, sex and age) for 32 patients. All of these are stored in a unique data file `warfarin_data.txt` using a standard format.

We use the MONOLIX GUI to select this datafile and define the content of each column.

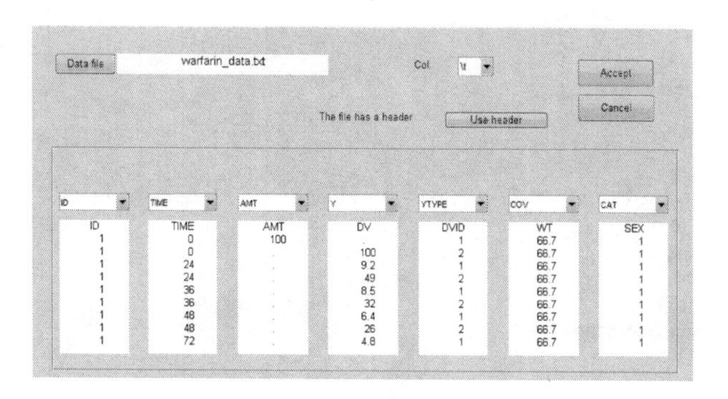

Model for the observations: The warfarin PK data we want to model is continuous longitudinal data. The model for the observations then consists of the structural PK model and the residual error model.

MONOLIX offers an extensive PK library for oral, iv bolus and infusion administration with 1, 2 and 3 compartment models, first and zero-order absorption processes, linear and nonlinear elimination, and various parametrizations. The PK model used in Section 7.1 for the warfarin data is a one-compartment model for oral administration assuming first-order absorption and linear elimination with parameters ka, V and Cl. We can find this model in the MONOLIX PK library under the name `oral1_1cpt_kaVCl`.

A constant residual error model was proposed for this data in (7.2). To implement this, it is possible to use the MONOLIX GUI to select the PK model from the MONOLIX PK library and a constant error model from several predefined error models (also including proportional, combined and exponential error models).

[3]Version 4.3 is used here and throughout the book.

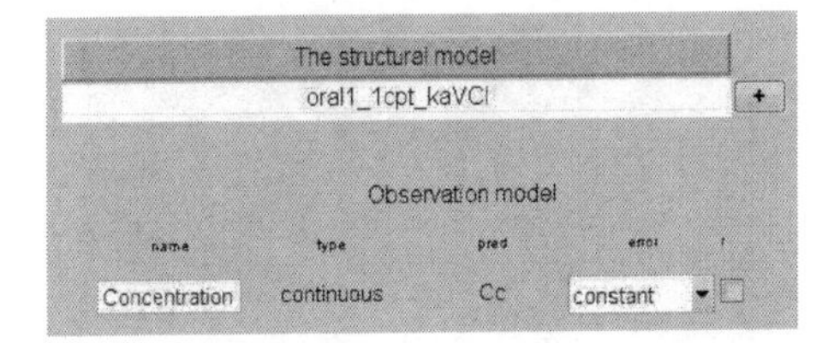

The very same PK model could also be implemented with MLXTRAN using instead the `pkmodel` function with arguments ka, V and Cl for characterizing the PK model. The output is the predicted plasmatic concentration C:

```
INPUT:
parameter = {ka, V, Cl}

EQUATION:
Cc = pkmodel(ka, V, Cl)

OUTPUT:
output = {Cc}
```

The residual error model can be defined in the script instead of the GUI.

```
INPUT:
parameter = {ka, V, Cl}

EQUATION:
Cc = pkmodel(ka, V, Cl)

DEFINITION:
Concentration = {type=continuous,
                 prediction=Cc,
                 errorModel=constant}
OUTPUT:
output = {Concentration}
```

Model for the individual parameters: The second step consists of defining a model for the individual PK parameters $\phi_i = (ka_i, V_i, Cl_i)$. As in (7.3), log-normal distributions are used for the three PK parameters, all considered mutually independent.

If we are using the GUI, predefined transforms are available for defining the parameter distributions: log, logit, probit, power and custom. Here, L stands for log-normal. The diagonal structure of the variance-covariance matrix Ω also needs to be defined.

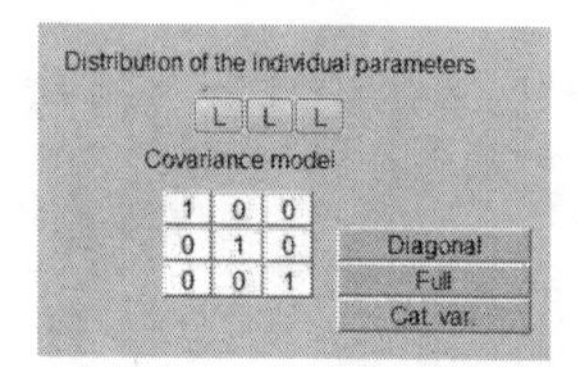

The model in (7.3) assumes a linear relationship between $\log(w_i/70)$ and $\log(V_i)$. We then need to transform the original "physiological" covariate w_i into a "statistical" covariate $c_i = \log(w_i/70)$.

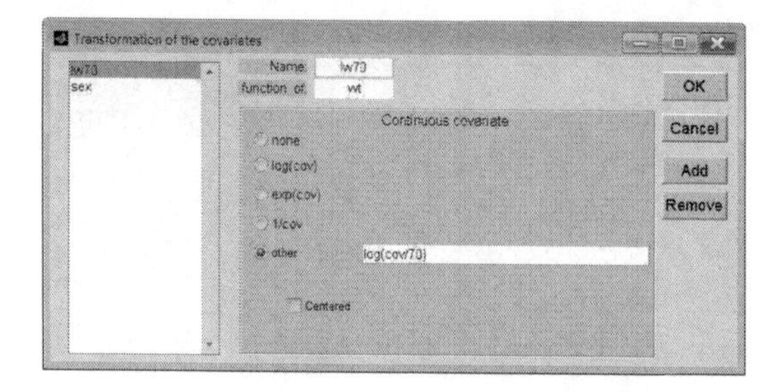

Here, only the predicted log-volume is considered to be a linear function of the transformed covariate.

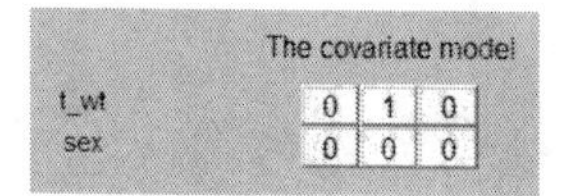

Once the data have been loaded and models implemented, it is then possible to perform various tasks, e.g., estimating the population parameters.

We start by choosing an initial value θ_0. For this, MONOLIX lets us visually compare the predictions obtained for the given parameter values and recorded observations. We can see that $ka = 1$, $V = 7$ and $Cl = 0.2$ give fairly good predictions for the observed concentrations. We can therefore use these as initial estimates.

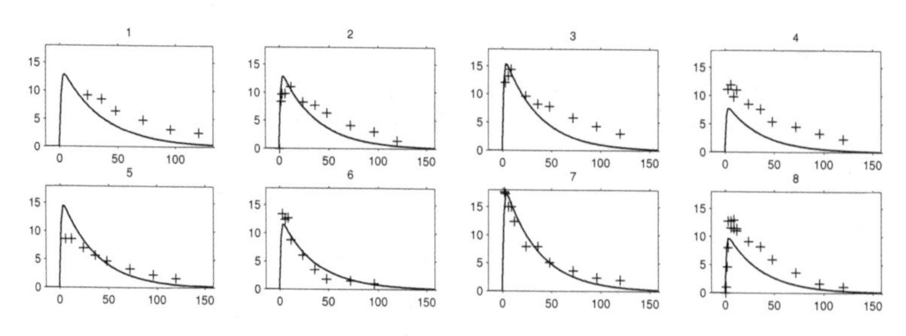

SAEM's default settings (number of iterations, number of Markov chains, simulated annealing) can be used as provided, or user modified.

The algorithms
New seed
123456
Numbers of iterations
K1
K2
auto
auto
Number of chains
2
auto
Simulated Annealing

The methods associated with the tasks we want to perform need to be selected, as well as the set of plots we want to output.

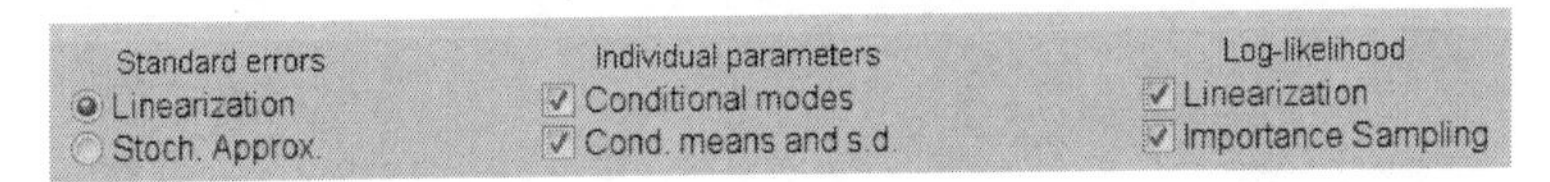

It is then possible to successively run individual tasks or else define a *workflow* (i.e., a sequence of tasks) to execute. All results are automatically stored as tables and plots in a folder associated with the project.

Bibliography

Aalen, O., Borgan, O., and Gjessing, H. (2008). *Survival and Event History Analysis: A Process Point of View*. Springer.

Aarons, L., Karlsson, M. O., Mentré, F., Rombout, F., Steimer, J.-L., and van Peer, A. (2001). Role of modelling and simulation in Phase I drug development. *European Journal of Pharmaceutical Sciences*, 13(2):115–122.

Agresti, A. (2007). *An Introduction to Categorical Data Analysis*, volume 423. Wiley Series in Probability and Statistics.

Agresti, A. (2010). *Analysis of Ordinal Categorical Data*, volume 656. Wiley Series in Probability and Statistics.

Albert, P. S. (1991). A two state Markov mixture model for a time series of epileptic seizure counts. *Biometrics*, 47(4):1371–1381.

Albert, P. S. and Follmann, D. A. (2004). Modeling repeated count data subject to informative dropout. *Biometrics*, 56(3):667–677.

Allassonnière, S., Kuhn, E., and Trouvé, A. (2010). Construction of Bayesian deformable models via a stochastic approximation algorithm: a convergence study. *Bernoulli*, 16(3):641–678.

Allenby, G. M. and Rossi, P. E. (1998). Marketing models of consumer heterogeneity. *Journal of Econometrics*, 89(1):57–78.

Alonso, A., Litière, S., and Molenberghs, G. (2008). A family of tests to detect misspecifications in the random-effects structure of generalized linear mixed models. *Computational Statistics & Data Analysis*, 52(9):4474–4486.

Alonso, A., Litière, S., and Molenberghs, G. (2010). Testing for misspecification in generalized linear mixed models. *Biostatistics*, 11(4):771–786.

Altman, R. M. (2007). Mixed hidden Markov models: an extension of the hidden Markov model to the longitudinal data setting. *Journal of the American Statistical Association*, 102(477):201–210.

Andersen, P. K. (2006). *Survival Analysis.* Wiley Reference Series in Biostatistics.

Andersen, S. W. and Millen, B. A. (2013). On the practical application of mixed effects models for repeated measures to clinical trial data. *Pharmaceutical Statistics*, 12(1):7–16.

Anisimov, V. V., Maas, H. J., Danhof, M., and Della Pasqua, O. (2007). Analysis of responses in migraine modelling using hidden Markov models. *Statistics in Medicine*, 26(22):4163–4178.

ANSES (French agency for food, environmental and occupational health & safety) (2011). Recommendations for carrying out statistical analyses of data from 90-day rat feeding studies in the context of marketing authorisation applications for organisms. Available at http://www.anses.fr/Documents/BIOT2009sa0285EN.pdf

Armbruster, D. A., Tillman, M. D., and Hubbs, L. M. (1994). Limit of detection (LOD)/limit of quantitation (LOQ): comparison of the empirical and the statistical methods exemplified with GC-MS assays of abused drugs. *Clinical Chemistry*, 40(7):1233–1238.

Baayen, R. H., Davidson, D. J., and Bates, D. M. (2008). Mixed-effects modeling with crossed random effects for subjects and items. *Journal of Memory and Language*, 59(4):390–412.

Baey, C., Didier, A., Lemaire, S., Maupas, F., and Cournède, P.-H. (2013). Modelling the interindividual variability of organogenesis in sugar beet populations using a hierarchical segmented model. *Ecological Modelling*, 263:56–63.

Baghishani, H. and Mohammadzadeh, M. (2012). Asymptotic normality of posterior distributions for generalized linear mixed models. *Journal of Multivariate Analysis*, 111:66–77.

Bagiella, E., Sloan, R. P., and Heitjan, D. F. (2000). Mixed-effects models in psychophysiology. *Psychophysiology*, 37(1):13–20.

Banerjee, S., Gelfand, A. E., and Carlin, B. P. (2003). *Hierarchical Modeling and Analysis for Spatial Data.* Chapman & Hall/CRC Monographs on Statistics and Applied Probability.

Bastogne, T., Samson, A., Vallois, P., Wantz-Mezieres, S., Pinel, S., Bechet, D., and Barberi-Heyob, M. (2010). Phenomenological modeling of tumor diameter growth based on a mixed effects model. *Journal of Theoretical Biology*, 262(3):544–552.

Bates, D. M. and DebRoy, S. (2004). Linear mixed models and penalized least squares. *Journal of Multivariate Analysis*, 91(1):1–17.

Bazzoli, C., Retout, S., and Mentré, F. (2010). Design evaluation and optimisation in multiple response nonlinear mixed effect models: PFIM 3.0. *Computer Methods and Programs in Biomedicine*, 98(1):55–65.

Beal, S. and Sheiner, L. (1980). The NONMEM system. *The American Statistician*, 34(2):118–119.

Bellio, R. and Brazzale, A. R. (2011). Restricted likelihood inference for generalized linear mixed models. *Statistics and Computing*, 21(2):173–183.

Bergstrand, M., Hooker, A. C., Wallin, J. E., and Karlsson, M. O. (2011). Prediction-corrected visual predictive checks for diagnosing nonlinear mixed-effects models. *The AAPS Journal*, 13(2):143–151.

Bergstrand, M. and Karlsson, M. (2009). Handling data below the limit of quantification in mixed effect models. *The AAPS Journal*, 11(2):371–380.

Bernal-Rusiel, J. L., Greve, D. N., Reuter, M., Fischl, B., and Sabuncu, M. R. (2013). Statistical analysis of longitudinal neuroimage data with linear mixed effects models. *NeuroImage*, 66:249–260.

Bertrand, J., Comets, E., Chenel, M., and Mentré, F. (2012). Some alternatives to asymptotic tests for the analysis of pharmacogenetic data using nonlinear mixed effects models. *Biometrics*, 68(1):146–155.

Birgé, L. and Massart, P. (2001). Gaussian model selection. *Journal of the European Mathematical Society*, 3(3):203–268.

Blundell, R., Griffith, R., and Windmeijer, F. (2002). Individual effects and dynamics in count data models. *Journal of Econometrics*, 108(1):113–131.

Bolker, B. M., Brooks, M. E., Clark, C. J., Geange, S. W., Poulsen, J. R., Stevens, M. H., and White, J.-S. S. (2009). Generalized linear mixed models: a practical guide for ecology and evolution. *Trends in Ecology & Evolution*, 24(3):127–135.

Bonate, P. L. (2011). *Pharmacokinetic-Pharmacodynamic Modeling and Simulation*. Springer.

Bondell, H. D., Krishna, A., and Ghosh, S. K. (2010). Joint variable selection for fixed and random effects in linear mixed-effects models. *Biometrics*, 66(4):1069–1077.

Box, G. E. P., Jenkins, G. M., and Reinsel, G. C. (2008). *Time Series Analysis: Forecasting and Control.* Wiley Series in Probability and Statistics.

Broström, G. and Holmberg, H. (2011). Generalized linear models with clustered data: fixed and random effects models. *Computational Statistics & Data Analysis*, 55(12):3123–3134.

Brown, H. and Prescott, R. (2006). *Applied Mixed Models in Medicine.* Wiley.

Buonaccorsi, J. P. (2010). *Measurement Error: Models, Methods, and Applications.* Chapman & Hall/CRC Interdisciplinary Statistics.

Bürger, J., Günther, A., de Mol, F., and Gerowitt, B. (2012). Analysing the influence of crop management on pesticide use intensity while controlling for external sources of variability with linear mixed effects models. *Agricultural Systems*, 111:13–22.

Burnham, K. and Anderson, D. (2002). *Model Selection and Multimodel Inference: A Practical Information-Theoretic Approach.* Springer.

Cappé, O., Moulines, E., and Rydén, T. (2005). *Inference in Hidden Markov Models.* Springer.

Carroll, R. J., Ruppert, D., Stefanski, L. A., and Crainiceanu, C. M. (2010). *Measurement Error in Nonlinear Models: A Modern Perspective, Second Edition.* Chapman & Hall/CRC Monographs on Statistics & Applied Probability.

Casella, G. (1985). An introduction to empirical Bayes data analysis. *The American Statistician*, 39(2):83–87.

Casella, G. and Berger, R. L. (1990). *Statistical Inference*, volume 70. Duxbury Press Belmont.

Celeux, G. and Diebolt, J. (1985). The SEM algorithm: a probabilistic teacher algorithm derived from the EM algorithm for the mixture problem. *Computational Statistics Quarterly*, 2(1):73–82.

Chan, P. L. S., Jacqmin, P., Lavielle, M., McFadyen, L., and Weatherley, B. (2011). The use of the SAEM algorithm in MONOLIX software for estimation of population pharmacokinetic-pharmacodynamic-viral dynamics parameters of maraviroc in asymptomatic HIV subjects. *Journal of Pharmacokinetics and Pharmacodynamics*, 38(1):41–61.

Chen, Y.-H. (2006). Computationally efficient Monte Carlo EM algorithms for generalized linear mixed models. *Journal of Statistical Computation and Simulation*, 76(9):817–828.

Chen, Z. and Dunson, D. B. (2003). Random effects selection in linear mixed models. *Biometrics*, 59(4):762–769.

Chi, Y.-Y. and Ibrahim, J. G. (2006). Joint models for multivariate longitudinal and multivariate survival data. *Biometrics*, 62(2):432–445.

Christensen, O. F. and Waagepetersen, R. (2002). Bayesian prediction of spatial count data using generalized linear mixed models. *Biometrics*, 58(2):280–286.

Claeskens, G. and Hart, J. (2009). Goodness-of-fit tests in mixed models. *Test*, 18(2):213–239.

Comets, E. and Brendel, K. (2010). Model evaluation in nonlinear mixed effect models, with applications to pharmacokinetics. *Journal de la Société Française de Statistique*, 151(1):106–128.

Comets, E., Brendel, K., and Mentré, F. (2008). Computing normalised prediction distribution errors to evaluate nonlinear mixed-effect models: the npde add-on package for R. *Computer Methods and Programs in Biomedicine*, 90(2):154–166.

Comets, E., Lavenu, A., and Lavielle, M. (2011). Saemix, an R version of the SAEM algorithm. *20th meeting of the Population Approach Group in Europe, Athens, Greece.* Abstr 2173.

Congdon, P. (2006). *Bayesian Statistical Modelling.* Wiley Series in Probability and Statistics.

Cooley, D., Nychka, D., and Naveau, P. (2007). Bayesian spatial modeling of extreme precipitation return levels. *Journal of the American Statistical Association*, 102(479):824–840.

Crawford, D. W., Jackson, E. L., and Godbey, G. (1991). A hierarchical model of leisure constraints. *Leisure Sciences*, 13(4):309–320.

Crawley, M. J. (2005). *Statistics: An Introduction Using R.* Wiley.

D'Argenio, D. Z. and Schumitzky, A. (1990). *ADAPT II. User's guide.* Biomedical Simulations Resource, University of Southern California, Los Angeles, pages 3–9.

Das, S. and Krishen, A. (1999). Some bootstrap methods in nonlinear mixed-effect models. *Journal of Statistical Planning and Inference*, 75(2):237–245.

Davidian, M. and Giltinan, D. M. (1995). *Nonlinear Models for Repeated Measurements Data.* Chapman & Hall/CRC Monographs on Statistics and Applied Probability.

Davidian, M. and Louis, T. A. (2012). Why statistics? *Science*, 336(6077):12.

Davison, A. C. (2003). *Statistical Models.* Cambridge Series in Statistical and Probabilistic Mathematics. Cambridge University Press.

De Gruttola, V. and Tu, X. M. (1994). Modelling progression of CD4-lymphocyte count and its relationship to survival time. *Biometrics*, 50(4):1003–1014.

Dekking, C., Kraaikamp, F. M., Lopuhaä, L. E., and Meester, H. P. (2005). *A Modern Introduction to Probability and Statistics. Understanding Why and How.* Springer.

Delattre, M. and Lavielle, M. (2012). Maximum likelihood estimation in discrete mixed hidden Markov models using the SAEM algorithm. *Computational Statistics & Data Analysis*, 56(6):2073–2085.

Delattre, M. and Lavielle, M. (2013). Coupling the SAEM algorithm and the extended Kalman filter for maximum likelihood estimation in mixed-effects diffusion models. *Statistics and Its Interfaces*, 6(4):519–532.

Delattre, M., Lavielle, M., and Poursat, M.-A. (2014). A note on BIC in mixed-effects models. *Electronic Journal of Statistics*, 8:456–475.

Delattre, M., Savic, R. M., Miller, R., Karlsson, M. O., and Lavielle, M. (2012). Analysis of exposure–response of CI-945 in patients with epilepsy: application of novel mixed hidden Markov modeling methodology. *Journal of Pharmacokinetics and Pharmacodynamics*, 39(3):263–271.

Delyon, B., Lavielle, M., and Moulines, E. (1999). Convergence of a stochastic approximation version of the EM algorithm. *Annals of Statistics*, 27(1):94–128.

Demidenko, E. (2005). *Mixed Models: Theory and Applications.* Wiley Series in Probability and Statistics.

Dempster, A. P., Laird, N. M., and Rubin, D. B. (1977). Maximum likelihood from incomplete data via the EM algorithm. *Journal of the Royal Statistical Society. Series B*, 39(1):1–38.

Diggle, P. and Kenward, M. G. (1994). Informative drop-out in longitudinal data analysis. *Journal of the Royal Statistical Society: Series C*, 43(1):49–93.

Dimova, R. B., Markatou, M., and Talal, A. H. (2011). Information methods for model selection in linear mixed effects models with application to HCV data. *Computational Statistics & Data Analysis*, 55(9):2677–2697.

Ditlevsen, S. and Gaetano, A. D. (2005). Mixed effects in stochastic differential equation models. *REVSTAT Statistical Journal*, 3:137–153.

Dobson, A. J. (2002). *An Introduction to Generalized Linear Models*. Chapman & Hall/CRC Texts in Statistical Science.

Donnet, S. and Samson, A. (2008). Parametric inference for mixed models defined by stochastic differential equations. *ESAIM: Probability and Statistics*, 12:196–218.

Donohue, M. C., Overholser, R., Xu, R., and Vaida, F. (2011). Conditional Akaike information under generalized linear and proportional hazards mixed models. *Biometrika*, 98(3):685–700.

Dornheim, H. and Brazauskas, V. (2011). Robust-efficient fitting of mixed linear models: methodology and theory. *Journal of Statistical Planning and Inference*, 141(4):1422–1435.

Drikvandi, R., Verbeke, G., Khodadadi, A., and Nia, V. P. (2013). Testing multiple variance components in linear mixed-effects models. *Biostatistics*, 14(1):144–159.

Dubois, A., Lavielle, M., Gsteiger, S., Pigeolet, E., and Mentré, F. (2011). Model-based analyses of bioequivalence crossover trials using the stochastic approximation expectation maximisation algorithm. *Statistics in Medicine*, 30(21):2582–2600.

Duchateau, L. and Janssen, P. (2008). *The Frailty Model. Statistics for Biology and Health*. Springer.

Durrett, R. (2010). *Probability: Theory and Examples*, volume 3. Cambridge University Press.

Efron, B. and Tibshirani, R. (1994). *An Introduction to the Bootstrap.* Chapman & Hall/CRC Monographs on Statistics and Applied Probability.

EFSA (European Food Safety Authority) (2007). EFSA review of statistical analyses conducted for the assessment of the MON 863 90-day rat feeding study. Available at http://www.efsa.europa.eu/en/efsajournal/pub/19r.htm.

EFSA, GMO Panel Working Group (2008). Safety and nutritional assessment of GM plants and derived food and feed: the role of animal feeding trials. *Food and Chemical Toxicology*, 46:S2–70.

Eidsvik, J., Martino, S., and Rue, H. (2009). Approximate Bayesian inference in spatial generalized linear mixed models. *Scandinavian Journal of Statistics*, 36(1):1–22.

Elashoff, R. M., Li, G., and Li, N. (2008). A joint model for longitudinal measurements and survival data in the presence of multiple failure types. *Biometrics*, 64(3):762–771.

Engle, R. F. (1984). Wald, likelihood ratio, and Lagrange multiplier tests in econometrics. *Handbook of Econometrics*, 2:775–826.

Fahrmeir, L. and Kaufmann, H. (1985). Consistency and asymptotic normality of the maximum likelihood estimator in generalized linear models. *The Annals of Statistics*, 13(1):342–368.

Fahrmeir, L., Tutz, G., and Hennevogl, W. (1994). *Multivariate Statistical Modelling Based on Generalized Linear Models*, volume 2. Springer.

Faraway, J. J. (2005). *Extending the Linear Model with R: Generalized Linear, Mixed Effects and Nonparametric Regression Models.* Chapman & Hall/CRC Texts in Statistical Science.

Faure, M. C., Sulpice, J.-C., Delattre, M., Lavielle, M., Prigent, M., Cuif, M.-H., Melchior, C., Tschirhart, E., Nüße, O., and Dupré-Crochet, S. (2013). The recruitment of p47phox and Rac2G12V at the phagosome is transient and phosphatidylserine dependent. *Biology of the Cell*, 105:1–18.

Fedorov, V. V. and Leonov, S. L. (2013). *Optimal Design for Nonlinear Response Models.* Chapman & Hall/CRC Biostatistics Series.

Fieuws, S., Verbeke, G., and Molenberghs, G. (2007). Random-effects models for multivariate repeated measures. *Statistical Methods in Medical Research*, 16(5):387–397.

Fitzmaurice, G., Davidian, M., Verbeke, G., and Molenberghs, G. (2008). *Longitudinal Data Analysis*. Chapman & Hall/CRC Handbooks of Modern Statistical Methods.

Fitzmaurice, G. M. (2003). Methods for handling dropouts in longitudinal clinical trials. *Statistica Neerlandica*, 57(1):75–99.

Fleming, T. R. and Harrington, D. P. (2011). *Counting Processes and Survival Analysis*, volume 169. Wiley.

Fong, Y., Rue, H., and Wakefield, J. (2010). Bayesian inference for generalized linear mixed models. *Biostatistics*, 11(3):397–412.

Fort, G. and Moulines, E. (2003). Convergence of the Monte Carlo expectation maximization for curved exponential families. *The Annals of Statistics*, 31(4):1220–1259.

Freedman, D. A. (2008). Survival analysis. *The American Statistician*, 62(2):110–119.

Freedman, D. A., Pisani, R., and Purves, R. (2007). *Statistics*. W. W. Norton & Company; 4th edition.

Friston, K., Stephan, K., Lund, T., Morcom, A., and Kiebel, S. (2005). Mixed-effects and fMRI studies. *NeuroImage*, 24(1):244–252.

Gabrielsson, J. L. and Weiner, D. L. (2007). *Pharmacokinetic and Pharmacodynamic Data Analysis: Concepts and Applications*. Swedish Pharmaceutical Press.

Gallant, A. R. (2009). *Nonlinear Statistical Models*. Wiley Series in Probability and Statistics.

Gardiner, C. W. (1996). *Handbook of Stochastic Methods: For Physics, Chemistry and the Natural Sciences*. Springer.

Gelman, A., Carlin, J. B., Stern, H. S., and Rubin, D. B. (2003). *Bayesian Data Analysis*. Chapman & Hall/CRC Texts in Statistical Science.

Giampaoli, V. and Singer, J. M. (2009). Likelihood ratio tests for variance components in linear mixed models. *Journal of Statistical Planning and Inference*, 139(4):1435–1448.

Gibbons, R. D. (2000). Mixed-effects models for mental health services research. *Health Services and Outcomes Research Methodology*, 1(2):91–129.

Gilks, W. W. R., Richardson, S., and Spiegelhalter, D. J. (1996). *Markov Chain Monte Carlo in Practice.* Chapman & Hall/CRC Interdisciplinary Statistics.

Gonzalez, A., Uhlendorf, J., Schaul, J., Cinquemani, E., Batt, G., and Ferrari-Trecate, G. (2013). Identification of biological models from single-cell data: a comparison between mixed-effects and moment-based inference. In *Proceedings of ECC – 12th European Control Conference*, pages 2652–2657.

González Manteiga, W., Lombardía, M. J., Martínez Miranda, M. D., and Sperlich, S. (2013). Kernel smoothers and bootstrapping for semiparametric mixed effects models. *Journal of Multivariate Analysis*, 114:288–302.

Greven, S. and Kneib, T. (2010). On the behaviour of marginal and conditional AIC in linear mixed models. *Biometrika*, 97(4):773–789.

Grewal, M. S. and Andrews, A. P. (2011). *Kalman Filtering: Theory and Practice Using MATLAB.* Wiley.

Gross, D., Shortle, J. F., Thompson, J. M., and Harris, C. M. (2013). *Fundamentals of Queueing Theory.* Wiley Series in Probability and Statistics.

Haldermans, P., Shkedy, Z., Van Sanden, S., Burzykowski, T., and Aerts, M. (2007). Using linear mixed models for normalization of cDNA microarrays. *Statistical Applications in Genetics and Molecular Biology*, 6:Art. 19.

Hall, D. B. (2004). Zero-inflated Poisson and binomial regression with random effects: a case study. *Biometrics*, 56(4):1030–1039.

Hammond, B., Lemen, J., Dudek, R., Ward, D., Jiang, C., Nemeth, M., and Burns, J. (2006). Results of a 90-day safety assurance study with rats fed grain from corn rootworm-protected corn. *Food and Chemical Toxicology*, 44(2):147–160.

Hartigan, J. A. (1975). *Clustering Algorithms.* Wiley Series in Probability and Mathematical Statistics.

Hastie, T., Tibshirani, R., and Friedman, J. (2011). *The Elements of Statistical Learning: Data Mining, Inference, and Prediction, Second Edition.* Springer Series in Statistics.

Hedeker, D. (2005). Generalized linear mixed models. *Encyclopedia of Statistics in Behavioral Science.*

Henderson, R., Diggle, P., and Dobson, A. (2000). Joint modelling of longitudinal measurements and event time data. *Biostatistics*, 1(4):465–480.

Holford, N. (1986). Clinical pharmacokinetics and pharmacodynamics of warfarin. understanding the dose-effect relationship. *Clinical Pharmacokinetics*, 11(6):483–504.

Holford, N., Ma, S., and Ploeger, B. (2010). Clinical trial simulation: a review. *Clinical Pharmacology & Therapeutics*, 88(2):166–182.

Holford, N. H. and Sheiner, L. B. (1981). Understanding the dose-effect relationship. *Clinical Pharmacokinetics*, 6(6):429–453.

Hosmer, D. W., Lemeshow, S., and May, S. (2008). *Applied Survival Analysis: Regression Modeling of Time to Event Data*. Wiley Series in Probability and Statistics.

Hu, C. and Sale, M. E. (2003). A joint model for nonlinear longitudinal data with informative dropout. *Journal of Pharmacokinetics and Pharmacodynamics*, 30(1):83–103.

Huang, X., Li, G., Elashoff, R. M., and Pan, J. (2011). A general joint model for longitudinal measurements and competing risks survival data with heterogeneous random effects. *Lifetime Data Analysis*, 17(1):80–100.

Huang, X. and Liu, L. (2007). A joint frailty model for survival and gap times between recurrent events. *Biometrics*, 63(2):389–397.

Huet, S., Bouvier, A., Poursat, M.-A., and Jolivet, E. (2003). *Statistical Tools for Nonlinear Regression: A Practical Guide with S-PLUS and R Examples*. Springer.

Hughes, J. P. (1999). Mixed effects models with censored data with application to HIV RNA levels. *Biometrics*, 55(2):625–629.

Hurwitz, J. and Peffley, M. (1987). How are foreign policy attitudes structured? a hierarchical model. *The American Political Science Review*, 81(4):1099–1120.

Ibrahim, J. G., Chen, M. H., and Sinha, D. (2005). *Bayesian Survival Analysis*. Springer Series in Statistics.

Ibrahim, J. G., Chu, H., and Chen, L. M. (2010). Basic concepts and methods for joint models of longitudinal and survival data. *Journal of Clinical Oncology*, 28(16):2796–2801.

Ibrahim, J. G., Zhu, H., Garcia, R. I., and Guo, R. (2011). Fixed and random effects selection in mixed effects models. *Biometrics*, 67(2):495–503.

Im, H. K., Gamazon, E. R., Stark, A. L., Huang, R. S., Cox, N. J., and Dolan, M. E. (2012). Mixed effects modeling of proliferation rates in cell-based models: Consequence for pharmacogenomics and cancer. *PLoS genetics*, 8(2):e1002525.

Jacqmin-Gadda, H., Thiébaut, R., Chêne, G., and Commenges, D. (2000). Analysis of left-censored longitudinal data with application to viral load in HIV infection. *Biostatistics*, 1(4):355–368.

Jiang, J. (2007). *Linear and Generalized Linear Mixed Models and Their Applications.* Springer Series in Statistics.

Joe, H. (2008). Accuracy of Laplace approximation for discrete response mixed models. *Computational Statistics & Data Analysis*, 52(12):5066–5074.

Kalbfleisch, J. D. and Prentice, R. L. (2011). *The Statistical Analysis of Failure Time Data.* Wiley Series in Probability and Statistics.

Karlsson, K. E., Plan, E. L., and Karlsson, M. O. (2011). Performance of three estimation methods in repeated time-to-event modeling. *The AAPS journal*, 13(1):83–91.

Karlsson, M. and Savic, R. (2007). Diagnosing model diagnostics. *Clinical Pharmacology & Therapeutics*, 82(1):17–20.

Kay, S. (1998). *Fundamentals of Statistical Signal Processing*, volume 2. Prentice-Hall.

Kelly, P. J. and Jim, L. L. (2000). Survival analysis for recurrent event data: an application to childhood infectious disease. *Statistics in Medicine*, 19(1):13–33.

Kinney, S. K. and Dunson, D. B. (2007). Fixed and random effects selection in linear and logistic models. *Biometrics*, 63(3):690–698.

Kirkpatrick, S. (1984). Optimization by simulated annealing: quantitative studies. *Journal of Statistical Physics*, 34(5-6):975–986.

Kjellsson, M. C., Ouellet, D., Corrigan, B., and Karlsson, M. O. (2011). Modeling sleep data for a new drug in development using Markov mixed-effects models. *Pharmaceutical Research*, 28(10):2610–2627.

Klein, J. P., van Houwelingen, H. C., Ibrahim, J. G., and Scheike, T. H. (2013). *Handbook of Survival Analysis*. Chapman & Hall/CRC Handbooks of Modern Statistical Methods.

Kleinbaum, D. G. (2011). *Survival Analysis*. Springer.

Klim, S., Mortensen, S. B., Kristensen, N. R., Overgaard, R. V., and Madsen, H. (2009). Population stochastic modelling (PSM) – an R package for mixed-effects models based on stochastic differential equations. *Computer Methods and Programs in Biomedicine*, 94(3):279–289.

Koch, G. G. and Reinfurt, D. W. (1971). The analysis of categorical data from mixed models. *Biometrics*, 27(1):157–173.

Kubokawa, T. (2011). Conditional and unconditional methods for selecting variables in linear mixed models. *Journal of Multivariate Analysis*, 102(3):641–660.

Kuhn, E. and Lavielle, M. (2004). Coupling a stochastic approximation version of EM with an MCMC procedure. *ESAIM: Probability and Statistics*, 8:115–131.

Kuhn, E. and Lavielle, M. (2005). Maximum likelihood estimation in nonlinear mixed effects models. *Computational Statistics & Data Analysis*, 49(4):1020–1038.

Laird, N. M. (2006). Missing data in longitudinal studies. *Statistics in Medicine*, 7(1-2):305–315.

Laird, N. M. and Ware, J. H. (1982). Random-effects models for longitudinal data. *Biometrics*, 38(4):963–974.

Lavielle, M. and Bleakley, K. (2011). Automatic data binning for improved visual diagnosis of pharmacometric models. *Journal of Pharmacokinetics and Pharmacodynamics*, 38(6):861–871.

Lavielle, M. and Mbogning, C. (2013). An improved SAEM algorithm for maximum likelihood estimation in mixtures of nonlinear mixed effects models. *Statistics and Computing*, online.

Lavielle, M. and Meza, C. (2007). A parameter expansion version of the SAEM algorithm. *Statistics and Computing*, 17(2):121–130.

Lavielle, M., Samson, A., Karina Fermin, A., and Mentré, F. (2011). Maximum likelihood estimation of long-term HIV dynamic models and antiviral response. *Biometrics*, 67(1):250–259.

Lawson, A. B. (2013). *Bayesian Disease Mapping: Hierarchical Modeling in Spatial Epidemiology*, volume 32. Chapman & Hall/CRC Interdisciplinary Statistics.

Lee, K., Lee, J., Hagan, J., and Yoo, J. K. (2012). Modeling the random effects covariance matrix for the generalized linear mixed models. *Computational Statistics & Data Analysis*, 56(6):1545–1551.

Lee, O. E. and Braun, T. M. (2011). Permutation tests for random effects in linear mixed models. *Biometrics*, 68(2):486–493.

Lee, W., Shi, J. Q., and Lee, Y. (2009). Approximate conditional inference in mixed effects models with binary data. *Computational Statistics & Data Analysis*, 54(1):173–184.

Lehmann, E. L. and Casella, G. (1998). *Theory of Point Estimation.* Springer Texts in Statistics.

Lesaffre, E. and Verbeke, G. (1998). Local influence in linear mixed models. *Biometrics*, 54(2):570–582.

Li, Z. and Zhu, L. (2013). A new test for random effects in linear mixed models with longitudinal data. *Journal of Statistical Planning and Inference*, 143(1):82–95.

Lian, H. (2012). A note on conditional Akaike information for Poisson regression with random effects. *Electronic Journal of Statistics*, 6:1–9.

Liang, H., Wu, H., and Zou, G. (2008). A note on conditional AIC for linear mixed-effects models. *Biometrika*, 95(3):773–778.

Lin, X. (2007). Estimation using penalized quasilikelihood and quasi-pseudo-likelihood in Poisson mixed models. *Lifetime Data Analysis*, 13(4):533–544.

Lindstrom, M. J. and Bates, D. M. (1988). Newton-Raphson and EM algorithms for linear mixed-effects models for repeated-measures data. *Journal of the American Statistical Association*, 83(404):1014–1022.

Lindstrom, M. J. and Bates, D. M. (1990). Nonlinear mixed effects models for repeated measures data. *Biometrics*, 46(3):673–687.

Littell, R. C., Milliken, G., Stroup, W., Wolfinger, R., and Schabenberger, O. (2006). *SAS for Mixed Models.* SAS Press.

Little, R. J. A. (1995). Modeling the drop-out mechanism in repeated-measures studies. *Journal of the American Statistical Association*, 90(431):1112–1121.

Little, R. J. A. and Rubin, D. B. (2002). *Statistical Analysis with Missing Data*. Wiley Series in Probability and Statistics.

Liu, C., Rubin, D. B., and Wu, Y. N. (1998). Parameter expansion to accelerate EM: The PX-EM algorithm. *Biometrika*, 85(4):755–770.

Louis, T. A. (1982). Finding the observed information matrix when using the EM algorithm. *Journal of the Royal Statistical Society: Series B*, 44(2):226–233.

Lunn, D. J., Thomas, A., Best, N., and Spiegelhalter, D. (2000). WinBUGS – a Bayesian modelling framework: concepts, structure, and extensibility. *Statistics and Computing*, 10(4):325–337.

Magnus, J. R. and Neudecker, H. (1999). *Matrix Differential Calculus with Applications in Statistics and Econometrics*. Wiley Series in Probability and Statistics.

Makowski, D. and Lavielle, M. (2006). Using SAEM to estimate parameters of models of response to applied fertilizer. *Journal of Agricultural, Biological, and Environmental Statistics*, 11(1):45–60.

Mari, A. (2002). Mathematical modeling in glucose metabolism and insulin secretion. *Current Opinion in Clinical Nutrition & Metabolic Care*, 5(5):495–501.

Maruotti, A. (2011). Mixed hidden Markov models for longitudinal data: an overview. *International Statistical Review*, 79(3):427–454.

Matos, L. A., Lachos, V. H., Balakrishnan, N., and Labra, F. V. (2013). Influence diagnostics in linear and nonlinear mixed-effects models with censored data. *Computational Statistics & Data Analysis*, 57(1):450–464.

Mbogning, C., Bleakley, K., and Lavielle, M. (2012). Between-subject and within-subject model mixtures for classifying HIV treatment response. *Progress in Applied Mathematics*, 4(2):148–166.

Mbogning, C., Bleakley, K., and Lavielle, M. (2014). Joint modeling of longitudinal and repeated time-to-event data with maximum likelihood estimation via the SAEM algorithm. *Journal of Statistical Computation and Simulation*, online.

McCulloch, C. E., Searle, S. R., and Neuhaus, J. M. (2008). *Generalized, Linear, and Mixed Models*. Wiley Series in Probability and Statistics.

McGilchrist, C. A. (1994). Estimation in generalized mixed models. *Journal of the Royal Statistical Society: Series B*, 56(1):61–69.

McLachland, G. J. and Peel, D. (2000). *Finite Mixture Models.* Wiley Series in Probability and Statistics.

McNeil, A. J. and Wendin, J. P. (2007). Bayesian inference for generalized linear mixed models of portfolio credit risk. *Journal of Empirical Finance*, 14(2):131–149.

Meintanis, S. G. and Portnoy, S. (2011). Specification tests in mixed effects models. *Journal of Statistical Planning and Inference*, 141(8):2545–2555.

Mentré, F., Duffull, S., Gueorguieva, I., Hooker, A. C., Leonov, S. L., Ogungbenro, K., and Retout, S. (2007). Software for optimal design in population pharmacokinetics and pharmacodynamics: a comparison. In *PAGE: Abstracts of the Annual Meeting of the Population Approach Group in Europe.* Abstr 1179.

Mentré, F. and Escolano, S. (2006). Prediction discrepancies for the evaluation of nonlinear mixed-effects models. *Journal of Pharmacokinetics and Pharmacodynamics*, 33(3):345–367.

Meyn, S. and Tweedie, R. L. (2009). *Markov Chains and Stochastic Stability.* Cambridge University Press.

Meza, C., Jaffrézic, F., and Foulley, J.-L. (2007). REML estimation of variance parameters in nonlinear mixed effects models using the SAEM algorithm. *Biometrical Journal*, 49(6):876–888.

Meza, C., Jaffrézic, F., and Foulley, J.-L. (2009). Estimation in the probit normal model for binary outcomes using the SAEM algorithm. *Computational Statistics & Data Analysis*, 53(4):1350–1360.

Meza, C., Osorio, F., and De la Cruz, R. (2010). Estimation in nonlinear mixed-effects models using heavy-tailed distributions. *Statistics and Computing*, 22(1):121–139.

Miller, R. G. (2011). *Survival Analysis.* Wiley Classics Library.

Min, Y. and Agresti, A. (2005). Random effect models for repeated measures of zero-inflated count data. *Statistical Modelling*, 5(1):1–19.

Molenberghs, G. and Kenward, M. G. (2007). *Missing Data in Clinical Studies.* Wiley Statistics in Practice.

Molenberghs, G. and Verbeke, G. (2005). *Models for Discrete Longitudinal Data.* Springer.

Muller, K. E. and Stewart, P. W. (2006). *Linear Model Theory: Univariate, Multivariate, and Mixed Models.* Wiley Series in Probability and Statistics.

Mun, J. and Lindstrom, M. J. (2013). Diagnostics for repeated measurements in linear mixed effects models. *Statistics in Medicine*, 32(8):1361–1375.

Nelder, J. A. and Lee, Y. (1991). Generalized linear models for the analysis of taguchi-type experiments. *Applied Stochastic Models and Data Analysis*, 7(1):107–120.

New, M. and Hulme, M. (2000). Representing uncertainty in climate change scenarios: a Monte-Carlo approach. *Integrated Assessment*, 1(3):203–213.

Ng, S. K., McLachlan, G. J., Wang, K., Ben-Tovim, L., and Ng, S. W. (2006). A mixture model with mixed effects components for clustering correlated gene-expression profiles. *Bioinformatics*, 22(14):1745–1752.

Nguyen, T. T., Bazzoli, C., and Mentré, F. (2011). Design evaluation and optimisation in crossover pharmacokinetic studies analysed by nonlinear mixed effects models. *Statistics in Medicine*, 31(11-12):1043–1058.

Nie, L. (2007). Convergence rate of MLE in generalized linear and nonlinear mixed-effects models: theory and applications. *Journal of Statistical Planning and Inference*, 137(6):1787–1804.

Nobre, J. S. S. and da Motta Singer, J. (2007). Residual analysis for linear mixed models. *Biometrical Journal*, 49(6):863–875.

Ntzoufras, I. (2011). *Bayesian Modeling Using WinBUGS*, volume 698. Wiley Series in Computational Statistics.

Nyberg, J., Ueckert, S., Strömberg, E. A., Hennig, S., Karlsson, M. O., and Hooker, A. C. (2012). PopED: An extended, parallelized, nonlinear mixed effects models optimal design tool. *Computer Methods and Programs in Biomedicine*, 108(2):789–805.

Oberg, A. and Davidian, M. (2000). Estimating data transformations in nonlinear mixed effects models. *Biometrics*, 56(1):65–72.

O'Brien, R. M., Hudson, K., and Stockard, J. (2008). A mixed model estimation of age, period, and cohort effects. *Sociological Methods Research*, 36(3):402–428.

O'Connell, M. and Krause, A. (2012). *A Picture Is Worth a Thousand Tables: Graphics in Life Sciences.* Springer.

O'Reilly, R. A. and Aggeler, P. M. (1968). Studies on coumarin anticoagulant drugs initiation of warfarin therapy without a loading dose. *Circulation*, 38(1):169–177.

Ott, J. (1979). Maximum likelihood estimation by counting methods under polygenic and mixed models in human pedigrees. *American Journal of Human Genetics*, 31(2):161–175.

Overgaard, R., Jonsson, N., Tornøe, C., and Madsen, H. (2005). Nonlinear mixed-effects models with stochastic differential equations: implementation of an estimation algorithm. *Journal of Pharmacokinetics and Pharmacodynamics*, 32(1):85–107.

Palmer, E. M., Horowitz, T. S., Torralba, A., and Wolfe, J. M. (2011). What are the shapes of response time distributions in visual search? *Journal of Experimental Psychology: Human Perception and Performance*, 37(1):58–71.

Parke, J. (1999). A procedure for generating bootstrap samples for the validation of nonlinear mixed-effects population models. *Computer Methods and Programs in Biomedicine*, 59(1):19–29.

Peng, H. and Lu, Y. (2012). Model selection in linear mixed effect models. *Journal of Multivariate Analysis*, 109(C):109–129.

Picchini, U. and Ditlevsen, S. (2010). Practical estimation of high dimensional stochastic differential mixed-effects models. *Computational Statistics & Data Analysis*, 55(3):1426–1444.

Picchini, U., Gaetano, A., and Ditlevsen, S. (2010). Stochastic differential mixed-effects models. *Scandinavian Journal of Statistics*, 37(1):67–90.

Pinheiro, J. and Bates, D. (2009). *Mixed-Effects Models in S and S-PLUS*. Springer.

Pinheiro, J. C. and Bates, D. M. (1995). Approximations to the log-likelihood function in the nonlinear mixed-effects model. *Journal of Computational and Graphical Statistics*, 4(1):12–35.

Pinheiro, J. C., Liu, C., and Wu, Y. N. (2001). Efficient algorithms for robust estimation in linear mixed-effects models using the multivariate t distribution. *Journal of Computational and Graphical Statistics*, 10(2):249–276.

Post, T., Freijer, J., Ploeger, B., and Danhof, M. (2008). Extensions to the Visual Predictive Check to facilitate model performance evaluation. *Journal of Pharmacokinetics and Pharmacodynamics*, 35(2):185–202.

Powers, D. A. and Xie, Y. (2008). *Statistical Methods for Categorical Data Analysis*. Emerald Group Publishing.

Proust, C. and Jacqmin-Gadda, H. (2005). Estimation of linear mixed models with a mixture of distribution for the random effects. *Computer Methods and Programs in Biomedicine*, 78(2):165–173.

Proust-Lima, C., Dartigues, J.-F. F., and Jacqmin-Gadda, H. (2011). Misuse of the linear mixed model when evaluating risk factors of cognitive decline. *American Journal of Epidemiology*, 174(9):1077–1088.

Rabe-Hesketh, S., Skrondal, A., and Pickles, A. (2005). Maximum likelihood estimation of limited and discrete dependent variable models with nested random effects. *Journal of Econometrics*, 128(2):301–323.

Rabiner, L. R. (1989). A tutorial on hidden Markov models and selected applications in speech recognition. *Proceedings of the IEEE*, 77(2):257–286.

Raftery, A. E. (1995). Bayesian model selection in social research. *Sociological Methodology*, 25:111–163.

Rao, C. R. and Toutenburg, H. (1999). *Linear Models: Least Squares and Alternatives*. Springer.

Reuter, M., Hennig, J., Netter, P., Buehner, M., and Hueppe, M. (2004). Using latent mixed Markov models for the choice of the best pharmacological treatment. *Statistics in Medicine*, 23(9):1337–1349.

Ribba, B., Kaloshi, G., Peyre, M., Ricard, D., Calvez, V., Tod, M., Cajavec-Bernard, B., Idbaih, A., Psimaras, D., Dainese, L., Pallud, J., Cartalat-Carel, S., Delattre, J.-Y., Honnorat, J., Grenier, E., and Ducray, F. (2012). A tumor growth inhibition model for low-grade glioma treated with chemotherapy or radiotherapy. *Clinical Cancer Research*, 18(18):5071–5080.

Ribbing, J., Nyberg, J., Caster, O., and Jonsson, E. (2007). The Lasso: a novel method for predictive covariate model building in nonlinear mixed effects models. *Journal of Pharmacokinetics and Pharmacodynamics*, 34(4):485–517.

Ritz, C. (2004). Goodness-of-fit tests for mixed models. *Scandinavian Journal of Statistics*, 31(3):443–458.

Ritz, C. and Streibig, J. C. (2008). *Nonlinear Regression with R (Use R!)*. Springer.

Rizopoulos, D. (2011). Fast fitting of joint models for longitudinal and event time data using a pseudo-adaptive Gaussian quadrature rule. *Computational Statistics & Data Analysis*, 56(3):491–501.

Rizopoulos, D. (2012). *Joint Models for Longitudinal and Time-To-Event Data: With Applications in R.* Chapman & Hall/CRC Biostatistics.

Robert, C. P. (2007). *The Bayesian Choice: From Decision-Theoretic Foundations to Computational Implementation.* Springer.

Robert, C. P. and Casella, G. (2004). *Monte Carlo Statistical Methods.* Springer Texts in Statistics.

Robert, C. P. and Casella, G. (2009). *Introducing Monte Carlo Methods with R.* Springer.

Rondeau, V., Mathoulin-Pelissier, S., Jacqmin-Gadda, H., Brouste, V., and Soubeyran, P. (2007). Joint frailty models for recurring events and death using maximum penalized likelihood estimation: application on cancer events. *Biostatistics*, 8(4):708–721.

Rosner, G. L. and Müller, P. (1997). Bayesian population pharmacokinetic and pharmacodynamic analyses using mixture models. *Journal of Pharmacokinetics and Biopharmaceutics*, 25(2):209–233.

Rowland, M. (2005). Editorial to the first issue dedicated to Lewis Sheiner. *Journal of Pharmacokinetics and Pharmacodynamics*, 32(2):157.

Russo, C., Aoki, R., and Paula, G. (2011). Assessment of variance components in nonlinear mixed-effects elliptical models. *TEST*, 21(3):519–545.

Samson, A., Lavielle, M., and Mentré, F. (2006). Extension of the SAEM algorithm to left-censored data in nonlinear mixed-effects model: application to HIV dynamics model. *Computational Statistics & Data Analysis*, 51(3):1562–1574.

Samson, A., Lavielle, M., and Mentré, F. (2007). The SAEM algorithm for group comparison tests in longitudinal data analysis based on nonlinear mixed-effects model. *Statistics in Medicine*, 26(27):4860–4875.

Savic, R. and Karlsson, M. (2009). Importance of shrinkage in empirical Bayes estimates for diagnostics: problems and solutions. *The AAPS Journal*, 11(3):558–569.

Savic, R. and Lavielle, M. (2009). Performance in population models for count data, part ii: a new SAEM algorithm. *Journal of Pharmacokinetics and Pharmacodynamics*, 36(4):367–379.

Savic, R. M., Mentré, F., and Lavielle, M. (2011). Implementation and evaluation of the SAEM algorithm for longitudinal ordered categorical data with an illustration in pharmacokinetics-pharmacodynamics. *The AAPS Journal*, 13(1):44–53.

Saville, B. R. and Herring, A. H. (2009). Testing random effects in the linear mixed model using approximate Bayes factors. *Biometrics*, 65(2):369–376.

Schelldorfer, J., Meier, L., Bühlmann, P., Winterthur, A. X. A., and Zürich, E. T. H. (2013). GLMMLasso: an algorithm for high-dimensional generalized linear mixed models using $\ell 1$ -penalization. *Journal of Computational and Graphical Statistics*, online.

Schluchter, M. D. (1992). Methods for the analysis of informatively censored longitudinal data. *Statistics in Medicine*, 11(14-15):1861–1870.

Schützenmeister, A. and Piepho, H.-P. (2012). Residual analysis of linear mixed models using a simulation approach. *Computational Statistics & Data Analysis*, 56(6):1405–1416.

Schwarz, G. (1978). Estimating the dimension of a model. *The Annals of Statistics*, 6(2):461–464.

Seber, G. A. F. and Wild, C. J. (2005). *Nonlinear Regression.* Wiley Series in Probability and Statistics.

Séralini, G., Cellier, D., and De Vendomois, J. (2007). New analysis of a rat feeding study with a genetically modified maize reveals signs of hepatorenal toxicity. *Archives of Environmental Contamination and Toxicology*, 52(4):596–602.

Serroyen, J., Molenberghs, G., Verbeke, G., and Davidian, M. (2009). Nonlinear models for longitudinal data. *The American Statistician*, 63(4):378–388.

Sharma, A. and Jusko, W. J. (1998). Characteristics of indirect pharmacodynamic models and applications to clinical drug responses. *British Journal of Clinical Pharmacology*, 45(3):229–239.

Sheiner, L. and Grasela, T. (1991). An introduction to mixed effect modeling: Concepts, definitions, and justification. *Journal of Pharmacokinetics and Pharmacodynamics*, 19(3):11S–24S.

Snoeck, E., Chanu, P., Lavielle, M., Jacqmin, P., Jonsson, E. N., Jorga, K., Goggin, T., Grippo, J., Jumbe, N. L., and Frey, N. (2010). A comprehensive hepatitis C viral kinetic model explaining cure. *Clinical Pharmacology & Therapeutics*, 87(6):706–713.

Song, X., Davidian, M., and Tsiatis, A. A. (2004). A semiparametric likelihood approach to joint modeling of longitudinal and time-to-event data. *Biometrics*, 58(4):742–753.

Spiegelhalter, D., Thomas, A., Best, N., and Lunn, D. (2003). WinBUGS user manual. *Cambridge: MRC Biostatistics Unit.*

Steimer, J.-L., Vozeh, S., Racine-Poon, A., Holford, N., and O'Neill, R. (1994). The population approach: rationale, methods, and applications in clinical pharmacology and drug development. In *Pharmacokinetics of Drugs*: volume 110 of *Handbook of Experimental Pharmacology*, pages 405–451. Springer-Verlag Berlin Heidelberg.

Stram, D. O. and Lee, J. W. (1994). Variance components testing in the longitudinal mixed effects model. *Biometrics*, 50(4):1171–1177.

Sutradhar, B. C. (2011). *Dynamic Mixed Models for Familial Longitudinal Data.* Springer.

Tempelman, R. J. and Gianola, D. (1996). A mixed effects model for overdispersed count data in animal breeding. *Biometrics*, 52(1):265–279.

Ten Have, T. R. and Localio, A. R. (1999). Empirical Bayes estimation of random effects parameters in mixed effects logistic regression models. *Biometrics*, 55(4):1022–1029.

Thai, H.-T., Mentré, F., Holford, N. H., Veyrat-Follet, C., and Comets, E. (2014). Evaluation of bootstrap methods for estimating uncertainty of parameters in nonlinear mixed-effects models: a simulation study in population pharmacokinetics. *Journal of Pharmacokinetics and Pharmacodynamics*, 41(1):15–33.

Thall, P. F. and Vail, S. C. (1990). Some covariance models for longitudinal count data with overdispersion. *Biometrics*, 46(3):657–671.

Therneau, T. M. (2000). *Modeling Survival Data: Extending the Cox Model.* Springer.

Tsiatis, A. A. and Davidian, M. (2004). Joint modeling of longitudinal and time-to-event data: an overview. *Statistica Sinica*, 14(3):809–834.

Uhlendorf, J., Miermont, A., Delaveau, T., Charvin, G., Fages, F., Bottani, S., Batt, G., and Hersen, P. (2012). Long-term model predictive control of gene expression at the population and single-cell levels. *Proceedings of the National Academy of Sciences*, 109(35):14271–14276.

Vaida, F. and Blanchard, S. (2005). Conditional Akaike information for mixed-effects models. *Biometrika*, 92(2):351–370.

Van der Laan, M. J. and Robins, J. M. (2003). *Unified Methods for Censored Longitudinal Data and Causality.* Springer.

Verbeke, G. and Lesaffre, E. (1996). A linear mixed-effects model with heterogeneity in the random-effects population. *Journal of the American Statistical Association*, 91(433):217–221.

Verbeke, G. and Molenberghs, G. (2000). *Linear Mixed Models for Longitudinal Data.* Springer.

Verbeke, G., Spiessens, B., and Lesaffre, E. (2001). Conditional linear mixed models. *The American Statistician*, 55(1):25–34.

Vock, D. M., Davidian, M., Tsiatis, A. A., and Muir, A. J. (2012). Mixed model analysis of censored longitudinal data with flexible random-effects density. *Biostatistics*, 13(1):61–73.

Vonesh, E. F. (1996). A note on the use of the Laplace's approximation for nonlinear mixed-effects models. *Biometrika*, 83(2):447–452.

Vonesh, E. F. and Chinchilli, V. M. (1997). *Linear and Nonlinear Models for the Analysis of Repeated Measurements.* CRC Press/Statistics: A Series of Textbooks and Monographs.

Vonesh, E. F., Chinchilli, V. M., and Pu, K. (1996). Goodness-of-fit in generalized nonlinear mixed-effects models. *Biometrics*, 52(2):572–587.

Wagner, H. and Tüchler, R. (2010). Bayesian estimation of random effects models for multivariate responses of mixed data. *Computational Statistics & Data Analysis*, 54(5):1206–1218.

Wakefield, J. C., Aarons, L., and Racine-Poon, A. (1998). *The Bayesian Approach to Population Pharmacokinetic/Pharmacodynamic Modelling. In Case Studies in Bayesian Statistics.* Springer.

Wald, A. (1949). Note on the consistency of the maximum likelihood estimate. *The Annals of Mathematical Statistics*, 20(4):595–602.

Wang, L., Zhang, B., Wolfinger, R. D., and Chen, X. (2008). An integrated approach for the analysis of biological pathways using mixed models. *PLoS Genet*, 4(7):e1000115+.

Wang, N. and Davidian, M. (1996). A note on covariate measurement error in nonlinear mixed effects models. *Biometrika*, 83(4):801–812.

Wang, X., Schumitzky, A., and D'Argenio, D. Z. (2007). Nonlinear random effects mixture models: maximum likelihood estimation via the EM algorithm. *Computational Statistics and Data Analysis*, 51(12):6614–6623.

Wei, G. C. G. and Tanner, M. A. (1990). A Monte Carlo implementation of the EM algorithm and the poor man's data augmentation algorithms. *Journal of the American Statistical Association*, 85(411):699–704.

West, B. T. and Galecki, A. T. (2012). An overview of current software procedures for fitting linear mixed models. *The American Statistician*, 65(4):274–282.

West, B. T., Welch, K. B., and Galecki, A. T. (2006). *Linear Mixed Models: A Practical Guide Using Statistical Software*. Chapman & Hall/CRC Press.

Wienke, A. (2010). *Frailty Models in Survival Analysis*, volume 37. Chapman & Hall/CRC Biostatistics Series.

Williams, R. (2006). Generalized ordered logit/partial proportional odds models for ordinal dependent variables. *Stata Journal*, 6(1):58–82.

Winkelmann, R. (2008). *Econometric Analysis of Count Data*. Springer.

Wolfinger, R. (1993). Laplace's approximation for nonlinear mixed models. *Biometrika*, 80(4):791–795.

Wolfinger, R. D. (1997). An example of using mixed models and proc mixed for longitudinal data. *Journal of Biopharmaceutical Statistics*, 7(4):481–500.

Wu, C. F. J. (1983). On the convergence properties of the EM algorithm. *The Annals of Statistics*, pages 95–103.

Wu, L. (2010). *Mixed Effects Models for Complex Data*. Chapman & Hall/CRC Monographs on Statistics and Applied Probability.

Wu, L., Hu, X. J., and Wu, H. (2008). Joint inference for nonlinear mixed-effects models and time to event at the presence of missing data. *Biostatistics*, 9(2):308–320.

Wu, M.-X., Yu, K.-F., and Liu, A.-Y. (2009). Estimation of variance components in the mixed effects models: a comparison between analysis of variance and spectral decomposition. *Journal of Statistical Planning and Inference*, 139(12):3962–3973.

Xiang, L., Yau, K. K., and Lee, A. H. (2012). The robust estimation method for a finite mixture of Poisson mixed-effect models. *Computational Statistics & Data Analysis*, 56(6):1994–2005.

Yang, Y., Kang, J., Mao, K., and Zhang, J. (2007). Regression models for mixed Poisson and continuous longitudinal data. *Statistics in Medicine*, 26(20):3782–3800.

Yau, K. K. W. and Kuk, A. Y. C. (2002). Robust estimation in generalized linear mixed models. *Journal of the Royal Statistical Society: Series B*, 64(1):101–117.

Yau, K. K. W., Wang, K., and Lee, A. H. (2003). Zero-inflated negative binomial mixed regression modeling of over-dispersed count data with extra zeros. *Biometrical Journal*, 45(4):437–452.

Zechner, C., Ruess, J., Krenn, P., Pelet, S., Peter, M., Lygeros, J., and Koeppl, H. (2012). Moment-based inference predicts bimodality in transient gene expression. *Proceedings of the National Academy of Sciences*, 109(21):8340–8345.

Zechner, C., Unger, M., Pelet, S., Peter, M., and Koeppl, H. (2014). Scalable inference of heterogeneous reaction kinetics from pooled single-cell recordings. *Nature Methods*, 11:197–202.

Zeileis, A., Kleiber, C., and Jackman, S. (2008). Regression models for count data in R. *Journal of Statistical Software*, 27(8):1–25.

Zeng, D., Lin, D., and Yin, G. (2005). Maximum likelihood estimation for the proportional odds model with random effects. *Journal of the American Statistical Association*, 100(470):470–483.

Zhang, B., Shen, X., and Mumford, S. L. (2011). Generalized degrees of freedom and adaptive model selection in linear mixed-effects models. *Computational Statistics & Data Analysis*, 56(3):574–586.

Zhang, D. and Davidian, M. (2001). Linear mixed models with flexible distributions of random effects for longitudinal data. *Biometrics*, 57(3):795–802.

Zuur, A. F. (2009). *Mixed Effects Models and Extensions in Ecology with R*. Springer.

Glossary

ADME absorption – distribution – metabolism – excretion

AFT accelerated failure time

AIC Akaike information criterion

ARMA autoregressive moving average process

BIC Bayesian information criterion

BSMM between-subject model mixture

cAIC conditional Akaike information criterion

cdf cumulative distribution function

CI confidence interval

CLT central limit theorem

CRD completely random dropout

CTS clinical trial simulation

CV coefficient of variation

DATXPLORE software for data visualization

DDE delayed differential equation

DDMoRe Drug and Disease MOdel REsources (European project supported by IMI)

d.f. degrees of freedom

EFSA European food safety authority

EKF extended Kalman filter

EM expectation-maximization algorithm

FIM Fisher information matrix

GLMM generalized linear mixed model

GMO genetically modified organism

GUI graphical user interface

HCV hepatitis C virus

HMM hidden Markov model

HOG high-osmolarity glycerol

ID informative dropout

i.i.d. independent and identically distributed

IIV inter-individual variability

IOV inter-occasion variability

IWRES individual weighted residuals

LLOD lower limit of detection

LLOQ lower limit of quantification

LRT likelihood ratio test

MAP maximum a posteriori

MAR missing at random

MBDD model based drug development

MCAR missing completely at random

MCEM Monte-Carlo EM algorithm

MCMC Markov chain Monte Carlo

MH Metropolis-Hastings algorithm

MLE maximum likelihood estimate

MLXPLORE software for model visualization and model exploration

MLXTRAN model coding language used by MONOLIX, MLXPLORE and Simulx

MNAR missing not at random

MONOLIX MOdèles NOn LInéaires à effets miXtes (platform for nonlinear mixed effects modeling)

nlme R and S+ package for Gaussian linear and nonlinear mixed-effects models

nlmem nonlinear mixed effects model

NONMEM NON-linear Mixed Effects Modeling (software package developed in the late 1970s at UCSF for population pharmacokinetic modeling)

NPDE normalized prediction distribution errors

ODE ordinary differential equation

PCA prothrombin complex activity

PD pharmacodynamics (study of the biochemical and physiological effects of drugs on the body)

pdf probability distribution function

PharmML pharmacometrics markup language

PI prediction interval

PK pharmacokinetics (describes how the body affects a specific drug after administration)

PKPD pharmacokinetics/pharmacodynamics

PWRES population weighted residuals

PX-SAEM parameter expansion version of SAEM

RD random dropout

r.s.e. relative standard error

SAEM stochastic approximation of EM algorithm

SDE stochastic differential equation

s.e. standard error

Simulx R and MATLAB function for the simulation of mixed effects models implemented in MLXTRAN and PharmML

TGI tumor growth inhibition model

ULOQ upper limit of quantification

VPC visual predictive check

WSMM within-subject model mixture

Index

9781032477350